ENDOCRINOLOGY RESEARCH AND CLINICAL DEVELOPMENTS

PITUITARY ADENOMA

PATHOPHYSIOLOGY, DIAGNOSIS AND TREATMENT OPTIONS

ENDOCRINOLOGY RESEARCH AND CLINICAL DEVELOPMENTS

Additional books in this series can be found on Nova's website under the Series tab.

Additional e-books in this series can be found on Nova's website under the eBooks tab.

ENDOCRINOLOGY RESEARCH AND CLINICAL DEVELOPMENTS

PITUITARY ADENOMA

PATHOPHYSIOLOGY, DIAGNOSIS AND TREATMENT OPTIONS

DIMITRIOS N. KANAKIS
EDITOR

NOVA BIOMEDICAL
New York

Library of Congress Cataloging-in-Publication Data

ISBN: 978-1-63484-985-2
Library of Congress Control Number: 2016934650

Published by Nova Science Publishers, Inc. † New York

To my Dear Parents Nikolao and Eleni

CONTENTS

FOREWORD

One hundred and thirty years have elapsed from the birth date of pituitary endocrinology in 1886, after Pierre Marie, a French neurologist, who described the clinical features of growth hormone excess and subsequently introduced the term "acromegaly."

Thanks to the pituitary research and development of new technologies during the last 30 years, a dramatic evolution occurred in diagnostics and introduction of novel clinical and neurosurgical therapeutic approaches. Application of modern techniques including immunohistochemistry and molecular pathology has largely contributed to a functional classification of pituitary adenomas. Accurate diagnosis, reliable prognostic and predictive markers have proven powerful tools for therapeutic outcomes. However, despite amazing advances that have enriched our understanding of fundamental mechanisms leading to pituitary tumorigenesis, even at the molecular level, many questions remain unanswered.

The editor brings together a group of authors, who provide a comprehensive text, which encompasses recent advances in the field of pituitary adenoma. The rich content of this book ranging from anatomy, morphogenesis and development of pituitary, through pathophysiology, pathogenesis and imaging, to clinical and surgical treatment of pituitary adenomas, covers a full spectrum of hot topics of interest.

I am fully convinced that this book will be useful for any scientist, who is interested in research and practice of pituitary endocrinology.

George Kontogeorgos, MD, PhD
Visiting Professor
University Toronto, Ontario, Canada
President, International Academy of Pathology

PREFACE

It was at the beginning of my medical education, when I first learned in the lessons of anatomy about the hypophysis and later in the lectures of physiology I further realized its important role in maintaining the physiological function of the entire human organism. In the next years, during the clinical courses of internal medicine I came across several pathological conditions which were related to this tiny but very fascinating organ. In addition, I noted for the first time that the majority of these disease entities are the result of hypophysis' neoplastic conversion in form of so called pituitary adenoma. Nowadays, it is well known that this tumor though benign can cause serious endocrinological problems, thus influence the daily activities of the patients.

Taking into account the aforementioned fact it becomes obvious that the hope of the affected persons for improvement of their quality of living relies in the field of research. However, and despite the remarkable advances of the last decades both in molecular biology/genetics but also in medicine the pathogenetic mechanism underlying the formation of pituitary adenoma remains still unclear, hence further investigation needs to be undertaken in order to discover and understand the potential pathways leading to its appearance. Subsequently, this could help the researchers to develop novel therapeutic methods and create proper drugs with fewer side effects.

The main purpose of this book is to provide the reader with all important information concerning pituitary adenoma and is oriented both towards medical students and young doctors who are interested in acquiring or recapitulating basic knowledge but also towards investigators whose intension is to explore the unresolved secrets of this tumor. Therefore, particular attention has been given in covering every aspect of this theme and simultaneously presenting the current data in a logical and comprehensible manner. In order to achieve this, the initial thought was to divide the book in four distinct parts, starting with general information about hypophysis and pituitary adenoma, continuing with the clinical symptomatology and the diagnostic approach of the tumor in the second and third section respectively and finally describing the treatment modalities that are currently in use.

At this point, I wish to show my gratitude to Nova Science Publisher both for the invitation to edit this book but also for its continuous and generous support. Further, I would like to express my cordial thanks to all authors one by one and in the order that they are referred in the book, namely Dr. D. Anestakis, Dr. J. Yovos, Dr. M. Yavropoulou, Dr. M. Tsolaki, Drs. O. Karapanou and S. Tsagarakis, Drs. D. Yoshida, A. T. Akio and A. Morita, Dr. W Saeger, Drs. A. Drevelegas, E. Papadopoulou and D. Chourmouzi, Dr. E. Moralidis,

Drs. C.-H. Kim and S.-Y. Jang, Dr. Y. Hayashi, Drs. S. Berkmann and J. Fandino, that accepted to participate in the book by writing a chapter according to their diagnostic, clinical and scientific expertise in the particular field. In fact, their substantial contribution led to the successful completion of this project. Last but not least, I am really grateful to Miss Rosalie Terzaki and Mr. Georgios Kalpakidis for their valuable technical assistance throughout the editing process.

In: Pituitary Adenoma
Editor: Dimitrios N. Kanakis

ISBN: 978-1-63484-985-2

Chapter 1

INTRODUCTION AND EPIDEMIOLOGY

Doxakis Anestakis*[*]*, MD, PhD
Teaching and Research Fellow, Department of Histopathology,
Laboratory of Forensic Medicine and Research Associate,
Laboratory of General Biology,
School of Health Sciences, Medical Faculty,
Aristotle University of Thessaloniki, Thessaloniki, Greece

ABSTRACT

The pituitary, a small bean-shaped gland at the base of the brain, maintains multiple homeostatic functions including metabolism, growth and reproduction. Pituitary adenomas represent approximately 10-12% of all adult primary intracranial neoplasms and 25% of surgically resected intracranial tumors, about half of these pituitary adenomas are hormonally active and develop in the anterior lobe of the pituitary gland. The peak incidence of pituitary tumors occurs between the ages of 30 and 60 years and they are equally distributed among the sexes in autopsy series. Only 3% to 7% of patients with pituitary adenomas are younger than 20 years old. Typical presenting manifestations include amenorrhea, infertility, visual field abnormalities, and headache. Diagnosis is often made with brain MRI, visual field testing, and serum hormone assay. Pituitary adenomas are classified based on upon anatomical, histological and functional criteria. Anatomically pituitary tumors are classified as microadenomas and macroadenomas. Histological classification utilizes an immunohistological characterization of the tumors in terms of their hormone production. Finally a classification with functional criteria includes secreting tumors, functioning tumors, or endocrine-active tumors and Non-functioning or endocrine-inactive pituitary tumors. About 50% of adenomas produce too much of one of the hormones.

Keywords: pituitary gland, history, epidemiology, classification, tumors, adenoma

[*] Corresponding author: Doxakis Anestakis, MD, PhD, Laboratory of Forensic Medicine, Aristotle University of Thessaloniki, PO Box: 325, 54124 Thessaloniki, Greece, E-mail: anestaki@auth.gr.

1. INTRODUCTION

The pituitary gland is a central endocrine organ that regulates basic physiological functions incuding growth, reproduction and metabolic homeostasis. It situates at the base of the brain, under the optic chiasm, inside a depression on the upper surface of the sphenoid bone, the sella turcica [1, 2].

It is a small neuro-endocrine organ with a diameter of only 1 centimeter, and a weight of about 0.5 gram. It is attached to the hypothalamus by the pituitary stalk and a portal system. The pituitary gland has three anatomical and functional parts, the posterior pituitary gland, which is of neuroectodermal origin, and the intermediate and anterior pituitary gland, which derives from the oral ectoderm [2].

The posterior pituitary gland (neurohypophysis) contains axons from neurons in the hypothalamus that secrete Vasopressin and Oxytocin. The neurohypophysis derives from neuroectoderm, an evagination of the neural tube at the base of the hypothalamus [1-3].

The intermediate gland (which is not present in humans) secretes Melanocyte Stimulating Hormone (MSH) [1, 3].

The anterior lobe (adenohypophysis) derives from buccal ectoderm, Rathke's pouch, which arises from the embryonic roof of the pharynx [3, 4].

The adenohypophysis is composed of three parts: a major anterior part, known as the pars distalis, a part surrounding much of the stalk, pars tuberalis and a vestigial part, pars intermedia, located next to the neurohypophysis. The anterior pituitary is devoid of a nerve supply, but has a unique blood supply, a portal system. The hypothalamohypophyseal portal system begins in a series of capillaries in the median eminence of the hypothalamus, and sends blood via veins to the anterior lobe, where it ends in a series of capillaries. This portal system carries neurohormones from the hypothalamus to the anterior pituitary, where they control the secretion of anterior lobe hormones [4].

The anterior pituitary consists of five different endocrine cell types, identified by antibodies against pituitary hormones and capable of production and secretion of pituitary hormones: [2, 4]

1. **Somatotroph cells.** These cells are acidophilic and produce growth hormone (GH).
2. **Lactotroph cells.** These cells are acidophilic and produce prolactin.
3. **Corticotroph cells.** These cells are basophilic and produce adrenocorticotrophic hormone (ACTH), pro-opiomelanocortin (POMC), melanocyte stimulating hormone (MSH) and endorphins.
4. **Thyreotrophic cells.** These cells are basophilic and produce thyrotropin (TSH).
5. **Gonadotrophic cells.** These cells are basophilic and produce luteinising hormone (LH) and follicle-stimulating hormone (FSH).

Specifically in response to releasing hormones secreted from the hypothalamus each cell type secretes its distinct hormone. Thyrotropin Releasing Hormone (TRH) stimulates Thyroid Stimulating Hormone (TSH) release from the thyrotropes. Gonadotropin Releasing Hormone (GnRH) stimulates release of Luteinising Hormone (LH) and Follicle- Stimulating Hormone (FSH) from gonadotropes. Growth hormone releasing hormone (GHRH) stimulates Growth Hormone (GH) release from the somatotropes and finally Corticotropin Releasing Hormone

(CRH) stimulates Adrenocorticotropin (ACTH) release from the corticotropes. A hypothalamic Prolactin Releasing Hormone (PRRH) has been characterised that binds to the G-protein coupled receptor hGR3[5], although subsequent studies have suggested that PRRH is only functional in females and only at high concentrations and that much of its function may be mediated by the hypothalamus [4-6].

TSH, LH, FSH and ACTH exert their effects through peripheral endocrine organs, whereas Prolactin and GH act directly on their target organs to regulate reproduction and growth respectively.

During adult life, the activity and size of the pituitary gland changes with age and in response to certain physiological events such as pregnancy. Accordingly the pituitary gland is subjected to a very complex regulation, consisting of hormonal regulation from the hypothalamus as well as feedback control from the peripheral target glands and other endocrine glands that regulate the activity and growth of the pituitary gland directly and indirectly through the hypothalamus. This plasticity of the pituitary gland, which is a consequence of the necessity to adapt to changing physiological needs, may be the reason why pituitary gland neoplasias are more frequent than tumors of other tissue [1, 6, 7].

2. The History

The earliest history of the pituitary gland dates back to Ancient Egypt (around 1365 BC) where a portrait, of the Pharaoh at the time (Akhenaten), shows signs of acromegaly. Galen, in 150 AD, was the first to describe the pituitary, and he proposed that its role was to drain the phlegm from the brain to the nasopharynx [8].

In 1543 the Belgian scientist Andreas Vesalius described the anatomy of pituitary gland for the first time. He believed that pituitary produces mucus, which is secreted from the brain into the nasal cavity. This is why pituitary was called the mucous gland (glandula pituitaria, pituita = mucus). The knowledge of pituitary anatomy and function, as well as of the characteristic changes in size and shape of the pituitary throughout the life and special physiologic conditions, is mandatory for the correct diagnosis and therefore these factors have to be taken into account before assessing pituitary abnormalities [2, 8].

In the early 18th century, De Haen described amenorrhea in a patient with a pituitary tumor. It was in 1742 that Joseph Lieutaud discovered the pituitary-portal blood system, known today as the hypothalamo-hypophysial axis. In 1772, Saucerotte was the first to describe acromegaly. In 1794, Frank distinguished diabetes insipidus from diabetes mellitus. Rathke described the formation of the gland in 1838. In 1887, Minkowski was the first to link the expansion of the pituitary gland to a number of clinical symptoms. Within a few years it was accepted that it was the anatomical growth of the gland that produced the symptoms [2, 6, 8].

In 1892, Vassale and Sacchi showed that by removing the pituitary gland (hypophysectomy) the water and mineral metabolism of the body were affected. In the same year, Massalongo attributed acromegaly to hyperfunction of the pituitary. The following year, Caton and Paul attempted surgical treatment to relieve the pressure from a pituitary tumor. In 1907, Schloffer became the first to operate on the pituitary via the nasal route [8].

In 1909, Aschner showed that a hypophysectomy in a growing animal caused dwarfism. Cushing and his team made the first experimental link between the pituitary and the reproductive organs in 1910. Glinski described post-partum necrosis of the pituitary gland in 1914. The following year Simmonds described pituitary cachexia [8, 9].

In 1924, the Soviet neurologist Nikolai Mikhailovich Itsenko reported two patients with pituitary adenoma. The resulting excessive adrenocorticotropic hormone secretion led to the production of large amounts of cortisol by the adrenal glands [10]. The disease associated with this increased secretion of cortisol was described by Harvey Cushing in 1932, after Cushing presented a unique case of a 23-year-old woman called Minnie G. Minnie's symptoms included painful obesity, amenorrhea, hypertrichosis (abnormal hair growth), underdevelopment of secondary sexual characteristics, hydrocephalus and cerebral tension [10, 11].

This combination of symptoms was not yet described for any medical disorder at the time. However, Cushing was confident that Minnie's symptoms were due to dysfunction of the pituitary gland, and resembled those associated with an adrenal tumor. Given this conviction, and his knowledge of the three anterior pituitary cell types, Cushing hypothesized that if acidophil hyperpituitarism (excess secretion from the acidophil cells) caused acromegaly, then an excess of basophil cells must be involved in another pituitary disorder that involves sexual dysfunction (amenorrhea in females and erectile dysfunction in males) and could explain Minnie's symptoms. Experimental evidence and case reports by Cushing led to his publication in 1932 on pituitary basophilism as the cause of Cushing's disease [11]. In this publication, the clinical symptoms of the disease, named after Harvey Cushing, were described. Out of the 12 cases with hypercortisolism described in Cushing's monograph on the pituitary body, 67% died within a few years after symptom presentation, whereas Minnie G. survived for more than 40 years after symptom presentation, despite the fact that she did not receive any treatments for a pituitary tumor. The prolonged survival led to the uniqueness of Minnie's case [10, 11]. The reason behind this survival remains a mystery, since an autopsy of Minnie was refused after her death.

However, the most likely explanation, proposed by J. Aidan Carney and based on statistical evidence, was that the basophil adenoma Minnie might have harbored underwent partial infarction, leading to symptom regression. The other hypothesis was that Minnie might have suffered from Primary Pigmented Nodular Adrenocortical Disease (PPNAD), which when associated with Cushing's syndrome (Carney complex) can infrequently cause spontaneous symptom regression of the latter [11].

3. Pituitary Tumors

1. Introduction and Epidemiology

Tumors are the result of failed growth control. The development of a tumor is a dynamic process that involves sequential acquisition of tumorigenic traits driven by selectional pressure. Accordingly tumor development often involves a series of changes to pathways providing growth signals or mediating growth inhibitory signals as well as controlling cell survival [3, 12]. Advanced tumor progression also requires increased angiogenesis and the acquisition of limitless replicative potential. In the pituitary gland, tumor development is often a gradual progression from hyperplasia, which is a general increase tissue size due to higher cell numbers, to neoplasia, which can be defined as an abnormal mass of cells produced by an autonomous growth of a tissue. Each cell type of the anterior lobe can give rise to pituitary tumors. They are the result of excessive proliferation and they can over-produce the specific hormones leading to endocrine syndromes, or they may be functionally silent [2, 9].

Neoplasias can be benign or malignant depending on their growth rate and invasiveness. A benign tumor which originates from glandular epithelium is called an adenoma, whereas a malignant tumor of the same origin is termed a carcinoma.

Different lesions may present as a mass within the sella turcica. In unselected autopsy series, the prevalence of pituitary tumors varies between 2 and 27%, with an average prevalence of 11% in a compilated series of 12411 patients [3, 6, 13].

About 10000 pituitary tumors are diagnosed each year in the United States. Almost all of these tumors are benign pituitary adenomas. Very few pituitary tumors are cancers (carcinomas) [13-15].

The actual number of pituitary tumors may be much higher than the number of tumors that are found each year. When examining people who have died or who have had imaging tests (like MRI scans) of their brain for other health problems, doctors have found that as many as one out of four people may have a pituitary adenoma without knowing it. These tumors are often small and never cause any symptoms or health problems, so very few of them would normally be diagnosed at all [16-18].

Pituitary tumors can occur at any age (including children), but they are most often found in older adults.

In patients operated for pituitary tumors, pituitary adenomas account for more than 90% of the tumors. Of other causes, the most common diagnosis is Rathke's cleft cyst (28%), craniopharyngioma (14%), metastatic carcinoma (12%), chordoma (11%) and meningioma (10%) [13, 14, 18, 19].

The vast majority of pituitary gland tumors are sporadic. Pituitary gland tumors are almost inevitably benign, but can nevertheless lead to death due to their localization just beneath the brain. Pathology from pituitary gland tumors normally arises from an excess of hormone secretion [12, 13].

4. Pituitary Adenomas

1. Introduction and Epidemiology

Pituitary adenomas represent approximately 10-12% of all adult primary intracranial neoplasms and 25% of surgically resected intracranial tumors, about half of these pituitary adenomas are hormonally active and develop in the anterior lobe of the pituitary gland [14]. Although classified as benign, they may cause significant morbidity in affected patients due to aberrant hormone secretion, as well as compressive effects on nearby tissues, such as the optic chiasm, or the healthy pituitary (hypopituitarism) [6, 14].

Table 1. Classification of Pituitary Adenomas According to Size

Microadenomas
Macroadenomas

Table 2. Classification of Pituitary Adenomas A ccording to Endocrine Function

Adenomas with *growth hormone excess*
Adenomas with *prolactin excess*
Adenomas with *growth hormone and prolactin excess*
Adenomas with *adrenocorticotropic hormone excess*
Adenomas with *thyrotropin hormone excess*
Adenomas with *follicle stimulating and luteinizing hormones excess*
Adenomas with *no apparent hormonal function*

Table 3. Classification of Pituitary Adenomas According to Histological Criteria

Chromophobic adenomas
Acidophilic adenomas
Basophilic adenomas

Pituitary adenomas exhibit a wide range of hormonal and proliferative behaviours [1]. They may be small, slowly growing and hormonally inactive, and might only be detected as radiographic "incidentalomas" or at postmortem examination. If, however, they produce hormones in excess, they can cause mood disorders, sexual dysfunction, infertility, obesity and disfigurement, hypertension, diabetes mellitus and accelerated heart disease. If untreated, hormone-excess syndromes can be lethal [20, 21].

Some pituitary adenomas grow rapidly, producing symptoms of an intracranial mass, loss of normal anterior pituitary hormone production, and visual-field disturbances due to stretching of the overlying optic chiasm. They can invade downward into paranasal sinuses, laterally into the cavernous sinuses (thereby disrupting coordinated eye movement) and upwards into the brain. They can cause death by invasion of the brain [20, 22, 23].

Pituitary adenomas are usually well demarcated and are separated from the adjacent compressed non-tumorous adenohypophysis by a pseudocapsule that consists of condensed reticulin fibers. Unlike many benign tumors of other locations, these lesions have no fibrous capsule. Some histologically benign tumors have an indistinct border, and clusters of adenoma cells may be found to spread deeply into the adjacent non-tumorous adenohypophysis [2, 22].

Typical presenting manifestations include amenorrhea, infertility, visual field abnormalities, and headache. Diagnosis is often made with brain MRI, visual field testing, and serum hormone assay [16, 17]. Pituitary adenomas are classified based on functional, histological criteria and according to their size (Table 1-3) [3, 23-25]:

1. *The classification of pituitary tumours according to their size includes* [12, 23, 25]:
   - **Microadenomas:** When the diameter is <10mm. Because these tumors are small, they rarely damage the rest of the pituitary or nearby tissues. But they can

cause symptoms if they make too much of a certain hormone. Many people actually have small adenomas that are never detected because they never grow large enough or secrete enough hormones to cause a problem.

A pituitary microadenoma is confined to the sella, and as such has no scope to produce symptoms due to mass effect. Thus they are most frequently diagnosed as the result of investigating hormonal imbalance (usually excess production of one or more hormones), while rarely they can be an incidental finding.

Microadenomas can occur in either sex. As many as 10% of the population may have a microadenoma, but most do not cause symptoms [14]. Prolactinomas, a subset of microadenomas, are diagnosed more frequently in women, possibly because of the more striking presenting features such as amenorrhea, galactorrhea, or both. In men, the diagnosis of inactive adenomas is often delayed until they have become macroadenomas and cause symptoms by compressing nearby structures. Microadenomas can occur at any age, but prevalence appears to increase with age [26].

Symptoms of a pituitary microadenoma may include the following: tiredness, headaches, vomiting, dizziness, vision problems, nausea, menstrual or breast changes, unexplained hair growth or loss [1, 13, 24, 26].

- **Macroadenomas:** When the diameter is >10mm. When the diameter is >40mm they are defined as large or giant pituitary adenomas [12]. Macroadenomas can affect a person's health in two ways. First, they can cause symptoms if they make too much of a certain hormone. Second, they can cause symptoms by pressing on normal parts of the pituitary or on nearby nerves, such as the optic nerves.

  Pituitary macrocadenomas are the most common suprasellar mass in adults, and responsible for the majority of transsphenoidal hypophysectomise [26]. Patients typically present with symptoms of local mass effect on adjacent structures (especially optic chiasm). Some may present hormonal imbalance, with symptoms of hypopituitarism (from compression) or secretion. The optic chiasm is located directly over the pituitary gland in 80% of individuals. The rest is divided between pre- and post-fixed chiasms. A pre-fixed optic chiasm is located anterior to its normal position over the tuberculum sellae, whereas a post-fixed chiasm is located over the dorsum sellae [5, 13, 26].

  A macroadenoma growing superiorly out of the pituitary fossa (or for that matter other pituitary region masses) will contact, elevate and compress the central part of the chiasm in most individuals. This central part carries fibers from the nasal retina, and thus results in the classical bitemporal hemianopsia. Patients typically complain of bumping into things or having car accidents, but as the macular fibres are often spared, they may not be aware of actual visual deficits [26].

  Some macroadenomas demonstrate invasive growth, and extension into the cavernous sinuses is characteristic. Prolactin secreting tumors are most frequently responsible for cavernous sinus extension, and typically prolactin level increase significantly when the tumor gains access to the sinus. Once in the sinus, these tumors are difficult to be completely resected [5]. They may compress cranial nerves resulting in deficits, although this is uncommon, seen in only 1-14% of cases [5, 13, 14, 27]. Most pituitary adenomas are microadenomas [13, 14].

2. *The clinical hormone-secreting types are [1, 3, 6, 26]:*
   - ***GH-secreting adenomas (or somatotropinomas):*** Growth hormone-producing tumors secrete too much growth hormone. GH-producing pituitary adenomas cause acromegaly and gigantism Acromegaly is a hormonal disorder that results from too much growth hormone (GH) in the body. Although pituitary gland normally produces GH, in acromegaly there is an excess of this hormone. Usually the excess GH comes from benign, or non-cancerous, tumors on the pituitary. These benign tumors are called adenomas [1, 3, 28].

     Acromegaly is most often diagnosed in middle-aged adults, although symptoms can appear at any age. If not treated, acromegaly can result in serious illness and premature death. Acromegaly is treatable in most patients, but because of its slow and often "sneaky" onset, it is often not diagnosed early or correctly. The most serious health consequences of acromegaly are: type 2 diabetes, high blood pressure, increased risk of cardiovascular disease, and arthritis. Patients with acromegaly are also at increased risk of developing colon polyps, which may develop into colon cancer if not removed [6, 28].

     When GH-producing tumors occur in childhood, the disease that results is called gigantism rather than acromegaly. A child's height is determined by the length of the so-called long bones in the legs. In response to GH, these bones grow in length at the growth plates areas near either end of the bone. Growth plates fuse after puberty, so the excessive GH production in adults does not result in increased height [28]. However, prolonged exposure to excess GH, before the growth plates fuse, causes increased growth of the long bones and thus increased height. Pediatricians may become concerned about this possibility if a child's growth rate suddenly and markedly increases beyond what would be predicted by previous growth and by the height of its parents [6, 26].
   - ***PRL-secreting adenomas (or prolactinomas):*** In this type of pituitary tumor, prolactin is overproduced. High prolactin levels can cause menstrual periods in women to be irregular or stop, and can cause galactorrhea (abnormal breast milk production). Men may experience impotence (erectile dysfunction) or a lack of interest in sex. Men may also have enlarged breasts, infertility, or a decrease in body hair. If these symptoms go unrecognized and progress, headaches and vision problems may occur next [5, 29].

     Prolactin (PRL) was characterized as recently as 1971 as a hormone distinct from growth hormone, which also has lactogenic activity. In humans, the predominant PRL species is a 23 kDa, 199-amino-acid, polypeptide synthesized and secreted by lactotroph cells in the anterior pituitary gland. Pituitary PRL production is under tonic inhibitory control by hypothalamic dopamine, in such a way that pituitary stalk interruption produces hyperprolactinemia [29]. The neuropeptides thyrotropin-releasing hormone (TRH) and vasoactive intestinal peptide (VIP) exert less important stimulatory effects on pituitary PRL release.

     Prolactin is essential for postpartum milk production and lactation. During pregnancy, increasing estrogen production stimulates the pituitary lactotrophs and causes increased PRL secretion. However, high estrogen levels inhibit PRL stimulation of the breasts, and, as a result, lactation does not occur until the estrogen levels decline postpartum [5, 9, 12, 29].

Prolactinomas are the most common hormonally active pituitary tumors. There is a marked female preponderance, and prolactinoma is relatively rare in men. Several studies have revealed small prolactinomas in approx 5% of autopsy pituitaries, most of which are undiagnosed during life [29]. From a clinical stand-point, prolactinomas may be divided arbitrarily into microprolactinomas (<10mm diameter) and macroprolactinomas (>10mm diameter) [5, 13, 14, 26]. This is a useful distinction that predicts tumor behavior and indicates appropriate management strategies.

Generally, microprolactinomas run a benign course. Some regress spontaneously, most stay unchanged for many years, and few expand to cause local pressure effects. Pooled data from seven studies, including 139 patients with untreated microprolactinomas, show documented tumor expansion in only nine patients (7%) [5, 13, 14]. In contrast, macroprolactinomas may present with pressure symptoms, often increase in size if untreated, and rarely disappear [26, 29].

Prolactinomas are usually sporadic tumors. Molecular genetics have shown nearly all to be monoclonal, suggesting that an intrinsic pituitary defect is likely to be responsible for pituitary tumorigenesis. Occasionally, prolactinoma may be part of a multiple endocrine neoplasia syndrome (MEN-1), but this occurs too infrequently to justify MEN-1 screening in every patient with a prolactinoma [5, 29].

- ***GH- and PRL-secreting adenomas (or mammosomatotroph adenomas):*** Mixed growth hormone GH- and PRL- secreting tumors are well recognized and give rise to acromegaly in association with hyperprolactinemia. Malignant prolactinomas are rare. A few cases have been described that have proved resistant to aggressive treatment with surgery, radiotherapy, dopamine agonists, and, occasionally, chemotherapy. In a small proportion, extracranial metastases in liver, lungs, bone, and lymph nodes have been documented [2, 27].
- ***ACTH-secreting adenomas (or corticotropinomas):*** ACTH stimulates the adrenal gland to make glucocorticoids (or steroids, which influence metabolism and act as anti-inflammatory and immunosuppressive agents). An oversupply of ACTH, such as that produced by this type of tumor, can cause Cushing's disease (one type of Cushing's syndrome) [1, 10, 11].

Cushing's syndrome results from prolonged exposure of tissues to excess of glucocorticoids. After Harvey Cushing's initial report in the early 20th century, Cushing's syndrome has been etiologically subdivided into adenocorticotropin hormone (ACTH)-independent (non-pituitary) and ACTH-dependent. Endogenous Cushing's syndrome is rare, with an overall incidence of approximately two to four new cases per million of population per year. ACTH-dependent Cushing's syndrome accounts for approximately 85% of endogenous cases. In the majority of these cases (80%), the cause is autonomous pituitary ACTH secretion and is referred as Cushing's disease [14]. In the remaining 20%, the ACTH secretion source is ectopic. Cushing's disease has a female to male preponderance (8:1), whereas the ectopic ACTH syndrome is more common in men (3:1) [13]. Ectopic corticotropin-releasing hormone (CRH) production causing Cushing's syndrome has also been described in 11 cases [13, 24].

Cushing's disease is characterized by obesity with central fat distribution, moon face, plethora, osteopenia, proximal muscle weakness, striae, hirsutism, acne, poor wound healing, easy bruisability, superficial fungal infections, hypertension, glucose intolerance, and gonadal dysfunction [11, 24].

Additional signs and symptoms may include: high blood pressure, abdominal obesity but with thin arms and legs, reddish stretch marks, a round red face, a fat lump between the shoulders, weak bones, acne, and fragile skin that heals poorly. Women may have more hair and irregular menstruation. Occasionally there may be changes in mood, headaches, and a chronic feeling of tiredness [26, 27, 30].

- ***TSH-secreting adenomas (or thyrotropinomas):*** Thyroid-stimulating hormone is produced by these tumors, which can become large and spread. TSH-secreting pituitary adenomas are benign tumors of the pituitary gland. They produce too much thyroid stimulating hormone (TSH), which causes the thyroid gland to enlarge and produce thyroid hormone in excess, leading to an overactive thyroid (hyperthyroidism). Patients typically present with signs and symptoms of hyperthyroidism, but these patients may also have headaches and loss of some of their field of vision, rarely, there are no symptoms (asymptomatic). Early diagnosis and correct treatment may prevent pituitary and heart complications and may improve cure rate. Patients may present with symptoms of hyperthyroidism including sweating, heat intolerance, shaky hands, palpitations, nervousness, increased stool frequency, weight loss, poor sleep quality, fatigue, and irregular periods. They may also present with headache, visual disturbance, an enlarged thyroid gland (goitre) and galactorrhea (inappropriate milky discharge from the breasts) [2, 6, 23].
- ***FSH- and LH-secreting adenomas (or gonadotropinomas):*** In women their main effects are on the ovaries, where they regulate ovulation (the release of eggs) and the production of the hormones estrogen and progesterone. In men, these hormones help regulate the testes' production of sperm and testosterone. Excess production can lead to abnormalities in these functions [2, 7, 24].
- ***Non-Functioning Pituitary Adenomas (NFPAs):*** They do not secrete an extra amount of hormone and, until they reach a certain size, the person does not have any symptoms [1, 31].

Not every pituitary tumor (adenoma) causes hormone-related symptoms. When blood testing does not reveal an abnormally high hormone level, we call this a non-functioning pituitary adenoma.

There are several possible reasons why non-functioning pituitary adenomas could arise, including: [31] The cellular production process of hormones typically involves making a much larger molecule, and then cutting it at the right places to make the hormone. In some cases, something is wrong with this cutting process and therefore a "functional" hormone is not made. It might be released into the bloodstream, but it is inactive and usually not detectable using standard blood tests.

In other cases, the tumor cells simply do not produce a hormone and thus classified as:

- *Silent somatotroph adenomas*
- *Silent lactotroph adenomas*
- *Silent thyrotroph adenomas*
- *Silent corticotroph adenomas*
- *Silent gonadotroph adenomas*

When the tumors are large enough, they may cause headaches and vision problems. The most common symptoms are due to the large tumor compressing nearby structures, leading to:

Vision Loss

- When large pituitary adenomas grow upward into the brain cavity, the tumor can elevate and compress the optic chiasm.
- A loss of the outer peripheral vision, called a bitemporal hemianopsia.

When severe, patients can only see what is directly in front of them, many patients do not become aware of their visual loss until it is quite severe.

Other Visual Problems

- Loss of visual acuity (blurry vision), especially if the adenoma grows forward and compresses an optic nerve.
- nability to perceive colors as brightly as usual [31].

About 50% of adenomas produce too much of more than one of the hormones (mixed tumors co-secreting GH with PRL, TSH or ACTH). The majority of NFPAs are derived from FSH- or LH-cells and are clinically silent [13, 14, 31]. From 25 to 90% of pituitary adenomas are prolactinomas. About 25% of them secrete growth hormone or growth hormone and prolactin. Excess prolactin may cause galactorrhea and excess growth hormone causes acromegaly clinically indistinguishable from sporadically occurring acromegaly [13, 14, 29, 31]. From the other types of pituitary adenomas the NFPAs constitute the 30% of adenomas, the somatotropinomas the 15-20%, the corticotropinomas the 5-15%, the thyrotropinomas and LH-FSH adenomas less than 1% [7, 13, 24]. There are limited data on the prevalence of pituitary tumors. Although classically considered to be rare, systematic assessments from autopsy and radiologic studies have shown a prevalence of 17% in the population [13, 14]. Pituitary tumors can be found in every age group, but their incidence tends to increase with age [24]. The peak incidence of pituitary tumors occurs between the ages of 30 and 60 years and they are equally distributed among the sexes in autopsy series. Functioning (also called secreting) tumors most frequently occur in younger adults. Only 3% to 7% of patients with pituitary adenomas are younger than 20 years old. Non-functioning (non-secreting) tumors tend to occur in older adults [14]. Women are diagnosed with pituitary tumors slightly more often than men. This may be a result of the tumor's interference with the menstrual cycle, which sometimes makes symptoms more obvious [13, 21, 24]. One-third is unassociated with hypersecretory syndromes, the majority of these produce but do not secrete the gonadotropins i.e., follicle-stimulating hormone and/or luteinizing hormone. Growth hormone (GH)-producing or adrenocorticotropic hormone (ACTH)-producing adenomas each account for 10-15% of pituitary adenomas. Adenomas producing thyrotropin (TSH) are rare [6, 12-14].

Pituitary macroadenomas constitute approximately 10% of all intracranial tumors overall [26]. The majority are clinically non-functioning and present as a result of either space-occupying effects or clinical hypopituitarism. Functioning tumours producing growth hormone, adrenocorticotrophic hormone or prolactin result in the classical endocrine conditions of acromegaly, Cushing's disease and galactorrhea/oligo/amenorrhea (impotence in the male) respectively [11, 28, 29, 31].

Non-functioning pituitary mass lesions may also produce modest hyperprolactinaemia as a result of disinhibition of the effects of hypothalamic dopamine on lactotroph cells [7, 18, 20]. The immunohistochemical staining often reflects the clinical phenotype, but provides additional information that together with the cytological and histological appearances of cells and tissue has an impact on the perceptions of potential aggressive behavior [2, 32].

Classification of pituitary adenomas according to their morphologic features has undergone a substantial change. On the basis of the staining properties of the cell cytoplasm, pituitary adenomas were previously defined as one of three morphologic entities: chromophobic, acidophilic, and basophilic adenomas. Chromophobic adenomas were assumed to be endocrinologically inactive tumors not capable of secreting hormones. Acidophilic adenomas were thought to secrete GH and to be associated with acromegaly or gigantism. Basophilic adenomas were regarded as ACTH-producing tumors accompanied by Cushing's disease. Since the tinctorial characteristics of adenoma cells cannot be correlated reliably with cell type, secretory activity, or cytogenesis, however, this basis for classification is no longer considered useful.

Progress in methodology, especially the introduction of immunohistochemistry and electron microscopy, has resulted in a new and more meaningful morphologic classification, which separates pituitary adenomas into distinct entities on the basis of hormone content, cellular composition, fine structural features, and cytogenesis [32, 33].

More recently, at a time when many thought that the yield from morphologic appraisal of pituitary tumors had peaked, the field of pituitary oncology was rejuvenated with the new and powerful applications of molecular science. The recent interface of molecular technology with conventional pathologic methods has provided novel insights into some of the most fundamental questions concerning the biology, pathogenesis, and cytogenesis of pituitary tumors. In this regard, the methodologies of in situ hybridization and the polymerase chain reaction (PCR) have been most informative. The former permits the visualization of mRNAs of interest directly within individual tumors cells, highlighting the differences in the processing, transcription, and expression of various genes that govern the secretory process among different pituitary tumor types. By facilitating the identification of specific genomic alterations within tumor tissue, the polymerase chain reaction has been instrumental in demonstrating certain mutations that may contribute to pituitary tumorigenesis. This technology is currently for a research interest only, but in the foreseeable future the emerging molecular strategies will be important for precisely in classifying and the prognosis of pituitary adenomas [11, 15, 26].

REFERENCES

[1] DeGroot LJ, Jameson J. Co-editors of Endocrinology, 5th edition. Elsevier Saunders, Philadelphia 2006.

[2] Ooi GT, Tawadros N, Escalona RM. Pituitary cell lines and their endocrine applications. *Mol Cell Endocrinol* 2004;228:1-21.

[3] Nussey S, Whitehead S. Endocrinology: An Integrated Approach. Chapter 7. Oxford: BIOS Scientific Publishers 2001.

[4] Yeung CM, Chan CB, Leung PS, Cheng CH. Cells of the anterior pituitary. *Int J Biochem Cell Biol* 2006;38:1441-1449.

[5] Hinuma S, Habata Y, Fujii R, Kawamata Y, Hosoya M, Fukusumi S, et al. A prolactin-releasing peptide in the brain. *Nature* 1998;393:272-276.

[6] Asa SL. Tumors of the pituitary gland. In: Rosai J (editor). Atlas of tumor pathology. 3rd Series, Fascicle 22. Armed Forces Institute of Pathology. Washington, DC 1998.

[7] Seal LJ, Small CJ, Kim MS, Stanley SA, Taheri S, Ghatei MA et al. Prolactin releasing peptide (PrRP) stimulates luteinizing hormone (LH) and follicle stimulating hormone (FSH) via a hypothalamic mechanism in male rats. *Endocrinology* 2000;141:1909-1912.

[8] Hyrtl J. Onomatologia Anatomica. Geschichte und Kritik der anatomischen Sprache der Gegenwart. Wien: Wilhelm Braumüller. K.K. Hof- und Unversitätsbuchhändler 1880.

[9] Donovan LE, Corenblum B. The natural history of the pituitary incidentaloma. *Arch Intern Med* 1995;155:181-183.

[10] Lanzino G, Maartens N, Laws ER Jr. Cushing's case XLV: Minnie G. *J Neurosurg* 2002;97:231-234.

[11] Cushing H. The basophil adenomas of the pituitary body. *Ann R Coll Surg Engl* 1969;44:180-181.

[12] Asa SL, Ezzat S. The pathogenesis of pituitary tumors. *Annu Rev Pathol* 2009;4:97-126.

[13] Yamada S. Epidemiology of pituitary tumors. In: Thapar K, Kovacs K, Scheithauer BW, Lloyd RV (editors). Diagnosis and management of pituitary tumors. Humana Press, Totawa 2001, pp 57-69.

[14] Daly AF, Tichomirowa MA, Beckers A. The epidemiology and genetics of pituitary adenomas. *Best Pract Res Clin Endocrinol Metab* 2009;23:543-554.

[15] Melmed S. Mechanisms for pituitary tumorigenesis: the plastic pituitary *J Clin Invest* 2003;112:1603–1618.

[16] Pisaneschi M, Kapoor G. Imaging the sella and parasellar region. *Neuroimaging Clin N Am* 2005;15:203-219.

[17] Scanarini M, Mingrino S. Functional classification of pituitary adenomas *Acta Neurochirurgica* 1980;52:195-202.

[18] Dudley KJ, Revill K, Clayton RN, Farrell WE. Pituitary tumours: all silent on the epigenetics front. *J Mol Endocrinol* 2009;42:461-468.

[19] Freda PU, Wardlaw S. Clinical review 110: Diagnosis and treatment of pituitary tumors *J Clin Endocrinol Metab* 1999;84:3859-3866.

[20] Aron DC, Howlett TA. Pituitary incidentalomas. *Endocrinol Metab Clin North Am* 2000;29:205-221.

[21] Fernandez A, Karavitaki N, Wass JA. Prevalence of pituitary adenomas: a community-based, cross-sectional study in Banbury (Oxfordshire, UK). *Clin Endocrinol* (Oxf) 2010;72:377-382.

[22] Herman V, Fagin J, Gonsky R, Kovacs K, Melmed S. Clonal origin of pituitary adenomas. *J Clin Endocrinol Metab* 1990;71:1427-1433.

[23] McDowell B, Wallace R, Carnahan R, Chrischilles EA, Lynch CF, Schlechte JA. Demographic differences in incidence for pituitary adenoma. *Pituitary* 2011;14:23-30.

[24] Fernandez A, Karavitaki N, Wass JA. Prevalence of pituitary adenomas: a community-based, cross-sectional study in Banbury (Oxfordshire, UK). *Clin Endocrinol* (Oxf) 2010;72:377-382.

[25] Chacko G, Chacko AG, Lombardero M, Mani S, Seshadri MS, Kovacs K, et al. Clinicopathologic correlates of giant pituitary adenomas. *J Clin Neurosci* 2009;16:660-665.

[26] Shruti P, Tanvi CD. Invasive Pituitary Macroadenoma: A Rare Case Report. *International Journal of Scientific Study* 2014;2:121-124.

[27] Korbonits M, Morris DG, Nanzer A, Kola B, Grossman AB. Role of regulatory factors in pituitary tumour formation. *Front Horm Res* 2004;32:63-95.

[28] Katznelson L, Laws R, Melmed S, Molitch E, Murad H., Utz A, Wass A. Acromegaly: An Endocrine Society Clinical Practice Guideline Journal of Clinical Endocrinology & Metabolism 2014;99:3933-3951.

[29] Klibanski A. Clinical practice. Prolactinomas. *N Engl J Med* 2010;362:1219-1226.

[30] Knosp E, Steiner E, Kitz K, Matula C. Pituitary adenomas with invasion of the cavernous sinus space: a magnetic resonance imaging classification compared with surgical findings. *Neurosurgery* 1993;33:610-617.

[31] Greenman Y, Ouaknine G, Veshchev I, Reider-Groswasser II, Segev Y, Stern N. Postoperative surveillance of clinically nonfunctioning pituitary macroadenomas: markers of tumour quiescence and regrowth. *Clin Endocrinol* (Oxf) 2003;58:763-769.

[32] Asa SL, Ryan N, Kovacs K, Singer W, Marangos PJ. Immunohistochemical localization of neuron-specific enolase in the human hypophysis and pituitary adenomas. *Arch Pathol Lab Med* 1984;108:40-43.

[33] Kasper M, Kasper M, Kern F, Heitz PU, Gudat F. Immunohistochemical studies on human pituitary gland and adenomas *J Hirnforsch* 1991;32:725-734.

In: Pituitary Adenoma
Editor: Dimitrios N. Kanakis

ISBN: 978-1-63484-985-2

Chapter 2

PITUITARY MORPHOGENESIS AND DEVELOPMENT: FROM PHYSIOLOGY TO DISEASE

John G. Yovos*, MD, PhD
Professor Emeritus of Medicine-Endocrinology, School of Health Sciences, Medical Faculty, Aristotle University of Thessaloniki, Thessaloniki, Greece

ABSTRACT

The developed pituitary gland comprises of three lobes: the anterior, the intermediate and the posterior lobe. The anterior and intermediate lobes derive from an invagination of the oral ectoderm forming the Rathke's pouch. These cells proliferate and subsequently undergo progressive terminal differentiation forming the 5 adult pituitary cell types of the anterior lobe, whereas the posterior lobe (or neurohypophysis) derives from a neuroectodermic projection, the infundibulum. In mammals, the intermediate lobe contains melanotrophs but is minimally present in humans. The molecular mechanisms of pituitary ontogenesis involve complex interactions between signaling molecules and pituitary transcription factors, which participate in a tightly regulated, spatially and temporally organized, procedure. Transcription factors, such as Prop1, Pou1f1 (Pit1), Hesx1, Lhx3 and Lhx4 regulate the entire morphogenesis interacting with DNA as co-activators or co-repressors. Genetic defects in pituitary Transcription Factors (TFs) are responsible for inherited abnormalities in pituitary development and some of these defects are associated with transient pituitary hyperplasia. Abnormal signaling from developmental molecules such as FGFs, BMPs, and master developing pathways (Wnt, Hedgehog, Notch) is being increasingly recognized in pituitary tumors. In this chapter we describe the current knowledge about the process of pituitary organogenesis, dysfunction and oncogenesis, compiling the data acquired from functional studies collected from deletions or mutations of the transcription factors in transgenic animals, as well as from the accumulated clinical experience.

---

* Corresponding author: John G. Yovos, MD, PhD, P.P. Germanou Str. 27, 54622 Thessaloniki, Greece, E-mail: giovos@med.auth.gr.

Keywords: Rathke pouch, ectodermal placode, adenohypophysis, neurohypophysis, Sonic hedgehog, wnt, Notch, transcription factors, somatotrophs, gonadotrophs, thyrotrophs, corticotrophs, lactotrophs, pituitary adenoma, growth factors

1. INTRODUCTION

The pituitary is an endocrine gland regulating an array of peripheral endocrine organs and functions relaying signals from the hypothalamus, which is the principal neural structure regulating homeostasis and integrates complex signals from other regions of the brain and the periphery maintaining the body's internal balance. Hypothalamus contains a group of specialized nuclei populated by magno- and parvocellular neuroendocrine tumors. Most of their axons end in the median eminence, releasing factors that control the release of hormones from pituitary endocrine cells. It is also likely to provide trophic stimuli for the maintenance and plasticity of the gland. The pituitary, in turn, releases a number of hormones in the circulation to regulate various processes such as growth, puberty, metabolism, stress responses, reproduction, and lactation. The gland is situated within the sella turcica of the sphenoid bone, at the base of the brain. The mature pituitary gland is composed of the adenohypophysis (consisting of the anterior and intermediate lobes) and the neurohypophysis (posterior lobe), which are functionally and morphologically distinct but interacting structures. The anterior lobe of the pituitary is populated by five different specialized hormone-producing cell types. In humans the intermediate lobe largely disappears during embryogenesis. Several studies have shown rather more complex cellular relationships since there are subpopulations within the same hormone cell types. The proportion of these co-expressing cells can alter under different physiological [1] or pathological conditions [2]. The processes determining cell fate, migration patterns, and final location of the different hormone-producing cells during development into the adult anterior lobe requires a finely regulated genetic program, and individual gene deletions can result in various abnormalities of the differentiated hormone phenotype [3-5]. The posterior lobe contains the terminal axonal projections of magnocellular neurons from the paraventricular and supraoptic nuclei of the hypothalamus and specialized supportive glial cells, the pituicytes, which surround the axonal projections. The magnocellular neurons synthesize and release oxytocin, required during parturition and lactation, and arginine vasopressin, which is involved in the regulation of osmotic balance. These peptide hormones are transported to the axon terminals within the posterior pituitary where they are released as required under hypothalamic control. Hypothalamic factors are rapidly transported via the dual (upper and lower) hypophyseal portal vascular plexus to the adenohypophysis where they regulate cell proliferation, hormone synthesis, and hormone release from all the pituitary cell types. Classically, these factors are thought of as specific secretagogues, defined by the specificity of receptors on their target cells. However, this is an over-simplification because there are a much larger number of peptides and other factors known to be co-expressed in subsets of these hypothalamic neurons [6]. These are also transported and released into portal blood, probably in much smaller quantities than the hypophysiotropic peptides, and may modulate the secretion of anterior pituitary hormones and possibly regulate anterior pituitary plasticity.

2. The Beginning

The pituitary gland of all vertebrates is an organ of mixed genesis. The posterior lobe (PL) of the gland derives from the neuroectoderm, which forms the diencephalon while the anterior (AL) and intermediate (IL) lobes originate from the dorsal bulging of the primary oral inlet, the Rathke's pouch (RP). These two parts of the gland closely interact both physiologically and developmentally. While morphological details as well as the organization of the gland vary among vertebrates, the general organization of the gland, its morphogenesis, and the molecular pathways involved in the development and functions of the differentiated distinct cell phenotypes are quite similar [7-10].

3. The Ectodermal Hypophyseal Placode

The ectodermal placode of the anterior pituitary is a thickening in the midline of the anterior neural ridge, which is located immediately anterior to the neural plate [11]. The posteriorly located midline part of the neural plate will be transformed to hypothalamus and the posterior lobe of pituitary (neurohypophysis) [12]. In mammals, the two areas that are involved in the formation of the pituitary gland are displaced ventrally from their anterior position during the process of head morphogenesis. As a result, the pituitary primordium displaced within the ectoderm at the roof of the oral cavity as the presumptive hypothalamus and neuropituitary and staying in contact with the hypophyseal placode, moves ventrally to form a part of ventral diencephalon. At approximately e9, the displaced placode begins to form the Rathke's pouch, the primordium of the anterior and intermediate lobe. By e10.5, a restricted region of the ventral diencephalon above the pouch gives rise to the infundibulum from which the posterior pituitary and pituitary stalk will derive. The juxtaposition of Rathke's pouch and the diencephalon is maintained throughout the early stages of pituitary morphogenesis. This relationship is necessary for tissue interactions between neural and oral ectoderm, which are critical for the initial stages of pituitary formation. By e10.5, the pouch is fully developed, and at e12.5 it is completely separated from the underlying oral ectoderm (Figure 1). The lumen of the pouch remains as a separator between the anterior and intermediate lobes in the mature gland. Several transcription factors expressed early in the ectodermal placode are required for later pituitary development. The paired-like homeodomain transcription factor.

Hesx1 is an important regulator of anterior development. The proteins Six3 and Six6 are also present in the placode. Finally, but not exhaustively, the homeodomain transcription factors Pitx1 and Pitx2 are also present at these early stages.

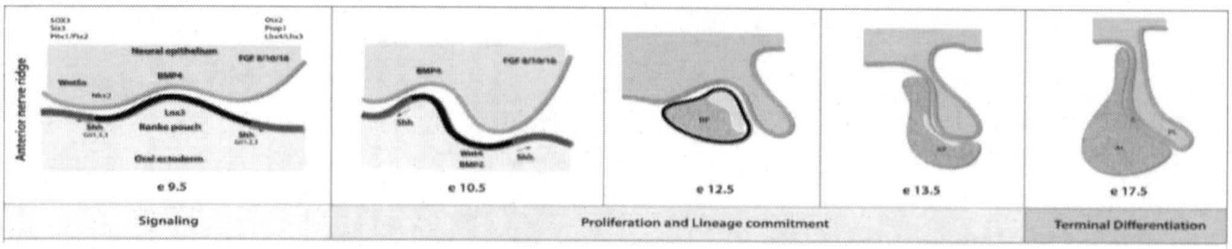

Figure 1. *Early pituitary morphogenesis.* The most anterior neural ridge gives rise to primordium of the anterior (AL) and intermediate (IL) lobes of the pituitary. The adjacent neural epithelium of the vental diencephalon (VD) develops into endocrine hypothalamus and the posterior lobe of the pituitary gland. VD, which expresses BMP4, FGF 8/10/18, and Wnt5a, makes direct contact with oral ectoderm and induces the formation of Rathke's pouch. Shh is expressed throughout the oral ectoderm except in the Rathke's pouch, creating a boundary between two ectodermal domains of Shh- and Shh+ cells. The opposing dorsal BMP4/FGF and ventral BMP2/Shh gradients determine the activation of specific genes and transcriptional factors such as Lnx3, Nkx2 and Pitx1/2 in each cell group according to their position in Rathke's pouch. The dorsal region of the Rathke's pouch becomes the intermediate lobe. The influndibulum grows downward and eventually becomes the posterior lobe (PL).

4. Cellular Differentiation and Signaling Molecules in the Developing Rathke Pouch

The Rathke's pouch is populated by proliferative progenitors that will gradually relocate ventrally, away from the lumen as they differentiate. A proliferative zone containing progenitors is maintained in the embryo, as well as, in the adults [15, 16]. An observed ventral re-localization is possibly associated with a passive movement of cells driven away by new proliferating cells. The phenotypic markers of the anterior pituitary primordium is directed by a complex morphogenetic procedure composed of signals emanating both from ventral diencephalon/infundibulum and from Rathke's pouch itself. The signals that are essential for the stratification of Rathke's pouch and for the timely and spatially organized process of endocrine cell type appearance are the same factors that are involved in the patterning of other organs, namely, Shh and members of FGF, BMP, Notch, and Wnt families of growth factors/morphogens [17]. The role of epidermal growth factor (EGF) signaling in pituitary development is not well documented. Although the signals from the diencephalon are essential for the regionalization within the pouch that allows the emergence of the different endocrine cell types [18-23], careful examination of the expression patterns of signaling molecules within the ventral diencephalon has revealed their presence for longer than previously thought (Figure 1) [24].

4.1. Sonic Hedgehog (Shh)

The secreted Shh plays an important role in cell patterning, as well as in the specification of different cell types and in the control of proliferation of numerous cell types. Three related transcription factors, Gli1, Gli2, and Gli3, acting downstream of the Shh pathway, are expressed in the ventral diencephalon and developing Rathke's pouch [17]. In mammals, during pituitary development, Shh is expressed in the ventral diencephalon and oral ectoderm but is excluded from the invaginating Rathke's pouch. The Shh downstream target gene

Patched1 is expressed in the developing pituitary, indicating that pituitary progenitors respond to the Shh signaling. Pituitary-specific blockage of this signaling by over-expressing the Shh antagonist Hip almost completely prevents Rathke's pouch growth and appearance of endocrine cell lineages. In contrast, Shh over-expression in the developing pituitary under the control of GSU regulatory element results in mild hyperplasia with expansion of ventral gonadotrope and thyrotrope cell lineages.

4.2. FGFs

The members of the fibroblast growth factors (FGFs) family are secreted molecules that bind to receptor tyrosine kinases resulting in activation of multiple signaling cascades through MAPK, PI3 kinase and phospholipase C, affecting, respectively, cell proliferation, survival and motility and play important roles in many aspects of morphogenesis and cell type differentiation, including anterior pituitary. Three members of this family, FGF8, -10, and -18, have been found in the ventral diencephalon and subsequently in the posterior lobe of pituitary during development [18, 19, 25, 26, 28]. FGF8 is an important component of signals originating from ventral diencephalon. It functions in the patterning of Rathke's pouch by maintaining proliferation and opposing the ventral BMP2 differentiation signal [18, 29]. During RP development the FGFs appear later than BMP4, from e9.5 up until at least e14.5 [18, 19]. FGFs are necessary for dorsal RP progenitor proliferation and maintenance. By analogy to other models, where FGFs act as chemo-attractants [30], they may also be involved in RP invagination [27].

4.3. BMPs

Bone morphogenetic proteins BMPs are secreted ligands, which bind to a serine-threonine receptor and activate an intracellular signaling pathway resulting in activation of SMADs and regulation of gene transcription. BMP signaling is crucial for the anterior pituitary development. At least two members of the BMP family, BMP4 and BMP2, participate in the development of the anterior pituitary. As noted above, BMP4 seems to be essential for the invagination of Rathke's pouch [31]. BMP4 is the earliest extrinsically required signaling molecule and its presence is critical for the continued progression of pituitary development [18, 31]. It is maintained in the infundibulum with a sharp ventral boundary up to at least e14.5 [18, 19, 24]. It remains to be determined whether BMP4, like FGF8, also regulates the expression or functions of Lhx3. Subsequent to the onset expression of BMP4 in ventral diencephalon, BMP2 starts to be expressed in RP at E10.5, first ventrally and then throughout, decreasing by e14.5 [18, 24]. It has shown that BMP2 is capable of inducing the expression of Isl1 and GSU, both of which are ventral markers of pituitary, and suppressing the expression of ACTH. The BMP2 signal together with a dorsal FGF8 signal appear to create opposing gradients that are suggested to generate temporally and spatially distinct patterns of transcription factor expression underlying cell lineage specification events [17-19]. BMP7 is first present in ventral mesenchyme at e10.5. The available data collectively suggest that BMP2 signaling provides a ventralizing positional procedure for pituitary development [18, 19]. It is worth noting that while BMP signaling is absolutely essential for the initiation of the cell type determination process, it has to be attenuated to achieve terminal differentiation. Normally, during anterior pituitary development the expression of BMP2 decreases dramatically after e14-15.

4.4. Notch

The Notch signaling pathway is an evolutionally conserved mechanism that regulates proliferation, apoptosis, cell fate determination, and morphogenesis. It has been described in the context of lateral inhibition and cell fate determination. Briefly, the membrane-bound ligands Delta-like or Jagged activate the trans-membrane receptor Notch on neighboring cells. Binding of the ligand allows for cleavage of the Notch intracellular domain (NICD) that can then translocate to the nucleus, where it displaces repressors that are otherwise associated with the transcription factor Rbp-J when the pathway is inactive. This in turn permits transcriptional activation of targets such as the Hes1 and bHLH transcription factors. Notch signaling is active during the early phases of pituitary development and it is required for infundibular morphogenesis as indicated by expression of Dll1, Jag1, Notch2, Notch3, as well as the direct downstream targets Hes1 and Hey1. Certain members of the Notch pathway are expressed in RP, becoming largely restricted to periluminal progenitors as the gland develops [32, 33]. Their expression becomes down-regulated in the future anterior pituitary at e13.5 as cells undergo lineage commitment [32-34]. Pituitary-specific inactivation of Rbp-J, which encodes a central mediator of the Notch signaling, leads to premature differentiation of progenitor cells as well as a streaming of the Pit1 lineage into corticotrope lineage. It has been shown that Rbp-J can bind to the evolutionally conserved recognition site in the first intron of the Prop1 gene and is recruited to this region during pituitary development, suggesting that Notch signaling directly activates Prop1 transcription and is required for maintaining high-level expression of Prop1, which is a necessary step for emergence of the Pit1 lineage. Conversely, regulation of Notch2 by Prop1 has also been suggested [32]. Finally, global impairment of endocrine differentiation results in up-regulation of Notch pathway components [35, 36]. These data collectively demonstrate that Notch signaling is required for generating diverse precursor pools and suggest that duration/intensity of Notch activity plays a critical role in lineage commitment [33]. In the later phases of pituitary development, Notch activity is attenuated, which is absolutely required for terminal differentiation of distinct cell lineages [33, 34]. Other components of the Notch pathway, including a subset of Notch-repressed neurogenic bHLH factors Mash1 and Math3, are expressed during pituitary development. It has also been shown that Mash1 and Math3 play critical roles in differentiation and functions of specific cell types.

4.5. Wnt

The canonical Wnt pathway is characterized by the central role of the intracellular protein β-catenin. In the absence of the ligand, β-catenin is targeted for degradation. When Wnt binds to the co-receptors LRP5/LRP6 and receptor Frizzled, cytoplasmic β-catenin can accumulate and translocate to the nucleus where it displaces the repressor Groucho, associated with the T-cell factor/lymphoid enhancer-binding factor (TCF/LEF) transcription factors. Wnt target genes that were silenced can now be activated. A second Wnt-activated pathway regulates planar cell polarity, affecting cell morphology and movement, and a third is the related non-canonical Wnt pathway, associated with intracellular Ca^{2+} release. Wnt signaling plays an important role in the control of proliferation of many cell types as well as in the patterning and in the maintenance of stem cell fate. During pituitary development, the Wnt/β-catenin pathway is active between e11.5 and e15.5, as indicated by expression of a direct downstream target Axin2, and is functionally required for Pit1 lineage determination and pituitary gland growth. Unlike in most other developmental processes regulated by the canonical Wnt pathway, induction of Pit1 expression is mediated by direct interactions between β-catenin and the tissue-specific paired-like homeodomain transcription factor Prop1, through an evolutionarily conserved Pit1 early enhancer [37-39]. The Prop1/β-catenin complex also acts as a transcriptional repressor for Hesx1, based on the recruitment of Groucho-related Tle, histone deacetylase (HDAC]) and Reptin co-repressors. Furthermore, β-catenin has been demonstrated to participate in Pitx2 activation [40, 41], which in turn stimulates progenitor proliferation, but the identity of the Wnt ligand is unknown [40]. Later on, β-catenin can interact with the transcription factor PROP1 and formation of this complex is important for emergence of endocrine lineages [38]. In conclusion, the Wnt canonical pathway may participate in progenitor proliferation and fate while dysregulation of the pathway is clearly linked to oncogenicity. Within RP, several Wnt ligands and members of the pathways are present and active [38, 42]. So far, two of them, Wnt4 and Wnt5a, have been reported to be specifically associated with the developmental events in the anterior pituitary. Wnt5a is expressed in the ventral diencephalon and infundibulum of mouse embryo since at least e9.5, while Wnt4 expression is detected in Rathke's pouch and sustained later through e14.5 [19]. Deletion of Wnt4, which is usually expressed transiently and exclusively in RP, causes a slight reduction in expression of the transcription factor Pit1 required for emergence of somatotropes, lactotropes and thyrotropes [42]. It seems that these two factors target independent, discrete, non-overlapping populations of pituitary precursors, and they play a role not in the specification of particular cell lineages but rather in the expansion of endocrine cell types. TCF4 is also expressed in (ventral diencephalon) VD and RP. Deletion of the gene results in a similar phenotype as Wnt5a ablation, but deletion of TCF/LEF factors is not necessarily comparable to loss of ligand or of β-catenin, because these actively repress transcription when the pathway is inactive. Both proteins are probably independently involved within VD in patterning and hence RP positioning. Whether other members of the Wnt family in combination with Wnt4,-5a play a role in lineage specification, as implicated by the pituitary specific deletion of the β-catenin gene, awaits further investigation. Other components of the Wnt/β-catenin signaling pathway, including frizzled2 (Fzd2), Lef1, Tcf3, and Tcf4, are expressed during pituitary development [43, 42]. Fzd2 is detectable in Rathke's pouch and infundibulum at e12.5 [43]. Tcf3 is expressed from e9.0 to e14.5 but is restricted from the Pit1-expressing caudomedial region of the gland. Tcf4 is detectable in early pituitary as well as in surrounding tissues and is markedly diminished by e13.5. Lef1 exhibits biphasic expression, initial transiently at e9.0 in Rathke's pouch and later reappearing at e13.5 in anterior and intermediate lobes of the gland [38].

5. Signaling Pathways and Transcriptional Regulators

A whole array of transcriptional regulators is required within RP for physiological development. Some of them are also present in VD, where they are necessary for infundibular morphogenesis and are indirectly involved in RP morphogenesis. Finally, others are exclusively present and required in VD and affect indirectly the developing pituitary (Figure 2).

5.1. Pitx

The Pitx proteins/transcription factors are morphogenetic regulators for different organs. They also participate in left–right asymmetry [44]. Pitx2 mutations are associated with *Axenfeld–Rieger syndrome*, mainly characterized by eye defects and pituitary abnormalities. Three bicoid-related Pitx transcription factors have been identified. Two of them, Pitx1 and Pitx2, exhibit overlapping and distinct expression patterns during pituitary development [45]. They are present in the hypophyseal placode, RP and later maintained in differentiated endocrine cells [46, 47]. They function redundantly and are required for maintenance of early RP progenitors [48]. Both transcription factors can recognize the same bicoid binding site and activate the promoters of multiple pituitary hormones including GSU, TSH, LH, FSH, GnRHr, PRL, and GH [49]. Genetic studies have demonstrated that they are required for cell proliferation, survival, and differentiation in a dosage-sensitive manner, with Pitx2 playing a more prominent role than Pitx1, and they function simultaneously to control Lhx3 expression [40, 50, 51]. Pitx1 has the ability to interact with the NH2-terminal transactivation domain of Pit1 [52] and to bind a cis-acting element of the POMC promoter [53]. In the pituitary, a definite pouch forms with induction of Lhx3, Hesx1, Pitx1, and GSU. Several studies have shown that Pitx1 and Pitx2 function in the same pathway to stimulate cell proliferation and survival. Over-expression of Pitx2 under the control of Pit1 or GSU regulatory elements leads to an increase in the number of somatotropes and gonadotropes, respectively [50, 40, 51]. Cell culture studies also show that the Wnt/β-catenin pathway can stimulate expression of Pitx2, which in turn regulates the expression of critical cell cycle regulators including Cyclin D1, D2 [15, 40, 54]. In addition to the early roles of Pitx2 in pituitary development, studies have shown that Pitx2 is necessary for expansion of the Pit1 lineages and differentiation of gonadotropes at later stages of pituitary organogenesis [51]. The requirement of Pitx1 and Pitx2 for terminal differentiation in the ventral cell types maybe explained, at least in part by the fact that both Pitx1 and Pitx2 are preferentially expressed in these cells [50].

5.2. Otx2

In mammals there are two related proteins, Otx1 and Otx2, and their requirement for the formation of anterior structures has been conserved throughout evolution from flies to mice [55]. In the mouse, Otx2 is expressed early in development, and in its absence gastrulation is impaired. As a consequence, mutant embryos lack anterior structures corresponding to the future head [56]. Later in development, it is still required for maintenance of the forebrain

[57, 58]. Although its role during pituitary development has not been precisely investigated, its requirement in anterior structures implies that it is also necessary for Rathke's pouch development. It is in particular necessary for correct Hesx1 expression in the forebrain [59]. Recently, mutations in Otx2 have been identified in patients with eye disorders such as anophthalmia or microphthalmia, with or without hypopituitarism.

5.3. LIM Homeodomain Transcription Factors

LHX proteins belong to the LIM-homeodomain transcription factors which are characterized by two tandem repeats of LIM domain located in the NH2-terminal of the DNA binding homeodomain. The LIM domain provides a protein-protein interaction interface that recruits cofactors mediating the LIM functions [60]. At least 12 members of the LIM family have been identified in mammals, and several of them are expressed in Rathke's pouch, including Isl1, Lhx2, Lhx3, and Lhx4. Isl1 is initially detected in the oral ectoderm at E8.5, throughout Rathke's pouch at e9.5, and then by e10.5 confined to the most ventral region of the pouch, apparently co-localized with GSU. Isl1 expression is induced by BMP2 and repressed by FGF8/FGF2, the opposing ventral and dorsal signals critical for pituitary development [18]. In e9.5 Isl1-/- embryos, the primitive pouch forms with aberrant thin epithelium, suggesting that Isl1 is necessary for proliferation and differentiation of pituitary progenitors [31]. Lhx2 is expressed throughout VD during RP development and required for infundibulum and posterior lobe formation [61]. In Lhx2 null mutants the infundibulum fails to evaginate and proliferate more. Additionally, BMP2 and FGF expression patterns are ventrally expanded. As a consequence, RP fails to expand dorsally and rather develop more rostrally. Importantly, cell differentiation is unaffected and all endocrine cell types are observed [61]. Lhx3 is expressed in the pituitary gland, motor neurons of the spinal cord and hindbrain, the retina, and the pineal gland. Lhx3 expression is first evident in Rathke's pouch at e9.5 and persists predominantly in the anterior and intermediate lobes of the adult pituitary. In Lhx3+/- mice, the pituitary gland is arrested after the formation of a definite Rathke's pouch with a failure to maintain Hesx1 expression and to induce Pit1. Except for some residual corticotropes, all other cell types in the anterior and intermediate lobes are completely absent [62]. A more extensive analysis of the Lhx3Cre/Cre mutants, reveal that Lhx3 is required for cell survival, consistent with the view that Lhx3 acts downstream of Pitx1 and Pitx2 in preventing cell apoptosis [63]. The function of Lhx3 is conserved in humans. Patients with loss-of-function mutations in Lhx3 have combined pituitary hormone deficiency [64-67]. In vitro studies have shown that Lhx3 can interact with other transcription factors found in pituitary and synergistically regulate the promoters of pituitary hormones and transcription factor genes. For example, Lhx3 with Pitx1 synergistically activates the promoter of GSU and with Pit1 regulates the promoter of PRL, Pit1 and TSH [68, 69]. A closed related gene, Lhx4, is also expressed in the invaginating pouch at e9.5. In contrast to Lhx3 that is expressed throughout adulthood, Lhx4 expression becomes restricted to the future anterior lobe of pituitary and diminished at e15.5. Lhx4 may participate, along with PROP1 in activation of Lhx3 expression [70]. In Lhx4+/- mice, there is increased cell death in e12.5 and e14.5 pituitary, and by e18.5 different cell types, including somatotropes, corticotropes, thyrotropes, and gonadotropes, are present, but with markedly reduced numbers leading to a hypoplastic anterior lobe. In addition to distinct roles of Lhx3 and Lhx4 in pituitary organogenesis, Lhx3 and Lhx4 act redundantly in the formation of a definitive pouch. However, while Lhx4-/- hypoplastic pituitaries contain all endocrine cell types, in Lhx3-/- mutants, deficiencies in all cell lineages are observed. This reflects the requirement for Lhx3 in the activation of several pituitary hormones, hypothalamic peptide receptors and transcription factors [71]. Additionally, expression of Notch2 is absent in Lhx3 mutants and this could underlie some of the differentiation defects [72]. Therefore, Lhx3 and Lhx4 are initially required for progenitor maintenance rather than proliferation and Lhx3 is also required for proper endocrine differentiation.

5.4. Hesx1

Hesx1 is a member of the paired-like homeodomain transcription factors. Hesx1 contains two repressor domains located in the NH2-terminal and homeodomain regions, respectively [73, 74]. The homeodomain recruits the NcoR/Sin3/HDAC corepressor complex. The NH2 terminus eh1 motif mediates the interaction with the Tle co-repressor, and their association is essential for Hesx1 function. Expression in the developing pituitary persists until e12, when Hesx1 is down-regulated simultaneously with the appearance of Prop1 transcripts and progressive differentiation of pituitary specific cell types. Hesx1 is expressed in RP progenitors until e13.5 [75, 76]. Its expression is activated by the Lim homeodomain transcription factor Lhx3, along with Pitx2 and Gata2/Gata3 [77], while it is down-regulated by the β-catenin/Prop1 complex [38]. Hesx1 is essential for correct development of the forebrain, and Hesx1 null mice display postnatal lethality probably caused by CNS defects comprising anophthalmia, a reduced prosencephalon and pituitary dysplasia. Human Hesx1 mutations are associated with Septo-optic dysplasia (SOD), a rare congenital syndrome characterized by variable CNS midline defects and hypopituitarism [78]. The development of RP in Hesx1 null embryos is characterized early on by a variable phenotype comprising multiple clefts, correlating with expanded infundibular Fgf10 expression, over-proliferation and often misplacement of the gland in the nasopharyngeal cavity, aspects of which are likely to be explained by loss of the gene in VD [74]. After birth, hypoplasia of the pituitary is observed and this is suggested to result from impaired hypothalamic control [79]. Despite these defects, endocrine cell differentiation occurs normally in Hesx1 mutants, but with increased numbers [74, 80]. Hesx1 is therefore an important regulator of early pituitary development and its interaction with Prop1 regulates RP development. Overproduction of both Hesx1 and Tle1 in Rathke's pouch results in near-complete absence of gonadotropes and three Pit1 lineages, probably by antagonizing the transactivation function of Prop1 on endogenous targets, suggesting that the interaction between Hesx1 and Tle is required for Hesx1 function and the temporal regulation of Hesx1/Tle complex is fundamental for pituitary organogenesis [74, 39]. In addition to Tle1, other members of the Tle family, including Tle3, Tle4, and Aes, are expressed during pituitary development. Tle3 is first detectable in the ventral diencephalon, and by e14.5, Tle3 is localized in the dorsal region of Rathke's pouch and later confined to the intermediate lobe. Tle4 is expressed in the developing infundibulum and posterior lobe and diminished by e16.5. Aes is transiently expressed in the dorsal region of Rathke's pouch from e12.5 to e16.5 and is possibly required for modeling the shape of pituitary gland. Inactivation of Aes leads to bifurcations of the pouch and severe pituitary dysmorphogenesis at birth [81].

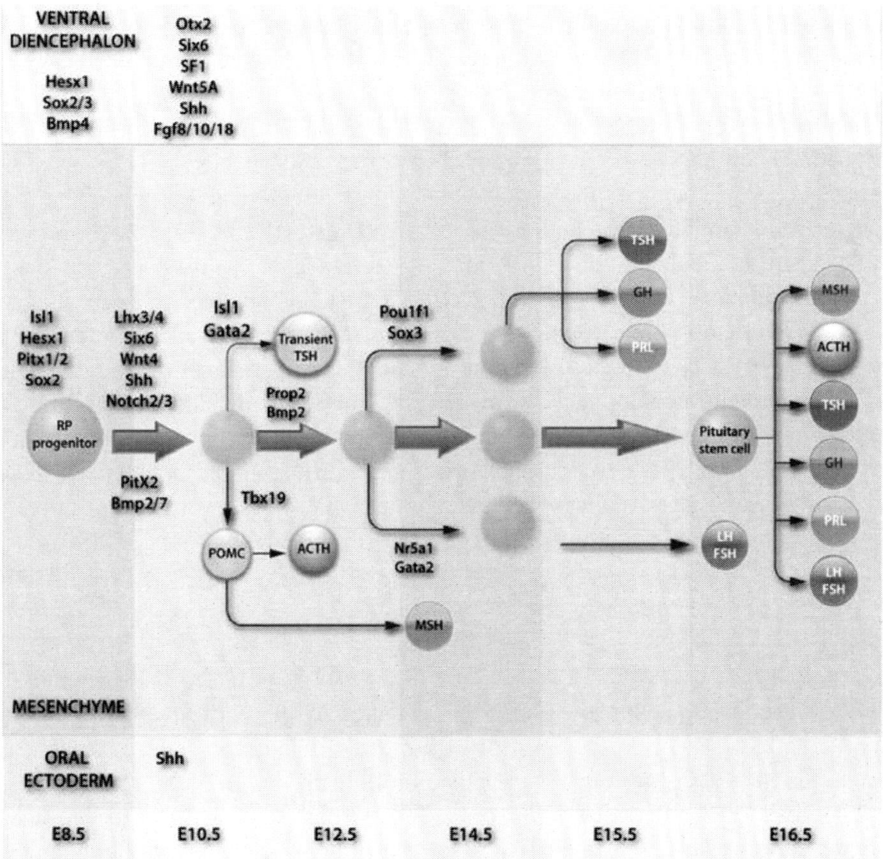

Figure 2. The outline of the time related developmental events in genes and transcription factors participating in human pituitary development with particular reference to pituitary cell differentiation.

5.5. Six Homeodomain Transcription Factors

In mammals, six members of the Six family have been identified, which belong to three subfamilies based on sequence conservation: (so) Six1, 2, (six4) Six4, 5, (optix) Six3, 6. Four of the Six genes, Six1, Six3, Six4, and Six6, are expressed in the developing pituitary. Six1 and Six4 are co-expressed in many embryonic primordium structures including Rathke's pouch [82]. Six1 is required for the development of many organs and plays an important role in regulating cell proliferation. A recent screen for target genes of Six1 and Six4, respectively, reveals that they regulate overlapping and distinct sets of genes, implying that Six1 and Six4 may share overlapping functions [83]. Indeed, inactivation of both Six1 and Six4 leads to more severe phenotypes than either single mutant with craniofacial and rib defects and general muscle hypoplasia [84]. Six1 regulates transcription of its target genes by recruiting cofactors via the Six domain. Six1 can either function as a repressor by interaction with Dach or Tle family members or as an activator by interaction with Eya proteins. Eya family proteins are characterized by a highly conserved COOH-terminal region known as the Eya domain, which mediates interactions with Six and Dach, as well as the less conserved

NH2-terminal transactivation domain [85, 86, 87]. Recent studies have shown that six1 plays a role in modulating proliferation of pituitary cells, while eya1 is required for lineage-specific differentiation. All the cell lineages except lactotropes are affected in eya1 mutants. Differentiation of corticotropes, melanotropes, and gonadotropes is completely impaired, whereas differentiation of somatotropes and thyrotropes initiates. The expression of GH and TSH, however, fails to be maintained probably due to progressive loss of pit1 expression. The closely related Six3 and Six6 are both expressed in VD and RP [88, 89], and Six6 expression is maintained in the adult pituitary [90]. Six3 is expressed in the most anterior part of the developing neural plate and later is restricted in retina precursor cells and pituitary. Six3 promotes cell proliferation and counteracts Wnt and BMP signaling and therefore specifying anterior identity [91, 92]. Six6 expression in pituitary exhibits a dorsal-ventral gradient at the early stage of pituitary development. At e13.5, the expression declines in the differentiated cells while remains persistent in periluminal cells. Deletion of Six6 results in hypoplastic pituitary and retina with reduced number of terminal differentiated cells due to defects in precursor cell proliferation. It has been suggested that Six6 promotes proliferation of progenitors by repressing expression of the cell cycle negative regulator p^{27kip1} [90].

5.6. Prop1

Prop1, a paired homeodomain transcription factor, is the earliest exclusive marker of pituitary formation and differentiation. Prop1 can bind to its recognition site and activate target gene via the COOH-terminal transactivation domain, whereas the NH2 terminus and the homeodomain of Prop1 act as repressors [39, 93], suggesting that Prop1 can function as both a transcriptional activator and a repressor. Prop1 can interact with β-catenin and this complex activates Pit1 expression [38]. There must, nevertheless, be another level of regulation for Pit1 activation as Prop1 is expressed from e10 while Pit1 is first detected at e13.5. It has been suggested that Prop1 probably just initiates Pit1 expression and is quickly down-regulated, because a maximum of only 9.7% of PIT1-expressing cells also express Prop1 [94]. Furthermore, it seems that Prop1is a transcriptional repressor for Hesx1, depending on the associated cofactors [38]. Expression of Prop1 is restricted in the developing pituitary. It is initially detected at e10 to e10.5, peaks at e12.5, and declines after e14.5. It has been shown recently that the Notch signaling is required for maintaining high levels of Prop1 expression at e12.5, a process mediated by an evolutionarily conserved Rbp-J binding site within the first intron of the Prop1 gene [33]. A homozygous mutation in the Prop1 homeodomain or targeted deletion of the Prop1 gene leads to a failure of Pit1 gene activation and loss of somatotropes, lactotropes, thyrotropes as well as delayed gonadotrope development. However, Hesx1 expression is maintained beyond its normal temporal limit [39, 95, 96]. Proliferation of the pituitary progenitors surrounding the lumen is not affected. However, they fail to migrate to the caudomedial region of the developing gland where Pit1 is normally expressed, resulting in an expansion of luminal structure and pituitary dysmorphogenesis [97-99, 38, 39]. Human PROP1 possesses similar function in pituitary development. Mutations in PROP1 are the leading cause of (combined pituitary hormone deficiency) CPHD in humans [65-67, 100] Genetic studies have demonstrated that temporal regulation of Prop1 expression is critical for proper pituitary development. Premature expression of Prop1 in Rathke's pouch proves to be deleterious leading to agenesis of the anterior pituitary gland probably by inhibiting the endogenous function of Hesx1 [74]. In contrast, persistent expression of Prop1 in thyrotropes and gonadotropes, under the control of GSU element, delays gonadotrope differentiation and leads to transient hypogonadotropic hypogonadism and increased susceptibility to pituitary adenomas [101, 102].

In summary, PROP1 is initially ubiquitously expressed in progenitors and confers a pituitary identity, while it is required later for morphogenesis of the pituitary anterior lobe.

5.7. Sox2/Sox3

The HMG box SoxB1 factors Sox2 and Sox3 are expressed throughout the CNS with particularly high levels of expression noted in the ventral diencephalon, including the infundibulum and presumptive hypothalamus [102, 103]. Sox2 is also expressed in Rathke's pouch. These factors generally, but not exclusively, promote an undifferentiated proliferative state [104]. Sox proteins act with co-factors, therefore, the specificity of their action often relies on their partner [s]. Moreover, there is redundancy within a sub-family. In VD, they have been shown to activate the same targets: Shh, as mentioned earlier [105], and also Six3 and Six6 [106, 107]. Sox2 is also required for pluripotent cell types in the early embryo, and homozygous null mutant mouse embryos die around implantation. In humans, heterozygous Sox2 loss-of-function mutations are associated with anophthalmia [108] and hypogonadotrophic hypogonadism [109], while both Sox3 deletions and duplications are linked to mild hypopituitarism [110]. Loss of Sox2 also significantly affects the number of GnRH neurons, therefore, the hypogonadotrophic hypogonadism displayed by human Sox2 lacking patients is likely to be of hypothalamic origin [111]. In RP, Sox2 is present from at least e9.5 and the protein is maintained in adult pituitary Stem Cells (SCs), along with a SoxE sub-family member, Sox9 [13, 112, 113]. Deletion of Sox2 in RP at e12.5 results in reduction of proliferation and, in consequence, endocrine cell deficits where later born cell types, in particular somatotropes, are more affected. Expression of the transcription factors Prop1 and Pit1 is down-regulated in Sox2 mutant embryos, but the molecular mechanisms underlying this are not known [111]. In conclusion, Sox2 is required within RP for progenitor proliferation. Targeted deletion of Sox3, which is situated on the X-chromosome, results a variable phenotype mainly characterized by hypopituitarism and craniofacial defects [103, 114, 115]. In Sox3/mutant mice, expression domain of Fgf8 and Bmp4 in the ventral diencephalon is expanded, which is accompanied by reduced proliferation and evagination of the infundibulum, leading to bifurcation of Rathke's pouch and anterior pituitary dysmorphology with extra clefts. There is a reduction in the levels of GH, LH, FSH, and TSH in the pituitary. The pituitary defect is suggested to result, at least in part, from a later requirement for Sox3 within the hypothalamus neurons [103, 115]. In humans, mutations in Sox3 are associated with X-linked mental retardation, variable learning deficits often associated with abnormal midline structures such as hypoplasia/agenesis of the corpus callosum and GH deficiency, and mutations in Sox2 are associated with abnormalities in the hypothalamo-pituitary and reproductive axes [109, 110, 116]. The similarity in the morphological abnormalities of Rathke's pouch between Sox3 mutants and mutants involving the Wnt pathway suggests their interplay during pituitary organogenesis. Other members of the SoxB1 family have also been reported to suppress β-catenin-mediated TCF signaling [117]. SOX2 has also been reported to inhibit WNT/β-catenin signaling in murine osteoblasts, where it represses the activity of aTCF responsive reporter, via an association of β-catenin with the C-terminal domain of SOX2 [118]. These experimental models suggest that interactions between the Sox proteins and β-catenin and the consequent effects on β-catenin target genes may be important for pituitary development.

5.8. Rx/Rax

Retina and anterior neural fold homeobox protein (Rx/Rax) is a paired-like homeodomain protein expressed early in the anterior neural plate. It plays a significant conserved role in eye morphogenesis. It is also maintained later in VD, and its deletion causes abnormal morphogenesis characterized by lack of infundibular evagination and down-regulation of Fgf10 expression from e10.5. Consequently, RP fails to develop beyond this stage and remains fused to oral ectoderm [145]. It is also important for later hypothalamic morphogenesis [146].

5.9. Pax6

Pax6 is a conserved member of a family of transcription factors containing a paired domain and a homeodomain. Pax6 is required for the development of the eye, olfactory system, brain, spinal cord, and pancreas. Pax6 is initially expressed in the anterior neural plate that will become telencephalon, diencephalon, eyes, and pituitary. During pituitary development, Pax6 is expressed in the oral ectoderm at e9.0, but is excluded from the Shh expressing region. By e10-e12, Pax6 expression is detected in the Rathke's pouch with an apparent dorsal/ventral gradient and becomes down-regulated at e13.5 and diminished when cells reach terminal differentiation at e17.5. Pax6 deficiency leads to a dorsal expansion of ventral GSU-expressing cell types, predominately thyrotropes, at the expense of dorsal cell types somatotropes and lactotropes. Thus the transient expression of Pax6 is required to establish the boundary between dorsal somatotropes/lactotropes and ventral thyrotropes/gonadotropes territories [147, 148]. The similar scheme of Pax6 in the dorsal/ventral patterning and specification of cell types is reiterated in CNS forebrain and spinal cord development (Table 1) [149].

6. Factors Regulating Cellular Differentiation

The definitive Rathke's pouch, formed by e11.5, initially contains undifferentiated proliferative progenitors. Gradually, these will differentiate and give rise to the five endocrine cell types present in the anterior pituitary. Naturally occurring mutations, but also studies on the role of specific genes during development, have led to the characterization of several transcription factors involved during endocrine differentiation. Regulated expression of these, both in time and space, is required to obtain the full set of endocrine cells at birth. The best studied/most representative among these factors are the following:

6.1. Pou1f1

Pou1f1 (previously Pit1) is a member of the POU homeodomain family of transcription factors characterized by two highly conserved protein domains, a Pou-specific domain and a Pou-DNA binding homeodomain. Pou1f1 (Pit1) is expressed relatively late during pituitary development. It becomes detectable by e13.5, reaches maximum expression by e16 and persists well into adulthood mainly in prospective somatotrope, lactotrope, and thyrotrope cells [119, 120]. It is required for the production of GH, PRL, and TSH, respectively, as well as for the expression of GHR Hr [121, 122]. Detailed analysis of Poufl (Pit1) regulatory regions has shown that it's early activation involves different enhancers, one of them bound by the giant zinc finger protein ATBF1 [123]. The presence of Pou1f1 binding sites within its own regulatory sequences suggests that Pou1f1 (Pit1) can be auto-regulated [124, 125]. The presence of normal GH, TSH, and PRL populations in the embryo shows that Pou1f1 (Pit1) is dispensable for their initial emergence but required for their postnatal expansion [126]. In postnatal endocrine cells, expansion is known to be under hypothalamic control, but there are also other signals involved locally in the gland. However, the postnatal phenotype is still unknown. It has been shown that Pou1f1 (Pit1) is able to inhibit the transcription factor Gata2 independently of its DNA binding properties, to prevent gonadotrope fate, whereas in thyrotropes, the two act in synergy to promote the thyrotrope fate [127]. This may explain how over-expression of Prop1, which activates Pou1f1 (Pit1), delays gonadotrope differentiation. In somatotropes, the Pou1f1 (Pit1) target gene Math3, encoding a bHLH transcription factor, allows terminal differentiation and is repressed by Notch signaling, probably preventing premature differentiation [33]. Pou1f1 (Pit1) therefore, functions more extensively being involved on the regulation of other cell types ensuring that the proper balance of endocrine cell types is achieved. Pou1f1 (Pit1) is reported to regulate its target genes by binding to response elements of their promoter regions and recruiting co-activator proteins, such as the cAMP response element-binding protein [128] and other transcription factors like Lhx3 to the transcriptional complex [129]. In humans, mutations in Pou1f1 are associated with GH, PRL, and variable TSH deficiency, with a hypoplastic anterior pituitary gland.

6.2. Gata2

Gata2 belongs to a family of six transcription factors characterized by the presence of at least one N-terminal transactivation domain and a zinc finger DNA binding domain. It has dual functions as a stem cell maintenance factor in some tissues [130], but also promotes differentiation in others [131]. Gata2 starts to be expressed at e10.5 in the ventral RP, where is induced by Bmp2 [127] along with α-GSU, the common subunit of LH, FSH, and TSH. It therefore forms prospective and definitive, gonadotropes and thyrotropes and its expression is maintained in the adult [127]. Gata2 has been shown in vitro to activate the Cga promoter [131] and also to induce TSH expression in synergy with Pou1f1 [Pit1] [127, 132]. Recent studies have shown that Gata2 may promote and be required for specification of the gonadotrope and thyrotrope lineages, respectively, in opposition and in synergy with Pou1f1 (Pit1) [127]. Also, these studies clearly highlight that Gata2 is required for the function of these cells in the postnatal gland.

6.3. Nr5a1

Nuclear receptor 5a1, encoded by the gene *Nr5a1* [also named steroidogenic factor-1, Sf1] is an orphan nuclear receptor involved as a trans-activating factor in steroid hormone biosynthesis. Phospholipid binding has been shown to increase its transactivation activity, although it is uncertain whether phospholipids should be considered as conventional ligands [134]. Nr5a1[Sf1] is expressed throughout the adrenal and reproductive axes during development and postnatal life, regulating several genes involved in sex determination, reproduction, and steroidogenesis, including in the hypothalamus and pituitary those encoding the GnRH receptor, LH, FSH, and GSU [135-138]. In the developing pituitary, Gata2 is capable of inducing Nr5a1 (Sf1) expression in the developing gonadotropes, with initial onset of expression at e13.5, therefore, after the initiation of GSU expression but before that of LHand FSH [127, 139]. It has been shown in vitro that interaction of Nr5a1(Sf1) with the transcription factors Egr1 and Pitx1 [61], and also more recently with β-catenin [140], is involved in activation of LH. Recently accumulated data show that pituitary expression of Nr5a1 (Sf1) is necessary for gonadotrope maturation, representing one of the functions of this factor in reproductive axis development. Mutations of Nr5a1 in humans are associated with 46XY sex reversal with adrenal failure, 46XY gonadal dysgenesis, and 46XX ovarian insufficiency and premature ovarian failure [141, 142].

6.4. Tbx19

Tbx19 (previously named as Tpit) is one of the 17 members of the T-Box family of transcription factors. The T-box is the DNA binding domain of these factors, and some of them also have a transactivation domain. For the Tbx19 (Tpit), transcriptional activation requires association with the co-activators of sarcoma virus/p160, but it can also interact with other partners [144]. Tbx19 (Tpit) is exclusively expressed in the developing pituitary, first at e12.5 in POMC-positive cells, then in corticotropes and melanotropes, where it is maintained in the adult gland [143]. It is capable of directly activating Pomc expression in association with Pitx1 [143]. Certain studies suggest that Tbx19 (Tpit) is required for the maturation and maintenance of corticotropes and melanotropes [3]. Interestingly, the studies also suggest that when it is over-expressed, Tbx19 (Tpit) may normally inhibit acquisition of these fates. TSH expression is normal, but the population of gonadotropin-expressing cells is greatly reduced. Different functions of Tbx19 (Tpit) may underline its ability to repress gonadotrope fate. This function is exerted by direct repression of Cga (GSU) expression, as well as, by a mutual antagonism between Tbx19 (Tpit) and Nr5a1 (Sf1), independent of DNA binding activity [3]. Therefore, Tbx19 (Tpit) promotes and is required for corticotrope and melanotrope fate while actively repressing gonadotrope identity. Mutations in Tbx19 (Tpit) are the commonest cause of isolated ACTH deficiency presenting in the neonatal period in humans (Table 1).

Table 1. Transcription factors participating in pituitary development and function

Gene	Expression	Pituitary phenotype
BMP4	VD	RP fails to form, embryonic lethal
FGF10	VD	Anterior pituitary agenesis due to increased apoptosis
FGF3	VD	Increased apoptosis leading to a complete loss of pituitary
FGF2	RP	Anterior pituitary agenesis due to increased apoptosis
Wnt4	RP	Hypoplastic pituitary with marked reduction of Pou1f1 lineages
Wnt5a	VD	Pituitary dysmorphogenesis. Cell differentiation occurs normally
Shh	VD, Oral ectoderm except RP	Pituitary hypoplasia with loss-of-expression of ventral transcription factors
Hesx1	VD, RP	Absence of pituitary or multiple oral ectoderm invagination
PitX1	RP	Decreased expression of LH, FSH, TSH, increased expression of POMC
Pitx2	RP	RP forms but fails to proliferate and differentiate at e12.5, lacks all cell types except corticotropes
Isl1	RP	RP forms but remains primitive, thin pouch wall, embryonic lethal
Lhx3	RP	Hypoplastic anterior pituitary with reduction of all cell types, increased apoptosis. Lhx3 and Lhx4 double KO fail to form a definite pouch
Lhx4	RP	Hypoplastic anterior pituitary with reduction of all cell types, increased apoptosis
Six6	RP	Hypoplastic pituitary
Six1	RP	No pituitary phenotype. Six1 and Eya1 double KO have smaller pituitaries
Prop1	RP	No Pit1 activation, lack three Pit1 lineages, reduced LH and FSH
Aes	RP	Pituitary dysmorphogenesis
Otx1	Postnatal	Transient dwarfism, delayed production of LH, FSH, and GH
Sox2	VD, Pituitary	Dysmorphic anterior lobe
Sox3	VD, RP	Reduced GH levels and dysmorphic anterior lobe

7. The Differentiation of Pituitary Cell

Initially, all Rathke's pouch cells express Isl1. The most ventral cells maintain the expression of this TF in response to BMP2, while FGF8 blocks Isl1 expression in the more dorsal cells. The presence of ISL1 activates αGSU, the common subunit of the heterodimeric hormones TSH, LH and FSH [18].

7.1. Gonadotropes

Both thyrotropes and gonadotropes express αGSU [the common subunit for TSH and gonadotrophins], the earliest marker of endocrine differentiation, appearing at e11.5. Therefore, early specification processes, comprising regulators of the Cga gene (encoding for αGSU), are shared between the two populations. Foxl2, a forkhead transcription factor, is the first marker of gonadotrope and thyrotrope commitment, expressed ventrally in RP at e10.5 [19], it persists in these two endocrine cell types until adulthood. Lhx3 and Lhx4 are required for its expression [150]. Gata2 is another important factor that is expressed by ventral cells.

This factor is necessary to restrict Pou1f1 activation in these cells and to ensure that a Pou1f1-independent cell lineage is established. GATA2 activates the expression of steroidogenic factor 1 (Sf1) [151, 152], which in turn stimulates αGSU and LHβgene expression, however, Gata2 does not significantly influence FSHβ expression [153]. However, a recent study showed that Gata2 and Gata4 increase FSHβ expression in vitro [154]. Although SF1 contributes to gonadotropic differentiation, the treatment of Sf1 knockout mice with GnRH completely restores the expression of gonadotrophins, demonstrating that SF1 is not the only TF involved [155]. PITX1 trans-activates αGSU, FSH β and LHβ [156], while Lhx3 up-regulates αGSU and FSHβ [157, 158], and HESX1 stimulates LHβ expression [153]. Animals and humans with Prop1 mutations usually have gonadotrophin deficiency. Functional studies suggest that Prop1 is important for FSHβ expression, even in adulthood [159]. It is possible that Prop1 participates in gonadotrope differentiation in a manner that is not well defined. In response to temporally and spatially organized TF expression, the gonadotropes complete differentiation by e17 [153].

7.2. Pou1f1-Specific Cells: Thyrotropes, Somatotropes and Lactotropes

The POU homeodomain protein Pou1f1 is exclusively expressed in the pituitary from e13.5 [160, 120]. Its expression is activated by Prop1 [38] and maintained in terminally differentiated somatotropes, lactotropes and thyrotropes, where it regulates expression of hormones and hypothalamic peptide receptors. Pou1f1 is also necessary for GH promoter hypomethylation, associated with active transcription, therefore, it also influences accessibility for other regulators [161]. In Pou1f1 mouse mutant embryos, emergence of endocrine cells takes place, but these are not maintained postnatally. Proliferation is reduced and apoptosis occurs, leading to GH, PRLand thyroid-stimulating hormone (TSH) deficiencies. The protein therefore appears to be necessary for postnatal expansion/survival probably in response to both hypothalamic and local signals [126]. In response to BMP2 signaling, Gata2 is activated and determines the gonadotropic and thyrotropic precursors. It has been suggested that Gata2 expression in thyrotropes is below the threshold necessary to block Pou1f1 activation, allowing the emergence of Gata2C/Pit1 cells [127]. The Pax6 ventral-dorsal gradient is important for distinguishing between the thyrotropic and somatotropic/lactotropic lineages [148]. In the absence of Pax6, thyrotropes occupy a larger region at the expense of lactotropes and somatotropes, and PRL and GH deficiencies result [120, 147, 148]. Thyrotropes are derived from two different populations. The first population appears in the rostral tip of the developing gland by e12, and this population is transient and independent of Pou1f1 expression [162]. The other population arises by e15.5 and is Pou1f1 dependent. This second population corresponds to the thyrotropes found in adulthood, suggesting that Pou1f1 is important for transactivating TSHb [163] and for maintaining this cellular lineage. Thyrotroph embryonic factor (Tef) is expressed exclusively in the rostral portion of the developing pituitary, where the thyrotropic precursors are located. Tef can bind to three different elements of the TSHb promoter, which leads to its effective transactivation [164]. Pitx1 and Pitx2 also collaborate in thyrotrope differentiation by acting synergistically with the αGSU/TSHb transactivation [165]. Lactotrope and somatotrope differentiation are completely dependent on Pou1f1 activation. These two cell types appear to arise from the same precursor, thus, secondary TFs restrict GH and PRL expression to their corresponding cell lineages [120]. In the embryo, PIT1 activates the expression of the bHLH factor Neuro D4 at e13.5. NeuroD4 is required for onset of somatotroph differentiation. In its absence, somatotroph numbers are very low in the embryo, although this improves postnatally. However, these cells never express the receptor for GH-releasing hormone [GHRH, hypothalamic peptide promoting GH secretion], resulting in dwarfism [33]. The Notch ligand Dlk1 is also expressed by somatotrophs and loss of the gene leads to a mild reduction in GH [166]. Cross-regulatory mechanisms between different cell types also control endocrine populations: after birth, the histone demethylase LSD1 acts as a co-activator on the Gh promoter, while it participates in Prl repression [35]. Pitx1 and Pitx2 co-operate with Pou1f1 to transactivate GH and PRL [156]. Among the elements that are important in determining somatotrope specificity, a small zinc finger protein, Zn-15, binds to the GH promoter, co-operating with Pou1f1 [167]. The retinoic acid receptor and the thyroid hormone nuclear receptor also cooperate with Pou1f1 in the regulation of GH gene expression [168, 169]. However, in lactotrope differentiation, the estrogen nuclear receptor synergistically partners with Pou1f1 [120]. Somatotrope and lactotrope differentiation finish at approximately e16 and e17 respectively [120].

7.3. Corticotropes

The most dorsal cells differentiate into corticotropes. This cell lineage is the most distinct among the pituitary cells [170]. In response to FGF8 signaling, corticotrope progenitors do not express any of the rostro-dorsal-specific TFs. Corticotrope differentiation depends on the interactions between PTX1, TPIT, NeuroD1 and LIF, which are all expressed just before pro-opiomelanocortin (POMC) expression is first detected and act synergistically at the level of the POMC promoter to transactivate this gene [154, 156, 171, 172]. PITX1 is also necessary for maintaining corticotrope-specific transcription [156]. The terminal differentiation of corticotropes depends on FGF8 down-regulation, which occurs by e14.5 [18]. Although Prop1 is not expressed in corticotropes, PROP1-deficient individuals may develop ACTH deficiencies. It has also been suggested that PROP1 is required for long-term maintenance of the corticotrope population, however, Nasonkin et al. [173] have shown that aged PROP1-deficient mice maintain ACTH production.

8. The Hypothalamo Pituitary Axis

The hormonal release of the anterior pituitary is under the influence of releasing hormones, which are secreted by the parvocellular neurons of the hypothalamus. CRH and TRH are synthesized by neurons in the paraventricular nucleus. GHRH is synthesized by neurons of the arcuate nucleus and the adjacent ventromedial nucleus. Somatostatin is mainly synthesized by neurons in the anterior periventricular nucleus. GnRH is synthesized by neurons located in the preoptic region. The parvocellular neurons project to the medial eminence where they release hormones that are conveyed to the anterior pituitary by the hypophysial-portal vasculature. The magnocellular neurons, the second set of neuroendocrine neurons of hypothalamus, are located in two nuclei of the anterior hypothalamus, the paraventricular and the supraoptic nuclei. They project their axons to the posterior pituitary where they release vasopressin and oxytocin directly into the general circulation. Induction and morphogenesis of the hypothalamus is regulated by Shh, Nodal, Bmp, and Wnt signals, as well as, by unidentified signals from Rathke's pouch [174-177]. Several studies have shown that the ventral diencephalon is essential for the formation of Rathke'spouch in part by producing signaling molecules including Fgf, Bmp, and Wnt. At a synchronized timing VD releases a number of hypothalamic specific factors that are required for pituitary functions. These factors, together with the signaling molecules and transcription factors are critical for pituitary development. The most important of these factors are summarized in (Table 2).

Table 2. Transcription factors participating in pituitary and hypothalamic development and function

Gene	Expression	Phenotypes
Pax6	RP	Dorsal expansion of ventral cell types at the expense of dorsal cell types. No GnRH-1 neurons
Sox3	Pituitary, VD	Reduced GH levels and dysmorphic anterior lobe
Hmx2.3	Hypothalamus	Reduced GHRH and GH production
Gsh1	Hypothalamus	Hypoplastic anterior pituitary, reduced production of GHRH, GH, PRL and LH
Otp	Hypothalamus	Reduced neuroblast proliferation, defective magnocellular and parvocellular
Sim1, 2	Hypothalamus	Magnocellular neurons and some parvocellular neurons fail to develop. Reduced TRH and Somatostatin (SS) neurons
Arnt2	Hypothalamus	Magnocellular neurons and some parvocellular neurons fail to develop
Brn2	Hypothalamus	Loss of posterior pituitary due to defects in survival of hypothalamus neurons
Ebf2	Hypothalamus	Defective GnRH-1 neurons migration
Nhlh2	Pituitary, Hypothalamus	Hypogonadal, reduced production of FSH, adult-onset obesity. Significant reduction of GnRH-1 neurons

9. Disorders of Pituitary Morphogenesis

Although the knowledge acquired from comparing genotype/phenotype analyses in mice and humans has many similarities, we should remain cautious in extrapolating exact mouse phenotypes to humans. Human studies are also hindered by the fact that clinical cases are too rare to generalize with confidence about phenotypic prevalence. Congenital hypopituitarism comprises a group of pathogenically different disorders. It may appear as isolated deficiency of a single pituitary hormone, for example idiopathic growth hormone deficiency (IGHD), ACTH deficiency, gonadotrophin deficiency (hypogonadotropic hypogonadism), TSH deficiency, or central diabetes insipidus. Alternatively, several pituitary hormone axes may be defective, resulting in a combined pituitary hormone deficiency (CPHD) that may also be associated with extra-pituitary defects such as optic nerve hypoplasia or midline forebrain abnormalities. Clinical features of hypopituitarism are often variable and may occur early in the neonatal period or later with growth failure or abnormal pubertal development. IGHD is by far the most common pituitary disease and may present with growth failure with an incidence ranging from 1 in 3,500 to 1 in 10,000 births [178-182]. At the more severe end of the spectrum, Septo-optical dysplasia (SOD) is a rare congenital anomaly with a prevalence of approximately 1 in 10,000 [195]. It is a genetically and phenotypically heterogeneous disorder characterized by a clinical triad of midline forebrain abnormalities, optic nerve hypoplasia, and hypopituitarism. Each of these components can occur in isolation or in combination. The majority of cases of hypopituitarism are idiopathic in origin, however, familial inheritance, which may be either dominant or recessive, accounts for between 5 and 30% of all cases [184]. The etiology of many cases still remains unknown and is likely to involve a combination of both genetic and environmental factors. Both genetic and environmental factors have been implicated in the etiology of SOD, for example [183, 185]. Environmental agents such as viral infections, vascular or degenerative changes, and exposure to alcohol or drugs have been implicated in the etiology of SOD. The condition presents more commonly in children born by younger mothers, and it clusters in geographical areas with a high frequency of teenage pregnancies [183, 186, 187]. Several genes causing abnormal pituitary function when mutated in the mouse have also been implicated in human pituitary development by the identification of mutations in their human orthologs in patients with various hypopituitary phenotypes. These can be broadly categorized into three groups:

1. Mutations in genes involved in early development and patterning of the forebrain and pituitary, these tend to result in syndromic forms of hypopituitarism in association with extra-pituitary defects affecting other tissues where they are expressed, most often the eyes, optic nerves, or midline forebrain structures.
2. Genes that are involved at initial stages of pituitary cell differentiation often resulting in CPHD.
3. Mutations in genes encoding specific hormone subunits or required for specification of particular cell types giving rise to isolated pituitary hormone deficiencies.

An outline of the clinical equivalency of genetic aberrations of various factors involved in the pituitary formation is given in Table 2. A detailed analysis of the aforementioned disorders is beyond the scope of this chapter.

10. Pituitary Adenomas

The pathogenesis of pituitary tumors remains controversial. The specific role and importance of intrinsic alterations of the pituitary cells themselves, dys regulation of hypothalamic hormones, and autocrine/paracrine action of locally produced growth factors are still elusive. Pituitary tumors are usually monoclonal benign adenomas that arise from expansion of single mutated precursor cells that possess certain proliferative advantage. Pituitary early progenitor cells that possess stem cell characteristics may differentiate into hormone-synthesizing pituitary cells. Pituitary adenomas probably arise from either early progenitor or fully differentiated hormone-expressing cells. Several tumor-inducing and tumor-promoting factors have been characterized in animal models, as well as in limited human tissue samples. These factors have been shown to possess proliferative potential to the precursor cell for adenoma formation and subsequent tumor growth, and include genetic or epigenetic abnormalities, paracrine growth factor disruptions and an altered intrapituitary microenvironment. These factors may be associated with pituitary-selective oncoprotein activation or tumor suppressor gene inactivation, or pituitary cell cycle dysregulation, all of which contribute to sustained cell proliferation. The initiating event remains unknown, although it has been shown that inactivated [188] or over-expressed cell cycle regulators are sufficient to induce pituitary oncogenesis [189]. Classic oncogene mutations are rarely encountered in pituitary tumors. Nevertheless, a considerable number of pituitary-specific cellular disruptions has been uncovered and affects oncogenes, transcription factors, tumor suppressors, cyclins, inactivating factors or proliferation inhibitors.

10.1. Hormonal Factors

Evidence Supporting a Hormonal Contribution Includes:

1. paradoxical pituitary hormone responses to exogenous hormonal stimulation that are characteristic of pituitary adenomas
2. the development of pituitary adenomas in situations of excessive hypothalamic hormone stimulation or reduced feedback suppression by target gland hormones, and
3. evidence of hypothalamic hormone production within the anterior pituitary that suggests a role for local excess stimulation. Studies in estrogen receptor β null mice have shown the requirement of estrogen receptor α for gonadotroph-cell adenoma development [190]. In fact, estrogen receptor α seems to be more abundantly expressed in large than small pituitary tumors. Strong arguments against a hormonal etiology, however, are the rarity of hyperplastic changes associated with adenomas, the lack of true adenomatous changes in the pituitary, even after long and sustained exposure to hypothalamic hormone stimulation in some instances, and the low frequency of recurrence after successful tumor resection. Additionally, some pituitary adenomas have been shown to lack hypothalamic hormone receptor synthesis.

10.2. Growth Factors and Receptors

Growth factors are polypeptides of several major families that regulate cell replication and functional differentiation by directly altering the expression of specific genes. They are considered to play an important role in the complex pathway of tumorigenesis. A number of oncogene products are similar to growth factors, their receptors, or enzymes that participate in the mitogenic process. In several systems, growth factors have been shown to interact with specific membrane receptors in regulating cell growth and gene expression in an autocrine or paracrine manner. Some of these factors are known to affect hormone production and some aremodulated by hormones. A few have been identified in the hypothalamus and are considered to play a physiological role in pituitary regulation. The pituitary is a site of both synthesis and action of growth factors [191]. A number of growth factors have been identified in adenohypophysial cells, including insulin-like growth factors-I and -II (IGF-I, IGF-II), EGF, nerve growth factor (NGF), transforming growth factor-α (TGF-α), transforming growth factor-β (TGF-β), and basic fibroblast growth factor (bFGF). Furthermore, bone morphogenetic protein and vascular endothelial growth factor families and Akt signaling pathways have been implicated in the pituitary oncogenic cascade. Wnt pathway inhibitors are also differentially expressed in pituitary adenomas versus normal pituitary tissue. Some of these are known to be released by pituitary cells in vitro. These substances may modulate hormone production as well as cell growth in human pituitary adenomas. The regulation of circulating or pituitary-derived growth factors and their respective receptors may, therefore, be important determinants of pituitary cell function and trophic hormone secretion. The relative significance of these different growth factors in human pituitary adenomas remains to be established although several have been implicated in the pathogenesis of these tumors.

10.3. Molecular Events

Evidence in favor of intrinsic pituitary cell defects accounting for the development of these lesions is based primarily on the monoclonal nature of these tumors. Mutations involving ras, p53, protein kinase C (PKC), c-erbB2 (neu), and retinoblastoma (Rb) genes are rare or absent in these neoplasms. Only a small fraction of adenomas have activating mutations of the Gsα. An obvious candidate gene is provided in multiple endocrine neoplasia type 1 (MEN-1), which is characterized by the development of pituitary adenomas. Loss of heterozygosity (LOH) at the MEN-1 gene locus is rare in sporadic adenomas and the recent cloning of the MEN-1 gene has allowed more specific analysis of the structure of this putative tumor suppressor in pituitary tumors. Although germ-line mutations and LOH are frequently encountered in familial adenomas, sporadic tumors exhibit a low frequency of mutations and LOH, and menin mRNA expression appears to be intact in most sporadic adenomas. A non-exhaustive list of well known genetic defects related to various types of pituitary adenomas is described in Table 3.

Table 3. Gene defects in various pituitary adenomas

Pituitary tumor	Gene	Defect
Corticotropinoma	Cyclin E, Pttg, Cyclin D1 p^{27Kip1} GR	↑ ↓ LOH
Prolactinoma	HmgA2 D2R	↑ ↓
Somatotropinoma	Gnas1, Gi2a FGFR4 AIP PRKAR1A, Sst2	Somatic mutation Alternative transcription Inactivating mutation ↓
Thyrotropinoma	TRβ	Inactivating mutation
Non-functioning adenomas	Gi2a, PKC ZAC	Somatic mutation LOH
All types	p16INK4a	Promoter methylation

FGFR4, fibroblast growth factor receptor 4, PKC, protein kinase C, Pttg, pituitary tumor transforminggene, LOH, loss of heterozygosity, D2R, dopamine receptor type 2, sst2, somatostatin receptor type 2, TR, thyroid hormone receptor, GR, glucocorticoid receptor, AIP, aryl hydrocarbon receptor interacting protein, PRKAR1A, type 1 alpha regulatory subunitof protein kinase A. ↓/↑ Decreased/Increasedexpression.

10.4. Signaling Mechanisms

Pathways involved in mitochondrial function, oxidative stress, mitogen-activated protein kinase signaling and cell cycle regulation have been implicated for adenoma formation. Clarification of these networks should result in a profound understanding of pituitary adenoma pathogenesis [192]. The pathophysiology of pituitary oncogenesis is characterized by a combination of abnormal cell proliferation coupled with an excessive hormone secretion.

a. Cyclins, Cyclin-Dependent Kinases (CDK), and CDK Inhibitors

The various phases of the cell cycle are regulated by cyclins that stimulate cyclin-dependent kinases (CDKs). When activated, these kinases phosphorylate and inactivate a crucial inhibitor of the cell cycle-retinoblastoma-associated protein (Rb), which is a tumor suppressor protein. The active, dephosphorylated form of Rb binds to E2F transcription factors, which restrains cell cycle progression through the G1 to S phase. This function of Rb acts to prevent replication of damaged DNA. Therefore, when phosphorylation is induced by complexes of cyclin and CDKs, Rb releases bound E2F transcription factors enabling the progression of the cell cycle. Although cyclins are over-expressed in nonfunctioning pituitary adenomas, the exact mechanism for this cell cycle aberration remains elusive. Although Rb is expressed in most nonfunctioning pituitary adenomas, approximately 25% of GH-secreting adenomas show hypermethylation of the Rb gene promoter with associated loss of expression [193]. Two families of CDK inhibitors-the Ink4a/Arf (p16, p15, p18) and cip/kip inhibitors (p21, p27, p57) - normally act as tumor suppressors by negatively regulating progression through the G1 and S phases of the cell cycle. These proteins inhibit CDK kinase activity, preventing phosphorylation and inactivation of pRb. In mice, deletion of p18 leads to gigantism, organomegaly, and pituitary intermediate lobe hyperplasia and adenomas, p18 protein levels are also attenuated in human adenomas [194]. A recent study in mice showed that disruption of the gene that encodes p27 results in a phenotype with increased body weight, organ hyperplasia and intermediate pituitary lobe tumors [188]. Furthermore, loss of p27 cooperates with over-expression of cyclin E to facilitate corticotroph oncogenesis [195]. The explanation of the increased proliferation is that the over-expression of corticotroph cyclin E levels leads to abnormal re-entry into the cell cycle of differentiated cells in an environment lacking the inhibitor p27. Dysfunction of p27 in pituitary oncogenesis may be due to disrupted translation of the protein. Glucocorticoid resistance of corticotroph adenoma cells is characteristic of Cushing disease. The failure of glucocorticoids to suppress proopiomelanocortin (POMC) gene expression leads to persistent ACTH synthesis and hypersecretion. The transcription activator Brg1, which is the catalytic subunit of the Sw1/Snf chromatin remodeling complex, normally functions to enable POMC repression, and in ACTH-secreting adenomas loss of Brg1 contributes to corticotroph glucocorticoid resistance [196]. In most corticotroph tumors and in pituitary carcinomas, both p27 and Brg1 levels are low or undetectable [196]. Another cell cycle regulator, encoded by pituitary tumor transforming gene 1 (*Pttg1*), controls the reliable separation of sister chromatids. *Pttg1* is a pro-angiogenic pituitary factor, and expression of this regulator is induced during initiation of estrogen-induced pituitary tumor formation [197]. Pituitary specific *Pttg1* over-expression results in focal pituitary hyperplasia and adenoma formation [189]. Maintenance of chromosomal stability requires tight control of intracellular cell-cycle dependent Pttg1 levels.

b. Dysfunctional Signaling Pathways

The G protein α (Gα) subunit, encoded by *GNAS*, is a key component of signal transduction pathways [198]. This factor activates adenylate cyclase, which induces the cyclic AMP (cAMP) and protein kinase A signaling pathway. The GTPase function of the Gα subunit is inactivated by *gsp* mutations of *GNAS* including amino acid substitutions at Arg201 or Gln227. These mutations are present in ~30% of GH-secreting adenomas, and they result in elevated somatotroph cAMP levels and hypersecretion of GH. Thus, constitutively induced somatotroph proliferation and GH secretion may occur independently of GH releasing hormone, and also may be associated with activation of downstream signaling factors including cAMP-response element binding factor activation [199]. Early postzygotic *gsp* mutations may give rise to an endocrine hypersecretory syndrome (McCune–Albright), which includes pigmented skin lesions, precocious puberty, hyperthyroidism, acromegaly and/or Cushing syndrome with bony fibrous dysplasia. This syndrome is associated with chromosome 20q13.2 mosaicism, which results in constitutively active Gα subunit and cAMP activation. Patients with McCune–Albright syndrome usually exhibit selective pituitary hyperplasia, rather than focal adenomas. Thus, cAMP is probably a common intracellular pathway for pituitary oncogenesis in certain cases.

c. Transcriptional Regulators

In transgenic mice, over-expression of an Hmga2 protein results in both GH-secreting and prolactin-secreting pituitary tumor formation, which appears to be mediated by enhanced E2F action [200]. In humans, re-arrangement and amplification of the Hmga2 gene expression seems to occur predominantly in prolactinomas, and Hmga2 mRNA abundance correlates with pituitary tumor size and proliferation markers [200]. These tumor growth effects may result from *Ccnb2* promoter induction, resulting in enhanced cyclin B2 levels and subsequent activation of the E2F transcription factor. Expression of several putative pituitary-selective tumor suppressor genes have been shown to be lost or down-regulated in pituitary adenomas. Several of these factors are inactivated by epigenetic mechanisms, and include Runt-related transcription factor 1, which up-regulates galectin-3, a pituitary tumor marker [201]. Expression of zinc finger protein Plagl1, a transcriptional co-regulator, appears to be lost in a subset of pituitary tumors and somatostatin analogs may in fact mediate anti-proliferative actions through Plagl1 [202]. Gadd45-γ and maternally imprinted Meg3 have been identified as pituitary-derived suppressor genes, and are silenced by methylation mechanisms especially in nonfunctioning pituitary tumors [203]. A dominant negative iso form of DNA-binding protein Ikaros is present in almost half of all pituitary adenomas and this molecule has been shown to regulate pituitary tumor cell chromatin remodeling and cell survival [204]. Ikaros also activates the POMC promoter and may serve as a systemic integrator of hypothalamic–pituitary signaling [205].

d. Small Non-Coding RNAs (Micro RNAs)

Micro RNAs act post-transcriptionally to regulate gene expression, mRNA translation and degradation. Although these molecules target both activating oncogenes and tumor suppressor genes, their exact role in pituitary oncogenesis has not yet been clarified. Expression of several miRNAs is down-regulated in ACTH-secreting pituitary tumors, including miR145, miR21, miR15 and miR16, while miR122 and miR493 are up-regulated in ACTH-expressing carcinomas [206, 207]. Suppression of miRlet-7 family members, as well as of miR15a/miR16, are conserved across most pituitary tumor subtypes. In nonfunctioning and in GH-secreting adenomas, Wee1-like protein kinase, which acts as a tumor suppressor protein, was shown to be regulated by miR128a, miR155 and miR516a-3p [208]. Clearly, pituitary tumor miRNAs are an emerging area of tumor research. In the last years several candidate factors have been implicated in the genesis and progression of pituitary adenomas. During the last decade several candidate factors have been implicated in the genesis and progression of pituitary adenomas. Abnormalities in the expression of cell cycle regulators, receptors, and growth factors and their signaling, as well as epigenetic mechanisms have been proposed to play a relevant role in cell transformation and clonal expansion. Nowadays, it becomes increasingly more apparent that no single factor might effectively explain oncogenesis in the pituitary.

CONCLUSION

Pituitary organogenesis during embryogenesis is a complex process that depends on both the activation and inactivation of different TFs at the appropriate times. The correct cellular migration in response to dorsal-ventral gradients enables each cell group to receive signals from distinct pathways, depending on the cell location. This process induces different responses and allows the determination of the five cell lineages that constitute the pituitary. Genetic studies, in combination with molecular and biochemical studies, have elucidated a primary diagram in which signaling molecules and transcription factors govern proper pituitary development and function. However, the large network required for these events remains incompletely defined. We still need a better understanding of how cell fates are specified in vivo, as embryonic progenitors exit the cell cycle, for efficient in vitro generation of all endocrine cell types. Generation of temporally regulated tissue-specific deletion of genes or hypomorphic allele of genes that are necessary for early embryonic development will reveal new functions. Genome-wide mutagenesis screen in mice and model organisms, combined with integrated genomic, proteomic, and bioinformatics approaches, will certainly uncover novel players in this elaborately regulated genetic program. Identification of required cofactors as well as downstream target genes of the transcription factors and complementary studies in epigenetic regulation of chromatin organization and nuclear architecture will delineate the molecular mechanisms underlying pituitary development, uncovering new principles of mammalian organogenesis. Significant advances have been made in recent years and we understand better as to how RP progenitors are controlled and how endocrine cells differentiate, and, importantly, we know that they form endocrine networks. Finally, the recent characterization of pituitary SCs opens the alternative possibility of direct somatic cell conversion into organ-specific SCs for use in regenerative medicine.

REFERENCES

[1] Shinkai, T, Sakurai, Y, Ooka, H. Age-related changes in the numbers of mammotrophs, somatotrophs and mammosomatotrophs in the anterior pituitary gland of female rats: a flow cytometric study. *Mech Ageing Dev*, 1995;83:125-131.

[2] Tierney, T, Robinson, IC. Increased lactotrophs despite decreased somatotrophs in the dwarf [dw/dw] rat: a defect in the regulation of lactotroph/somatotroph cell fate? *J Endocrinol*, 2002;175:435-446.

[3] Pulichino, AM, Vallette-Kasic, S, Tsai, JP, Couture, C, Gauthier, Y, Drouin, J. Tpit determines alternate fates during pituitary cell differentiation. *Genes Dev*, 2003;17:738-747.

[4] Himes, AD, Raetzman, LT. Premature differentiation and aberrant movement of pituitary cells lacking both Hes1 and Prop1. *Dev Biol*, 2009;325:151-161.

[5] Raetzman, LT, Cai, JX, Camper, SA. Hes1 is required for pituitary growth and melanotrope specification. *Dev Biol*, 2007;304:455-466.

[6] Hokfelt, T, Meister, B, Villar, MJ, Ceccatelli, S, Corts, R, Schalling, M, et al. Colocalization of messenger substances with special reference to the hypothalamic arcuate and paraventricular nuclei. *Prog Clin Biol Res*, 1990;342:257-264.

[7] Treier, M, Rosenfeld, MG. The hypothalamic-pituitary axis: codevelopment of two organs. *Curr Opin Cell Biol*, 1996;8:833-843.

[8] Sheng, HZ, Westphal, H. Early steps in pituitary organogenesis. *Trends Genet*, 1999;15:236-240.

[9] Burrows, HL, Douglas, KR, Seasholtz, AF, Camper, SA. Genealogy of the anterior pituitary gland: Tracing a family tree. *Trends Endocrinol Metab*, 1999, 10:343-352.

[10] Dasen, JS, Rosenfeld, MG. Combinatorial codes in signaling and synergy: lessons from pituitary development. *Curr Opin Genet Dev*, 1999;9:566-574.

[11] Kouki, T, Imai, H, Aoto, K, Eto, K, Shioda, S, Kawamura, K, et al. Developmental origin of the rat adenohypophysis prior to the formation of Rathke's pouch. *Development*, 2001;128:959-963.

[12] Couly, G, Le Douarin, NM. The fate map of the cephalic neural primordium at the presomitic to the 3-somite stage in the avian embryo. *Development*, 1998;103 Suppl: 101-113.

[13] Fauquier, T, Rizzoti, K, Dattani, M, Lovell-Badge, R, Robinson, IC. SOX2-expressing progenitor cells generate all of the major cell types in the adult mouse pituitary gland. *Proc Natl Acad Sci USA*, 2008;105:2907-2912.

[14] Gleiberman, AS, Michurina, T, Encinas, JM, Roig, JL, Krasnov, P, Balordi, F, et al. Genetic approaches identify adult pituitary stem cells. *Proc Natl Acad Sci USA*, 2008;105:6332-6337.

[15] Baek, SH, Kioussi, C, Briata, P, Wang, D, Nguyen, HD, Ohgi, KA, et al. Regulated subset of G1 growth-control genes in response to derepression by the Wnt pathway. *Proc Natl Acad Sci USA*, 2003;100:3245-3250.

[16] Bailey, JS, Rave-Harel, N, McGillivray, SM, Coss, D, Mellon, PL. Activin regulation of the follicle-stimulating hormone beta-subunit gene involves Smads and the TALE homeodomain proteins Pbx1 and Prep1. *Mol Endocrinol*, 2004;18:1158-1170.

[17] Dasen, JS, Rosenfeld, MG. Signaling and transcriptional mechanisms in pituitary development. *Annu Rev Neurosci*, 2001;24:327-355.

[18] Ericson, J, Norlin, S, Jessell, TM, Edlund, T. Integrated FGF and BMP signaling controls the progression of progenitor cell differentiation and the emergence of pattern in the embryonic anterior pituitary. *Development*, 1998;125:1005-1015.

[19] Treier, M, Gleiberman, AS, O'Connell, SM, Szeto, DP, McMahon, JA, McMahon, AP, et al. Multistep signaling requirements for pituitary organogenesis in vivo. *Genes Dev*, 1998;12:1691-1704.

[20] Ferrand, R. [Experimental study of the factors in cytological differentiation of the adenohypophysis in the chick embryo]. *Arch Biol [Liege]*, 1972;83:297-371.

[21] Kawamura, K, Kikuyama, S. Induction from posterior hypothalamus is essential for the development of the pituitary proopiomelacortin [POMC] cells of the toad [Bufo japonicus]. *Cell Tissue Res*, 1995;279:233-239.

[22] Daikoku, S, Chikamori, M, Adachi, T, Maki, Y. Effect of the basal diencephalon on the development of Rathke's pouch in rats- a study in combined organ-cultures. *Dev Biol*, 1982;90:198-202.

[23] Watanabe, YG. Effects of brain and mesenchyme upon the cytogenesis of rat adenohypophysis in vitro. I. Differentiation of adrenocorticotropes. *Cell Tissue Res*, 1982;227:257-266.

[24] Davis, SW, Camper, SA. Noggin regulates Bmp4 activity during pituitary induction. *Dev Biol*, 2007;305:145-160.

[25] Maruoka, Y, Ohbayashi, N, Hoshikawa, M, Itoh, N, Hogan, BL, Furuta, Y. Comparison of the expression of three highly related genes, Fgf8, Fgf17 and Fgf18, in the mouse embryo. *Mech Dev*, 1998;74:175-177.

[26] Treier, M, O'Connell, S, Gleiberman, A, Price, J, Szeto, DP, Burgess, R, Chuang, PT, McMahon, AP, Rosenfeld, MG. Hedgehog signaling is required for pituitary gland development. *Development*, 2001;128:377-386.

[27] Friedl, P, Gilmour, D. Collective cell migration in morphogenesis, regeneration and cancer. *Nature Reviews. Molecular Cell Biology*, 2009;10:445–457.

[28] Xu, J, Liu, Z, Ornitz, DM. Temporal and spatial gradients of Fgf8 and Fgf17 regulate proliferation and differentiation of midline cerebellar structures. *Development*, 2000;127:1833-1843.

[29] Norlin, S, Nordstrom, U, Edlund, T. Fibroblast growth factor signaling is required for the proliferation and patterning of progenitor cells in the developing anterior pituitary. *Mech Dev*, 2000;96:175-182.

[30] Friedl, P, Gilmour, D. Collective cell migration in morphogenesis, regeneration and cancer. *Nat Rev Mol Cell Biol*, 2009;10:445-457.

[31] Takuma, N, Sheng, HZ, Furuta, Y, Ward, JM, Sharma, K, Hogan, BL, et al.1998 Formation of Rathke's pouch requires dual induction from the diencephalon. *Development*, 1998;125:4835-4840.

[32] Raetzman, LT, Ross, SA, Cook, S, Dunwoodie, SL, Camper, SA, Thomas, PQ. Developmental regulation of Notch signaling genes in theembryonic pituitary: Prop1 deficiency affects Notch2 expression. *Dev Biol*, 2004;265:329-340.

[33] Zhu, X, Zhang, J, Tollkuhn, J, Ohsawa, R, Bresnick, EH, Guillemot, F, et al. Sustained Notch signaling in progenitors is required for sequential emergence of distinct cell lineages during organogenesis. *Genes Dev*, 2006;20:2739-2753.

[34] Raetzman, LT, Wheeler, BS, Ross, SA, Thomas, PQ, Camper, SA. Persistent expression of Notch2 delays gonadotrope differentiation. *Mol Endocrinol*, 2006;20:2898-2908.

[35] Wang, J, Scully, K, Zhu, X, Cai, L, Zhang, J, Prefontaine, GG, et al. Opposing LSD1 complexes function in developmental gene activation and repression programmes. *Nature*, 2007;446:882-887.

[36] Welcker, JE, Hernandez-Miranda, LR, Paul, FE, Jia, S, Ivanov, A, Selbach, M, et al. Insm1 controls development of pituitary endocrine cells and requires a SNAG domain for function and for recruitment of histone-modifying factors. *Development*, 2013;140:4947-4958.

[37] DiMattia, GE, Rhodes, SJ, Krones, A, Carriere, C, O'Connell, S, Kalla, K, et al. The Pit-1 gene is regulated by distinct early and late pituitary-specific enhancers. *Dev Biol*, 1997;182:180-190.

[38] Olson, LE, Tollkuhn, J, Scafoglio, C, Krones, A, Zhang, J, Ohgi, KA, et al. Homeodomain-mediated beta-catenin-dependent switching events dictate cell-lineage determination. *Cell*, 2006;125:593-605.

[39] Sornson, MW, Wu, W, Dasen, JS, Flynn, SE, Norman, DJ, O'Connell, SM, et al. Pituitary lineage determination by the Prophet of Pit-1 homeodomain factor defective in Ames dwarfism. *Nature*, 1996;384:327-333.

[40] Kioussi, C, Briata, P, Baek, SH, Rose, DW, Hamblet, NS, Herman, T, et al. Identification of a Wnt/Dvl/β-catenin/Pitx2 pathway mediating cell-type-specific proliferation during development. *Cell*, 2002;111:673-685.

[41] Ai, D, Wang, J, Amen, M, Lu, MF, Amendt, BA, Martin, JF. Nuclear factor 1 and T-cell factor/LEF recognition elements regulate Pitx2 transcription in pituitary development. *Mol Cell Biol*, 2007;27:5765-5775.

[42] Potok, MA, Cha, KB, Hunt, A, Brinkmeier, ML, Leitges, M, Kispert, A, et al. 2008 WNT signaling affects gene expression in the ventral diencephalon and pituitary gland growth. *Dev Dyn*, 2008;237:1006-1020.

[43] Douglas, KR, Brinkmeier, ML, Kennell, JA, Eswara, P, Harrison, TA, Patrianakos, AI, et al. Identification of members of the Wnt signaling pathway in the embryonic pituitary gland. *Mamm Genome*, 2001;12:843-851.

[44] Soukup, V, Horacek, I, Cerny, R. Development and evolution of the vertebrate primary mouth. *J Anat*, 2013;222:79-99.

[45] Gage, PJ, Suh, H, Camper, SA. The bicoid-related Pitx gene family in development. *Mamm Genome*, 1999;10:197-200.

[46] Gage, PJ, Camper, SA. Pituitary homeobox 2, a novel member of the bicoid-related family of homeobox genes, is a potential regulator of anterior structure formation. *Hum Mol Genet*, 1997;6:457-464.

[47] Lanctot, C, Lamolet, B, Drouin, J. The bicoid-related homeoprotein Ptx1 defines the most anterior domain of the embryo and differentiates posterior from anterior lateral mesoderm. *Development*, 1997;124:2807-2817.

[48] Charles, MA, Suh, H, Hjalt, TA, Drouin, J, Camper, SA, Gage, PJ. PITX genes are required for cell survival and Lhx3 activation. *Mol Endocrinol*, 2005;19:1893-1903.

[49] Tremblay, JJ, Goodyer, CG, Drouin, J. Transcriptional properties of Ptx1 and Ptx2 isoforms. *Neuroendocrinology*, 2000;71:277-286.

[50] Charles, MA, Suh, H, Hjalt, TA, Drouin, J, Camper, SA, Gage, PJ. PITX genes are required for cell survival and Lhx3 activation. *Mol Endocrinol*, 2005;19:1893-1903.

[51] Suh, H, Gage, PJ, Drouin, J, Camper, SA. Pitx2 is required at multiple stages of pituitary organogenesis:pituitary primordium formation and cell specification. *Development*, 2002;129:329-337.

[52] Szeto, DP, Ryan, AK, O'Connell, SM, Rosenfeld, MG. P-OTX:a PIT-1-interacting homeodomain factor expressed during anterior pituitary gland development. *Proc Natl Acad Sci USA*, 1996;93:7706-7710.

[53] Lamonerie, T, Tremblay, JJ, Lanctot, C, Therrien, M, Gauthier, Y, Drouin, J. Ptx1, a bicoid-related homeo box transcription factor involved in transcription of the pro-opiomelanocortin gene. *Genes Dev*, 1996;10:1284-1295.

[54] Briata, P, Ilengo, C, Corte, G, Moroni, C, Rosenfeld, MG, Chen, CY, et al. The Wnt/beta-catenin3Pitx2 pathway controls the turnover of Pitx2 and other unstable mRNAs. *Mol Cell*, 2003;12:1201-1211.

[55] Boncinelli, E, Morgan, R. Downstream of Otx2, or how to get a head. *Trends Genet*, 2001;17:633-636.

[56] Acampora, D, Mazan, S, Lallemand, Y, Avantaggiato, V, Maury, M, Simeone, A, et al. Forebrain and midbrain regions are deleted in Otx2/mutants due to a defective anterior neuroectoderm specification during gastrulation. *Development*, 1995;121:3279-3290.

[57] Kurokawa, D, Kiyonari, H, Nakayama, R, Kimura-Yoshida, C, Matsuo, I, Aizawa, S. Regulation of Otx2 expression and its functions in mouse forebrain and midbrain. *Development*, 2004;131:3319-3331.

[58] Kurokawa, D, Takasaki, N, Kiyonari, H, Nakayama, R, Kimura-Yoshida, C, Matsuo, I, et al. Regulation of Otx2 expression and its functions in mouse epiblast and anterior neuroectoderm. *Development*, 2004;131:3307-3317.

[59] Rhinn, M, Dierich, A, Le Meur, M, Ang, S. Cell autonomous and non-cell autonomous functions of Otx2 in patterning the rostral brain. *Development*, 1999;126:4295-4304.

[60] Hunter, CS, Rhodes, SJ. LIM-homeodomain genes in mammalian development and human disease. *Mol Biol Rep*, 2005;32:67-77.

[61] Zhao, Y, Mailloux, CM, Hermesz, E, Palkovits, M, Westphal, H. A role of the LIM homeobox gene Lhx2 in the regulation of pituitary development. *Dev Biol*, 2010;337;313-323.

[62] Sheng, HZ, Zhadanov, AB, Mosinger, B, Jr. Fujii, T, Bertuzzi, S, Grinberg, A, et al. Specification of pituitary cell lineages by the LIM homeobox gene Lhx3. *Science*, 1996;272:1004-1007.

[63] Zhao, Y, Morales, DC, Hermesz, E, Lee, WK, Pfaff, SL, Westphal, H. Reduced expression of the LIM-homeobox gene Lhx3 impairs growth and differentiation of Rathke's pouch and increases cell apoptosis during mouse pituitary development. *Mech Dev*, 2006;123:605-613.

[64] Bhangoo, AP, Hunter, CS, Savage, JJ, Anhalt, H, Pavlakis, S, Walvoord, EC, et al. A novel LHX3 mutation presenting as combined pituitary hormonal deficiency. *J Clin Endocrinol Metab*, 2006;91:747-753.

[65] Cohen, LE, Radovick, S. Other transcription factors and hypopituitarism. *Rev Endocr Metab Disorders*, 2002;3:, 301-311.

[66] Cushman, LJ, Showalter, AD, Rhodes, SJ. Genetic defects in the development and function of the anterior pituitary gland. *Ann Med*, 2002;34:179-191.

[67] Mullis, PE. Genetic control of growth. *Eur J Endocrinol*, 2005;152:11-31.
[68] Bach, I, Carriere, C, Ostendorff, HP, Andersen, B, Rosenfeld, MG. A family of LIM domain-associated cofactors confer transcriptional synergism between LIM and Otx homeodomain proteins. *Genes Dev*, 1997;11:1370-1380.
[69] Sloop, KW, Parker, GE, Hanna, KR, Wright, HA, Rhodes, SJ. LHX3 transcription factor mutations associated with combined pituitary hormone deficiency impair the activation of pituitary target genes. *Gene*, 2001;265:61-69.
[70] Raetzman, LT, Ward, R, Camper, SA. Lhx4 and Prop1 are required for cell survival and expansion of the pituitary primordia. *Development*, 2002;129:4229-4239.
[71] Prince, KL, Walvoord, EC, Rhodes, SJ. The role of homeodomain transcription factors in heritable pituitary disease. *Nature Reviews. Endocrinology*, 2011;7:727-737.
[72] Ellsworth, BS, Butts, DL, Camper, SA. Mechanisms underlying pituitary hypoplasia and failed cell specification in Lhx3-deficient mice. *Dev Biol*, 2008;313:118-129.
[73] Brickman, JM, Clements, M, Tyrell, R, McNay, D, Woods, K, Warner J, et al. Molecular effects of novel mutations in Hesx1/HESX1 associated with human pituitary disorders. *Development*, 2001;128:5189-5199.
[74] Dasen, JS, Barbera, JP, Herman, TS, Connell, SO, Olson, L, Ju, B, et al. Temporal regulation of a paired-like homeodomain repressor/TLE corepressor complex and a related activator is required for pituitary organogenesis. *Genes Dev*, 2001;15:3193-3207.
[75] Hermesz, E, Mackem, S, Mahon, KA. Rpx: a novel anterior-restricted homeobox gene progressively activated in the prechordal plate, anterior neural plate and Rathke's pouch of the mouse embryo. *Development*, 1996;122:41-52.
[76] Thomas, P, Beddington, R. Anterior primitive endoderm may be responsible for patterning the anterior neural plate in the mouse embryo. *Curr Biol*, 1996;6:1487-1496.
[77] Chou, SJ, Hermesz, E, Hatta, T, Feltner, D, El-Hodiri, HM, Jamrich, M, et al. Conserved regulatory elements establish the dynamic expression of Rpx/HesxI in early vertebrate development. *Dev Biol*, 2006;292:533-545.
[78] Dattani, MT, Martinez-Barbera, JP, Thomas, PQ, Brickman, JM, Gupta, R, Martensson, IL, et al. Mutations in the homeobox gene HESX1/Hesx1 associated with septooptic dysplasia in human and mouse. *Nat Genet*, 1998;19:125-133.
[79] Gaston-Massuet, C, Andoniadou, CL, Signore, M, Sajedi, E, Bird, S, Turner, JM, et al. Genetic interaction between the homeobox transcription factors HESX1 and SIX3 is required for normal pituitary development. *Dev Biol*, 2008;324:322-333.
[80] Sajedi, E, Gaston-Massuet, C, Andoniadou, CL, Signore, M, Hurd, PJ, Dattani, M, et al. 2008 DNMT1 interacts with the developmental transcriptional repressor HESX1. *Biochim Biophys Acta*, 2008;1783:131-143.
[81] Brinkmeier, ML, Potok, MA, Cha, KB, Gridley, T, Stifani, S, Meeldijk, J, et al. TCF and Groucho-related genes influence pituitary growth and development. *Mol Endocrinol*, 2003;17:2152-2161.
[82] Kawakami, K, Sato, S, Ozaki, H, Ikeda, K. Six family genes—structure and function as transcription factors and their roles in development. *Bioessays*, 2000;22:616-626.
[83] Ando, Z, Sato, S, Ikeda, K, Kawakami, K. Slc12a2 is a direct target of two closely related homeobox proteins, Six1 and Six4. *FEBS Lett*, 2005;272:3026-3041.

[84] Grifone, R, Demignon, J, Houbron, C, Souil, E, Niro, C, Seller, MJ, et al. Six1 and Six4 homeoproteins are required for Pax3 and Mrf expression during myogenesis in the mouse embryo. *Development*, 2005;132:2235-2249.

[85] Brugmann, SA, Pandur, PD, Kenyon, KL, Pignoni, F, Moody, SA. Six1 promotes a placodal fate within the lateral neurogenic ectoderm by functioning as both a transcriptional activator and repressor. *Development*, 2004;131:5871-5881.

[86] Heanue, TA, Reshef, R, Davis, RJ, Mardon, G, Oliver, G, Tomarev, S, et al. Synergistic regulation of vertebrate muscle development by Dach2, Eya2, Six1, homologs of genes required for Drosophila eye formation. *Genes Dev*, 1999;13:3231-3243.

[87] Li, X, Oghi, KA, Zhang, J, Krones, A, Bush, KT, Glass, CK, et al. Eya protein phosphatase activity regulates Six1-Dach-Eya transcriptional effects in mammalian organogenesis. *Nature*, 2003;426:247-254.

[88] Jean, D, Bernier, G, Gruss, P. Six6 [Optx2] is a novel murine Six3- related homeobox gene that demarcates the presumptive pituitary/hypothalamic axis and the ventral optic stalk. *Mech Dev*, 1999;84:31-40.

[89] Larder, R, Clark, DD, Miller, NL, Mellon, PL. Hypothalamic dysregulation and infertility inmice lacking the homeodomain protein Six6. *J Neurosci*, 2011;31:426-438.

[90] Li, X, Perissi, V, Liu, F, Rose, DW, Rosenfeld, MG. Tissue-specific regulation of retinal and pituitary precursor cell proliferation. *Science*, 2002;297:1180-1183.

[91] Gestri, G, Carl, M, Appolloni, I, Wilson, SW, Barsacchi, G, Andreazzoli, M. Six3 functions in anterior neural plate specification by promoting cell proliferation and inhibiting Bmp4 expression. *Development*, 2005;132:2401-2413.

[92] Lagutin, OV, Zhu, CC, Kobayashi, D, Topczewski, J, Shimamura, K, Puelles, L, et al. Six3 repression of Wnt signaling in the anterior neuroectoderm is essential for vertebrate forebrain development. *Genes Dev*, 2003;17:368-379.

[93] Showalter, AD, Smith, TP, Bennett, GL, Sloop, KW, Whitsett, JA, Rhodes, SJ. Differential conservation of transcriptional domains of mammalian Prophet of Pit-1 proteins revealed by structural studies of the bovine gene and comparative functional analysis of the protein. *Gene*, 2002;291:211-221.

[94] Yoshida, S, Kato, T, Susa, T, Cai, LY, Nakayama, M, Kato, Y. PROP1 coexists with SOX2 and induces PIT1-commitment cells. *Biochem Biophys Res Commun*, 2009;385:11-15.

[95] Gage, PJ, Brinkmeier, ML, Scarlett, LM, Knapp, LT, Camper, SA, Mahon, KA. 1996 The Ames dwarf gene, df, is required early in pituitary ontogeny for the extinction of Rpx transcription and initiation of lineage-specific cell proliferation. *Mol Endocrinol*, 1996;10:1570-1581.

[96] Nasonkin, IO, Ward, RD, Raetzman, LT, Seasholtz, AF, Saunders, TL, Gillespie, PJ, et al. Pituitary hypoplasia and respiratory distress syndrome in Prop1 knockout mice. *Hum Mol Genet*, 2004;13:2727-2735.

[97] Andersen, B, Pearse, RV, 2nd, Jenne, K, Sornson, M, Lin, SC, Bartke, A, Rosenfeld, MG. The Ames dwarf gene is required for Pit-1 gene activation. *Dev Biol*, 1995;172:495-503.

[98] Gage, PJ, Lossie, AC, Scarlett, LM, Lloyd, RV, Camper, SA. Ames dwarf mice exhibit somatotrope commitment but lack growth hormone- releasing factor response. *Endocrinology*, 1995;136:1161-1167.

[99] Ward, RD, Raetzman, LT, Suh, H, Stone, BM, Nasonkin, IO, Camper, SA. Role of PROP1 in pituitary gland growth. *Mol Endocrinol*, 2005;19:698-710.

[100] Wu, W, Cogan, JD, Pfaffle, RW, Dasen, JS, Frisch, H, O'Connell, SM, et al. Mutations in PROP1 cause familial combined pituitary hormone deficiency. *Nat Genet*, 1998;18: 147-149.

[101] Cushman, LJ, Watkins-Chow, DE, Brinkmeier, ML, Raetzman, LT, Radak, AL, Lloyd, RV, et al. Persistent Prop1 expression delays gonadotrope differentiation and enhances pituitary tumor susceptibility. *Hum Mol Genet*, 2001;10:1141-1153.

[102] Vesper, AH, Raetzman, LT, Camper, SA. Role of prophet of Pit1 [PROP1] in gonadotrope differentiation and puberty. *Endocrinology*, 2006;147:1654-1663.

[103] Rizzoti, K, Brunelli, S, Carmignac, D, Thomas, PQ, Robinson, IC, Lovell-Badge, R. SOX3 is required during the formation of the hypothalamo-pituitary axis. *Nat Genet*, 2004;36:247-255.

[104] Sarkar, A, Hochedlinger, K. A gutsy way to grow: intestinal stem cells as nutrient sensors. *Cell*, 2011;147: 487-489.

[105] Zhao, L, Zevallos, SE, Rizzoti, K, Jeong, Y, Lovell-Badge, R, Epstein, DJ. Disruption of SoxB1-dependent Sonic hedgehog expression in the hypothalamus causes septo-optic dysplasia. *Dev Cell*, 2012;22:585-596.

[106] Lee, B, Rizzoti, K, Kwon, DS, Kim, SY, Oh, S, Epstein, DJ, et al. Direct transcriptional regulation of Six6 is controlled by SoxB1 binding to a remote forebrain enhancer. *Dev Biol*, 2012;366:393-403.

[107] Lee, B, Song, H, Rizzoti, K, Son, Y, Yoon, J, Baek, K, et al. Genomic code for Sox2 binding uncovers its regulatory role in Six3 activation in the forebrain. *Developmental Biology*, 2013;381:491-501.

[108] Fantes, J, Ragge, NK, Lynch, SA, McGill, NI, Collin, JR, Howard-Peebles, PN, et al. Mutations in SOX2 cause anophthalmia. *Nat Genet*, 2003;33:461-463.

[109] Kelberman, D, Rizzoti, K, Avilion, A, Bitner-Glindzicz, M, Cianfarani, S, Collins, J, et al. 2006 Mutations within Sox2/SOX2 are associated with abnormalities in the hypothalamo–pituitary–gonadal axis in mice and humans. *J Clin Invest*, 2006;116:2442-2455.

[110] Laumonnier, F, Ronce, N, Hamel, BC, Thomas, P, Lespinasse, J, Raynaud, M, et al. Transcription factor SOX3 is involved in X-linked mental retardation with growth hormone deficiency. *Am J Hum Genet*, 2002;71:1450-1455.

[111] Jayakody, SA, Andoniadou, CL, Gaston-Massuet, C, Signore, M, Cariboni, A, Bouloux, PM, et al. SOX2 regulates the hypothalamic-pituitary axis at multiple levels. *J Clin Invest*, 2012;122:3635-3646.

[112] Andoniadou, CL, Matsushima, D, Mousavy Gharavy, SN, Signore, M, Mackintosh, AI, Schaeffer, M, et al. 2013 Sox2[C] stem/progenitor cells in the adult mouse pituitary support organ homeostasis and have tumor-inducing potential. *Cell Stem Cell*, 2013;13:433-445.

[113] Rizzoti, K, Akiyama, H, Lovell-Badge, R. Mobilized adult pituitary stem cells contribute to endocrine regeneration in response to physiological demand. *Cell Stem Cell*, 2013;13:419-432.

[114] Weiss, J, Meeks, JJ, Hurley, L, Raverot, G, Frassetto, A, Jameson, JL. Sox3 is required for gonadal function, but not sex determination, in males and females. *Mol Cell Biol*, 2003;23:8084-8091.

[115] Rizzoti, K, Lovell-Badge, R. SOX3activity during pharyngeal segmentation is required for craniofacial morphogenesis. *Development*, 2007;134:3437-3448.

[116] Solomon, NM, Ross, SA, Morgan, T, Belsky, JL, Hol, FA, Karnes, PS, et al. 2004 Array comparative genomic hybridisation analysis of boys with X linked hypopituitarism identifies a 3.9 Mb duplicated critical region at Xq27 containing SOX3. *J Med Genet*, 2004;41:669-678.

[117] Kan, L, Israsena, N, Zhang, Z, Hu, M, Zhao, LR, Jalali, A, et al. Sox1 acts through multiple independent pathways to promote neurogenesis. *Dev Biol*, 2004, 269:580-594.

[118] Mansukhani, A, Ambrosetti, D, Holmes, G, Cornivelli, L, Basilico, C. Sox2 induction by FGF and FGFR2 activating mutations inhibits Wnt signaling and osteoblast differentiation. *J Cell Biol*, 2005;168:1065-1076.

[119] Bodner, M, Castrillo, JL, Theill, LE, Deerinck, T, Ellisman, M, Karin, M. The pituitary-specific transcription factor GHF-1 is a homeobox-containing protein. *Cell*, 1988;55:505-518.

[120] Simmons, DM, Voss, JW, Ingraham, HA, Holloway, JM, Broide, RS, Rosenfeld, MG, et al. Pituitary cell phenotypes involve cell-specific Pit-1 mRNA translation and synergistic interactions with other classes of transcription factors. *Genes Dev*, 1990;4: 695-711.

[121] Rhodes, SJ, DiMattia, GE, Rosenfeld, MG. Transcriptional mechanisms in anterior pituitary cell differentiation. *Curr Opin Genet Dev*, 1994;4:709-717.

[122] Andersen, B, Rosenfeld, MG. POU domain factors in the neuroendocrine system: lessons from developmental biology provide insights into human disease. *Endocr Rev*, 2001;22:2-35.

[123] Qi, Y, Ranish, JA, Zhu, X, Krones, A, Zhang, J, Aebersold, R, et al. Atbf1 is required for the Pit1 gene early activation. *Proc Natl Acad Sci USA*, 2008;105:2481-2486.

[124] Andersen, B, Rosenfeld, MG. Pit-1 determines cell types during development of the anterior pituitary gland. A model for transcriptional regulation of cell phenotypes in mammalianorganogenesis. *J Biol Chem*, 1994;269:29335-29338.

[125] Rhodes, SJ, Chen, R, DiMattia, GE, Scully, KM, Kalla, KA, Lin, SC, et al. A tissue-specific enhancer confers Pit-1-dependent morphogen inducibility and autoregulation on the pit-1 gene. *Genes Dev*, 1993;7:913-932.

[126] Ward, RD, Stone, BM, Raetzman, LT, Camper, SA. Cell proliferation and vascularization in mouse models of pituitary hormone deficiency. *Mol Endocrinol*, 2006;20:1378-1390.

[127] Dasen, JS, O'Connell, SM, Flynn, SE, Treier, M, Gleiberman, AS, Szeto, DP, et al. Reciprocal interactions of Pit1 and GATA2 mediate signaling gradient-induced determination of pituitary cell types. *Cell*, 1999;97:587-598.

[128] Xu, L, Lavinsky, RM, Dasen, JS, Flynn, SE, McInerney, EM, Mullen, TM, et al. 1998 Signal-specific co-activator domain requirements for Pit-1 activation. *Nature*, 1998;395:301-306.

[129] Sloop, KW, Dwyer, CJ, Rhodes, SJ. An isoform-specific inhibitory domain regulates the LHX3LIM homeodomain factor holoprotein and the production of a functional alternate translation form. *J Biol Chem*, 2001;276:6311-36319.

[130] Huang, TS, Hsieh, JY, Wu, YH, Jen, CH, Tsuang, YH, Chiou, SH, et al. Functional network reconstruction reveals somatic stemness genetic maps and dedifferentiation-

like transcriptome reprogramming induced by GATA2. *Stem Cells*, 2008, 26, 1186-1201.

[131] Morceau, F, Schnekenburger, M, Dicato, M, Diederich, M. GATA-1: friends, brothers, and coworkers. *Ann NY Acad Sci*, 2004;1030:537-554.

[132] Steger, DJ, Hecht, JH, Mellon, PL. GATA-binding proteins regulate the human gonadotropin-subunit gene in the placenta and pituitary gland. *Mol Cell Biol*, 1994;14:5592-5602.

[133] Gordon, DF, Woodmansee, WW, Black, JN, Dowding, JM, Bendrick-Peart, J, Wood, WM, et al. Domains of Pit-1 required for transcriptional synergy with GATA-2on the TSH gene. *Mol Cell Endocrinol*, 2002;196:53-66.

[134] Urs, AN, Dammer, E, Kelly, S, Wang, E, Merrill, Jr. AH, Sewer, MB. Steroidogenic factor-1 is a sphingolipid binding protein. *Mol Cell Endocrinol*, 2007;265-266:174-178.

[135] Barnhart, KM, Mellon, PL. The orphan nuclear receptor, steroidogenic factor-1, regulates the glycoprotein hormone-subunit gene in pituitary gonadotropes. *Mol Endocrinol*, 1994;8:878-885.

[136] Brown, P, Mcneilly, AS. Steroidogenic factor-1 [SF-1] and the regulation of expression of luteinising hormone and follicle stimulating hormone -subunits in the sheep anterior pituitary in vivo. *Int J Biochem Cell Biol*, 1997;29:1513-1524.

[137] Ngan, ES, Cheng, PK, Leung, PC, Chow, BK. Steroidogenic factor-1 interacts with a gonadotrope-specific element within the first exon of the human gonadotropin-releasing hormone receptor gene to mediate gonadotrope-specific expression. *Endocrinology*, 1999;140:2452-2462.

[138] Tremblay, JJ, Drouin, J. Egr-1 is a downstream effector of Gn RH and synergizes by direct interaction with Ptx1 and SF-1 to enhance luteinizing hormone gene transcription. *Mol Cell Biol*, 1999;19:2567-2576.

[139] Ingraham, HA, Lala, DS, Ikeda, Y, Luo, X, Shen, WH, Nachtigal, MW, et al. The nuclear receptor steroidogenic factor 1 acts at multiple levels of the reproductive axis. *Genes Dev*, 1994;8:2302-2312.

[140] Salisbury, TB, Binder, AK, Grammer, JC, Nilson, JH. Maximal activity of the luteinizing hormone-subunit gene requires-catenin. *Mol Endocrinol*, 2007, 21, 963-971.

[141] Lin, L, Achermann, JC. Steroidogenic factor-1 [SF-1, Ad4BP, NR5A1] and disorders of testis development. *Sex Dev*, 2008;2:200-209.

[142] Lourenco, D, Brauner, R, Lin, L, De Perdigo, A, Weryha, G, Muresan, M, et al. Mutations in NR5A1 associated with ovarian insufficiency. *N Engl J Med*, 2009;360:1200-1210.

[143] Lamolet, B, Pulichino, AM, Lamonerie, T, Gauthier, Y, Brue, T, Enjalbert, A, et al. A pituitary cell-restricted T box factor, Tpit, activates POMC transcription in cooperation with Pitx homeoproteins. *Cell*, 2001;104:849-859.

[144] Naiche, LA, Harrelson, Z, Kelly, RG, Papaioannou, VE. T-box genes in vertebrate development. *Annu Rev Genet*, 2005;39:219-239.

[145] Medina-Martinez, O, Amaya-Manzanares, F, Liu, C, Mendoza, M, Shah, R, Zhang, L, et al. Cell-autonomous requirement for rx function in the mammalian retina and posterior pituitary. *PLoS ONE*, 2009;4:e4513.

[146] Lu, F, Kar, D, Gruenig, N, Zhang, ZW, Cousins, N, Rodgers, HM, et al. Rax is a selector gene for mediobasal hypothalamic cell types. *J Neurosci*, 2013;33:259-272.

[147] Bentley, CA, Zidehsarai, MP, Grindley, JC, Parlow, AF, Barth-Hall, S, Roberts, VJ. Pax6 is implicated in murine pituitary endocrine function. *Endocrine*, 1999;10:171-177.

[148] Kioussi, C, O'Connell, S, St-Onge, L, Treier, M, Gleiberman, AS, Gruss, P, et al. Pax6 is essential for establishing ventraldorsal cell boundaries in pituitary gland development. *Proc Natl Acad Sci USA*, 1999;96:14378-14382.

[149] Simpson, TI, Price, DJ. Pax6: a pleiotropic player in development. *Bioessays*, 2002;24:1041-1051.

[150] Ellsworth, BS, Egashira, N, Haller, JL, Butts, DL, Cocquet, J, Clay, CM, et al. FOXL2 in the pituitary: molecular, genetic, and developmental analysis. *Mol Endocrinol*, 2006;20:2796-2805.

[151] Steger, DJ, Hecht, JH, Mellon, PL. 1994 GATA-binding proteins regulate the human gonadotropin a-subunit gene in the placenta and pituitary gland. *Mol Cell Biol*, 1994; 14:5592-5602.

[152] Zhao, X, Teng, R, Asanuma, K, Okouchi, Y, Johkura, K, Ogiwara, N, et al. Differentiation of mouse embryonic stem cells into gonadotrope-like cells in vitro. *J Soc Gynecol Investig*, 2005;12:257-262.

[153] Brown, P, McNeilly, AS. Transcriptional regulation of pituitary gonadotrophin subunit genes. *Rev Reprod*, 1999;4:117-124.

[154] Lo, A, Zheng, W, Gong, Y, Crochet, JR, Halvorson, LM. 2011 GATA transcription factors regulate LHb gene expression. *J Mol Endocrinol*, 2011;47:45-58.

[155] Ikeda, Y, Luo, X, Abbud, R, Nilson, JH, Parker, KL. The nuclear receptor steroidogenic factor 1 is essential for the formation of the ventromedial hypothalamic nucleus. *Mol Endocrinol*, 1995;9:478-486.

[156] Tremblay, JJ, Lanctot, C, Drouin, J. The pan-pituitary activator of transcription, Ptx1 [pituitary homeobox 1], acts in synergy with SF-1 and Pit1 and is an upstream regulator of the Lim–homeodomain gene Lim3/Lhx3. *Mol Endocrinol*, 1998;12:428-441.

[157] Bach, I, Rhodes, SJ, Pearse, RV, II, Heinzel, T, Gloss, B, Scully, KM, et al. P-Lim, a LIM homeodomain factor, is expressed during pituitary organ and cell commitment and synergizes with Pit-1. *PNAS*, 1995;92:2720-2724.

[158] West, BE, Parker, GE, Savage, JJ, Kiratipranon, P, Toomey, KS, Beach, LR, et al. Regulation of the folliclestimulating hormone beta gene by the LHX3 LIM-homeodomain transcription factor. *Endocrinology*, 2004;145:4866-4879.

[159] Aikawa, S, Sato, T, Ono, T, Kato, T, Kato, Y. High level expression of Prop-1 gene in gonadotropic cell lines. *J Reprod Dev*, 2006;52:195-201.

[160] Li, S, Crenshaw, EB, III, Rawson, EJ, Simmons, DM, Swanson, LW, Rosenfeld, MG. Dwarf locus mutants lacking three pituitary cell types result from mutations in the POU-domain gene pit-1. *Nature*, 1990;347:528-533.

[161] Massah, S, Hollebakken, R, Labrecque, MP, Kolybaba, AM, Beischlag, TV, Prefontaine, GG. 2014 Epigenetic characterization of the growth hormone gene identifies SmcHD1 as a regulator of autosomal gene clusters. *PLoS ONE*, 2014;9:e97535.

[162] Turton, JP, Strom, M, Langham, S, Dattani, MT, Le Tissier, P. Two novel mutations in the POU1F1 gene generate null alleles through different mechanisms leading to combined pituitary hormone deficiency. *Clin Endocrinol* (Oxf), 2012;76:387-393.

[163] Lin, SC, Li, S, Drolet, DW, Rosenfeld, MG. Pituitary ontogeny of the Snell dwarf mouse reveals Pit-1-independent and Pit-1-dependent origins of the thyrotrope. *Development*, 1994;120:515-522.

[164] Drolet, DW, Scully, KM, Simmons, DM, Wegner, M, Chu, KT, Swanson, LW, et al. 1991 TEF, a transcription factor expressed specifically in the anterior pituitary during embryogenesis, defines a new class of leucine zipper proteins. *Genes Dev*, 1991;5: 1739-1753.

[165] Drouin, J, Lamolet, B, Lamonerie, T, Lanctot, C, Tremblay, JJ. The PTX family of homeodomain transcription factors during pituitary developments. *Mol Cell Endocrinol*, 1998;140:31-36.

[166] Cheung, LY, Rizzoti, K, Lovell-Badge, R, Le Tissier, PR. Pituitary phenotypes of mice lacking the Notch signalling ligand delta-like 1 homologue. *Journal of Neuroendocrinology*, 2013;25:391-401.

[167] Lipkin, SM, Naar, AM, Kalla, KA, Sack, RA, Rosenfeld, MG. Identification of a novel zinc finger protein binding a conserved element critical for Pit-1-dependent growth hormone gene expression. *Genes Dev*, 1993;7:1674-1687.

[168] Schaufele, F, West, BL, Baxter, JD. Synergistic activation of the rat growth hormone promoter by Pit-1 and the thyroid hormone receptor. *Mol Endocrinol*, 1992;6:656-665.

[169] Palomino, T, Barettino, D, Aranda, A. Role of GHF-1 in the regulation of the rat growth hormone gene promoter by thyroid hormone and retinoic acid receptors. *J Biol Chem*, 1998;273:27541-27547.

[170] Reynaud, R, Chadli-Chaieb, M, Vallette-Kasic, S, Barlier, A, Sarles, J, Pellegrini-Bouiller, I, et al. A familial form of congenital hypopituitarism due to a PROP1 mutation in a large kindred: phenotypic and in vitro functional studies. *J Clin Endocrinol Metab*, 2004;89:5779-5786.

[171] Poulin, G, Turgeon, B, Drouin, J. NeuroD1/b2 contributes to cellspecific transcription of the proopiomelanocortin gene. *MolCell Biol*, 1997;17:6673-6682.

[172] Yano, K, Bauchat, JR, Liimatta, MB, Clemmons, DR, Duan, C. Downregulation of protein kinase C inhibits insulin-like growth factor I-induced vascular smooth muscle cell proliferation, migration, and gene expression. *Endocrinology*, 1999;140:4622-4632.

[173] Nasonkin, IO, Ward, RD, Bavers, DL, Beuschlein, F, Mortensen, AH, Keegan, CE, et al. 2011 Aged PROP1 deficient dwarf mice maintain ACTH production. *PLoS ONE*, 2011;6:e28355.

[174] Daikoku, S, Chikamori, M, Adachi, T, Maki, Y. Effect of the basal diencephalon on the development of Rathke's pouch in rats: a study in combined organ cultures. *Dev Biol*, 1982;90:198-202.

[175] Kapsimali, M, Caneparo, L, Houart, C, Wilson, SW. Inhibition of Wnt/Axin/beta-catenin pathway activity promotes ventral CNS midline tissue to adopt hypothalamic rather than floorplate identity. *Development*, 2004;131:5923-5933.

[176] Ohyama, K, Ellis, P, Kimura, S, Placzek, M. Directed differentiation of neural cells to hypothalamic dopaminergic neurons. *Development*, 2005;132:5185-5197.

[177] Wilson, SW, Houart, C. Early steps in the development of the forebrain. *Dev Cell*, 2004;6:167-181.

[178] Parkin, JM. Incidence of growth hormone deficiency. *Arch Dis Child*, 1974;49:904-905.

[179] Vimpani, GV, Vimpani, AF, Lidgard, GP, Cameron, EH, Farquhar, JW. Prevalence of severe growth hormone deficiency. *Br Med J*, 1977;2:427-430.
[180] Lindsay, R, Feldkamp, M, Harris, D, Robertson, J, Rallison, M. Utah Growth Study: growth standards and the prevalence of growth hormone deficiency. *J Pediatr*, 1994; 125:29-35.
[181] Bao, XL, Shi, YF, Du, YC, Liu, R, Deng, JY, Gao, SM. Prevalence of growth hormone deficiency of children in Beijing. *Chin Med J [Engl]*, 1992;105:401-405.
[182] Thomas, M, Massa, G, Craen, M, de Zegher, F, Bourguignon, JP, Heinrichs, C, et al. Prevalence and demographic features of childhood growth hormone deficiency in Belgium during the period 1986-2001. *Eur J Endocrinol*, 2004, 151, 67-72.
[183] Patel, L, McNally, RJ, Harrison, E, Lloyd, IC, Clayton, PE. Geographical distribution of optic nerve hypoplasia and septo-optic dysplasia in Northwest England. *J Pediatr*, 2006, 148, 85-88.
[184] Phillips, 3rd JA, Cogan, JD. Genetic basis of endocrine disease. 6. Molecular basis of familial human growth hormone deficiency. *J Clin Endocrinol Metab*, 1994, 78, 11-16.
[185] Wales, JK, Quarrell, OW. Evidence for possible Mendelian inheritance of septo-optic dysplasia. *Acta Paediatr*, 1996;85:391-392.
[186] Murray, PG, Paterson, WF, Donaldson, MD. Maternal age in patients with septo-optic dysplasia. *J Pediatr Endocrinol Metab*, 2005;18:471-476.
[187] McNay, DE, Turton, JP, Kelberman, D, Woods, KS, Brauner, R, Papadimitriou, A, et al. HESX1 mutations are an uncommon cause of septooptic dysplasia and hypopituitarism. *J Clin Endocrinol Metab*, 2007;92: 691-697.
[188] Kiyokawa, H, Kineman, RD, Manova-Todorova, KO, Soares, VC, Hoffman, ES, Ono, M, et al. 1996 Enhanced growth of mice lacking the cyclin-dependent kinase inhibitor function of p27(Kip1). *Cell*, 1996, 85, 721-732.
[189] Abbud, RA, Takumi, I, Barker, EM, Ren, SG, Chen, DY, Wawrowsky, K, et al. 005 Early multipotential pituitary focal hyperplasia in the alpha-subunit of glycoprotein hormone-driven pituitary tumor-transforming gene transgenic mice. *Mol Endocrinol*, 2005;19:1383-1391.
[190] Fan, X, Gabbi, C, Kim, HJ, Cheng, G, Andersson, LC, Warner, M, et al. Gustafsson JA 2010 Gonadotropin-positive pituitary tumors accompanied by ovarian tumors in aging female ERbeta-/- mice. *Proc Natl Acad Sci USA*, 2010;107:6453-6458.
[191] Ezzat, S, Melmed, S. The role of growth factors in the pituitary. *J Endocrinol Invest*, 1990;13:691-698.
[192] Tanase, CP, Neagu, M, Albulescu, R. Key signaling molecules in pituitary tumors. *Expert Rev Mol Diagn*, 2009;9:859-877.
[193] Simpson, DJ, Hibberts, NA, McNicol, AM, Clayton, RN, Farrell, WE. Loss of pRb expression in pituitary adenomas is associated with methylation of the RB1 CpG island. *Cancer Res*, 2000;60:1211-1216.
[194] Hossain, MG, Iwata, T, Mizusawa, N, Qian, ZR, Shima, SW, Okutsu, T, et al. Expression of p18(INK4C) is down-regulated in human pituitary adenomas. *Endocr Pathol*, 2009;20:114-121.
[195] Roussel-Gervais, A, Bilodeau, S, Vallette, S, Berthelet, F, Lacroix, A, Figarella-Branger, D, et al. Cooperation between Cyclin E and p27(Kip1) in pituitary tumorigenesis. *Mol Endocrinol*, 2010;24:1835-1845.

[196] Bilodeau, S, Vallette-Kasic, S, Gauthier, Y, Figarella-Branger, D, Brue, T, Berthelet, F, et al.. Role of Brg1 and HDAC2 in GR trans-repression of the pituitary POMC gene and misexpression in Cushing disease. *Genes Dev*, 2006;20:2871-2886.
[197] Heaney, AP, Horwitz, GA, Wang, Z, Singson, R, Melmed, S. Early involvement of estrogen-induced pituitary tumor transforming gene and fibroblast growth factor expression in prolactinoma pathogenesis. *Nat Med*, 1999;5:1317-1321.
[198] Landis, CA, Masters, SB, Spada, A, Pace, AM, Bourne, HR, Vallar, L. GTPase inhibiting mutations activate the alpha chain of Gs and stimulate adenylyl cyclase in human pituitary tumours. *Nature*, 1989;340:692-696.
[199] Bertherat, J, Chanson, P, Montminy, M. 1995 The cyclic adenosine 3', 5'-monophosphate-responsive factor CREB is constitutively activated in human somatotroph adenomas. *Mol Endocrinol*, 1995;9:777-783.
[200] Fedele, M, Visone, R, De Martino, I, Troncone, G, Palmieri, D, Battista, S. HMGA2 induces pituitary tumorigenesis by enhancing E2F1 activity. *Cancer Cell*, 2006;9:459-471.
[201] Zhang, HY, Jin, L, Stilling, GA, Ruebel, KH, Coonse, K, Tanizaki, Y, et al. 2009 RUNX1 and RUNX2 upregulate Galectin-3 expression in human pituitary tumors. *Endocrine*, 2009;35:101-111.
[202] Theodoropoulou, M, Tichomirowa, MA, Sievers, C, Yassouridis, A, Arzberger, T, Hougrand, O, et al. Tumor ZAC1 expression is associated with the response to somatostatin analog therapy in patients with acromegaly. *Int J Cancer*, 2009;125:2122-2126.
[203] Zhang, X, Gejman, R, Mahta, A, Zhong, Y, Rice, KA, Zhou, Y, et al. 2010 Maternally expressed gene 3 (MEG3) noncoding ribonucleic acid: isoform structure, expression, and functions. *Endocrinoloigy*, 2010;151:939-947.
[204] Ezzat, S, Yu, S, Asa, SL. 2005 The zinc finger Ikaros transcription factor regulates pituitary growth hormone and prolactin gene expression through distinct effects on chromatin accessibility. *Mol Endocrinol* 2005;19:1004-1011.
[205] Ezzat, S, Mader, R, Yu, S, Ning, T, Poussier, P, Asa, SL. 2005 Ikaros integrates endocrine and immune system development. *J Clin Invest*, 2005;115:1021-1029.
[206] Amaral, FC, Torres, N, Saggioro, F, Neder, L, Machado, HR, Silva, WA, Jr, et al. 2009 Micro RNAs differentially expressed in ACTH-secreting pituitary tumors. *J Clin Endocrinol Metab*, 2009;94:320-323.
[207] Bottoni, A, Zatelli, MC, Ferracin, M, Tagliati, F, Piccin, D, Vignali, C, et al. Identification of differentially expressed micro RNAs by microarray: a possible role for micro RNA genes in pituitary adenomas. *J Cell Physiol*, 2007;210:370-377.
[208] Butz, H, Likó, I, Czirják, S, Igaz, P, Khan, MM, Zivkovic, V, et al. 2010 Down-regulation of Weel kinase by a specific subset of micro RNA in human sporadic pituitary adenomas. *J Clin Endocrinol Metab*, 2010;95:E181-E191.

In: Pituitary Adenoma
Editor: Dimitrios N. Kanakis

ISBN: 978-1-63484-985-2

Chapter 3

THE ROLE OF INTRACELLULAR SIGNALING PATHWAYS NOTCH, HEDGEHOG, AND WNT IN THE PATHOGENESIS OF PITUITARY ADENOMAS

Maria P. Yavropoulou**, *MD, MSc, PhD
Endocrinologist, School of Health Sciences, Medical Faculty,
Aristotle University of Thessaloniki, Thessaloniki, Greece

ABSTRACT

Pituitary adenomas are usually benign tumors that cause symptoms by compression of surrounding structures or impaired hormone secretion. Treatment either surgical or medical depends on the tumor subtype and degree of compression. However, a significant proportion of patients do not achieve optimal control of mass effects or hormonal hypersecretion. Unraveling the pathogenesis of pituitary adenomas is the critical step in the quest of new subcellular treatment targets that will decrease morbidity and mortality related to these tumors. A large diversity of pathogenetic mechanisms has been described so far including deregulation of cell cycle, molecular pathways and angiogenesis. Major signaling pathways such as Notch, Wnt and Hedgehog, which are mainly active in the early phase of pituitary organogenesis and are essential for the development of somatotrophs, lactotrophs thyrotrophs and corticotrophs, have been implicated in the pathogenesis of pituitary adenomas. In this chapter we outline novel data regarding the role of Notch, Wnt and Hedgehog regulatory networks in pituitary development and pathogenesis of pituitary adenomas.

Keywords: Notch signaling, Hedgehog signaling, Wnt signaling, non-functioning pituitary adenomas, somatotropinomas

* Corresponding author: Maria Yavropoulou, MD, PhD, Laboratory of Clinical and Molecular Endocrinology, 1st Department of Internal Medicine, AHEPA University Hospital, S. Kyriakidi Str. 1, 54636 Thessaloniki, Greece, Tel: +302310 993187, Fax: +302310 994608, E-mail: margia@med.auth.gr, Webpage: http://www.maria-yavropoulou.eu/

1. Introduction

Pituitary adenomas are among the most frequent intracranial tumors. Series of radiological and autopsy studies suggest a prevalence as high as up to 22.5% [1]. Although the majority of pituitary adenomas are benign and malignancy occurs rarely, they usually behave as an expanding mass causing compression and excessive hormone secretion or insufficiency [2]. Surgical resection remains the first line treatment for most of the pituitary tumors except for prolactinomas, which efficiently respond to medical treatment. Despite the recent advances in molecular genetics, the molecular pathogenesis of pituitary adenomas remains largely unknown, and the current classification of clinically functional and nonfunctional tumors does not reflect possible molecular distinctions between the subtypes.

Over the past 30 years, studies of developmental biology have identified the role of evolutionarily highly conserved intracellular signaling pathways such as Wnt, Notch and Hedgehog in pituitary development and disease. Through these pathways specific secreted proteins control differentiation and function of recipient cells in a paracrine and/or autocrine manner. Tight concerted actions of these signals lead to specific cell fates and the formation of distinct cell populations in the developing pituitary, while in adult pituitary they regulate proliferation and hormonal secretion of pituitary cells.

In this chapter we outline the recent knowledge regarding the role of Notch, Hedgehog and Wnt signaling pathways in the development of pituitary and their involvement in the pathogenesis of pituitary adenomas.

2. The Notch Signaling and Its Components

Notch signaling pathway regulates cell fate through lateral inhibition and formation of boundaries, both of which represent patterning processes of critical importance in the regulation of spacing of different cell types within tissues [3, 4]. Its function involves juxtacrine cellular signaling, where both the signal sending and receiving cells are affected through ligand-receptor crosstalk. Upon activation by specific ligands Notch regulates a variety of cell types during specification, patterning, and morphogenesis through effects on differentiation, proliferation, survival and apoptosis [5].

During "lateral inhibition," Notch signaling, having mainly a permissive role, contributes to binary cell fate choices in populations of developmentally equivalent cells, by inhibiting one of the fates in some cells and allowing them to later adopt an alternative one. Notch may also regulate the adoption of a third cell fate at the border of neighboring populations of different cell types [6, 7].

The formation of boundaries takes place between distinct cell populations and promotes the exhibition of discrete physiological functions in specific organs and tissues [8]. Embryogenesis undergoes a variety of boundary formations and Notch signaling is a critical regulator of this process [9].

2.1. Ligands-Receptors

There are four Notch receptors in mammals (Notch1, Notch2, Notch3, Notch4) and five classic DSL (Delta/Serrate/Lag-2) ligands, Jagged1, Jagged 2, Delta-like 1, Delta-like 3 and Delta-like 4.

Notch receptors are single-pass, trans-membrane proteins composed of a functional extracellular domain (NECD), a trans-membrane domain and an intracellular domain (NICD). Notch ligands are also trans-membrane proteins in the signal-sending cells and both ligands and receptors require a catalytic process to become active. Some of the Delta–like ligands can undergo cleavage in the membrane by a specific metalloprotease, and thus act not only in neighboring cells but in distant tissues as well.

2.2. The Intracellular Cascade

Ligand binding leads to the cleavage of Notch receptors by a TNF-a converting enzyme (TACE), which belongs to the ADAM family of disintegrin and metalloproteases. The clipping of the extracellular domain creates a membrane-tethered intermediate called Notch extracellular truncation (NEXT), which is a substrate for an intra-membrane cleaving protease, γ-secretase. After the γ-secretase-induced cleavage, NICD is free to enter into the nucleus where it interacts with the CSL (CBF1/Suppressor of Hairless/LAG-1) DNA-binding protein (RPBJ in Drosophila) and activates transcription of target genes. The CSL protein is bound to transcriptional co-repressors in the absence of NICD. The formation of the NICD-CSL complex displaces transcriptional co-repressors and recruits co-activators such as MAML (mammalian Mastermind/Lag-3) and MED8 (Mediator of RNA polymerase II transcription subunit 8), promoting the transcription of target genes. The downstream effectors of canonical Notch signaling are the transcription factors Hairy Enhancer of Split (HES) 1, 5, 6 and 7 and HES-related with YRPW motif (HEY) 1, 2 and HEY L [10]. (Figure 1)

HES belong to a family of basic helix-loop-helix (bHLH) genes and participate in the regulation of cell fate decision and boundary formation. Some of them have been implicated in specific disorders in humans. In particular, HES1 is essential for Notch-induced T-cell acute lymphoblastic leukemia [11]. On the other hand, HES7 that is both a direct target of Notch signaling pathway and part of a negative feedback mechanism required to attenuate Notch signaling [12], was found mutated and non-functional in a family with autosomal recessive spondylocostal disorder.

Co-activators and co-repressors that are recruited during activation of Notch signaling are shared with other signaling pathways, and thus over-expression of NICD can affect the transcription of genes that are regulated by proteins apart from Notch pathway. The nuclear environment is the key that will define which targets are available to Notch-CSL-induced activation [10, 13, 14].

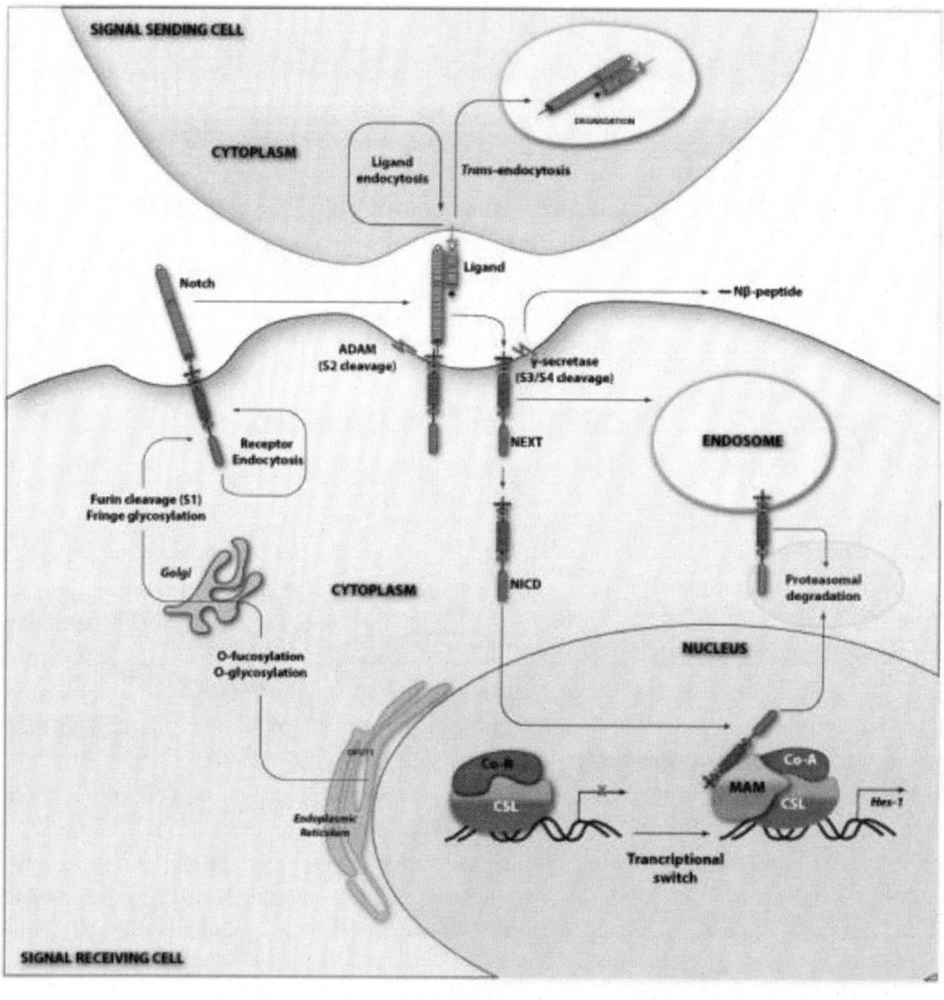

Figure 1. The Notch receptor is synthesized as a single trans-membrane receptor that is glycosylated and undergoes proteolytic cleavage at site 1 (S1), yielding a bipartite heterodimeric receptor, that is held together by non-covalent interaction and is expressed on the cell surface of a `signal-receiving cell.' Activation begins when a ligand presented by the signal sending cell interacts with the receptor. Conformational changes exposes site 2 (S2) in Notch receptor for cleavage by ADAM metalloproteases, generating the membrane-anchored Notch extracellular truncation (NEXT) fragment, a substrate for the γ-secretase complex. Gamma-Secretase then cleaves NEXT progressively from site 3 (S3) to site 4 (S4) to release the Notch intracellular domain (NICD) and Nβ peptide. NICD then enters the nucleus where it associates with the DNA-binding protein CSL. The transcriptional co-activator MAML then recognizes the NICD/CSL interface, and this tri-protein complex recruits additional co-activators to activate transcription. In the absence of NICD, CSL may associate with ubiquitous co-repressor proteins and histone deacetylases to repress transcription of target genes [10].

3. The Notch Signaling and the Pituitary Gland

3.1. The Role of Notch Signaling in the Development of the Pituitary Gland

The development of the pituitary gland is based on the interaction between the neural ectoderm, which becomes the posterior pituitary, and the oral ectoderm fated to become the Rathke's pouch (anterior pituitary) [15, 16]. The definitive Rathke's pouch initially contains undifferentiated proliferative progenitors. Gradually, these will differentiate and give rise to the five endocrine cell types present in the anterior pituitary.

During pituitary development, Notch signaling components are expressed in the invaginating pouch. Then they are quickly down-regulated from the differentiating zone ventrally but are maintained dorsally around the lumen of Rathke's pouch [17, 18]. NOTCH 2 is expressed in the periluminal cells of Rathke's pouch that are undergoing rapid proliferation but not in the differentiated cells that express αGSU (α-subunit of glycoprotein) and are able to secrete glycoprotein hormones, such as TSH, FSH and LH [19]. NOTCH 2 expression decreases as pituitary development proceeds, indicating that it may need to be absent for cell differentiation to occur. The time and location of NOTCH 2 expression appears coincident with the expression of PROP 1 (prophet of pituitary transcription factor), which precedes and is required for the expression of PIT 1 (Pou domain transcription factor 1), the master transcription factor of pituitary development and hormone expression [20]. Mutations in PROP 1 gene have been associated with deficiencies in LH, FSH, GH, prolactin, and TSH. NOTCH 2 expression is not detectable in PROP 1 mutant pituitaries [17]. There are several Notch family members expressed in the pituitary in similar spatiotemporal patterns to NOTCH 2, although their expression is maintained in PROP 1 mutants. These include NOTCH 3, DELTA-LIKE 1, and HES 1. HES1 expression overlaps with NOTCH 2 expression in undifferentiated cells in Rathke's pouch [17]. The normal location of NOTCH 2 expression at the juncture between highly proliferating and differentiating cells, and the lack of expression in PROP 1 mutants, make it a plausible candidate for explaining the profound organ disorganization characteristic of PROP 1 mutant mice [21].

According to recent data, Notch signaling in the pituitary controls the transition from proliferation to differentiation and potentially, through lateral inhibition, influences the differentiation of cells into the five hormone producing cell types. NOTCH 2 knockout mice display early embryonic lethality, and there is potential for redundancy of NOTCH 2 and NOTCH 3 function because of their overlapping expression patterns [22]. Thus, it is difficult to discern the function of NOTCH 2 in pituitary development with simple loss of function approaches. Certain studies have shown that persistent expression of activated NOTCH 2 interferes with the development of gonadotropes and, to a lesser extent, of thyrotropes [22].

Moreover, fully differentiated gonadotropes extinguish NOTCH 2 transgene expression, suggesting that NOTCH 2 can inhibit cell differentiation in the pituitary gland, similarly to what it does in the nervous system and pancreatic endocrine cells. In contrast, the proliferation of pituitary cells expressing activated NOTCH 2 does not seem to be affected.

In the adult gland, components of the Notch signaling pathway are expressed by cells in the same locations proposed to contain progenitor/stem cells [23].

Exclusive deletion of Rbp-j (Rbp-J-/-) in Rathke's pouch [18] results in premature differentiation of corticotropes. Such a phenotype is also observed when HES 1 gene is deleted, and is correlated with decreased proliferation [18, 24], although one study also reported increased cell death [25].

In RBP-J-/- embryos in Drosophila, PROP 1 expression, which is a direct target of RBP-J [18], is not increased. As a consequence, PIT 1 fails to be expressed. It appears that Notch signaling is required to prevent early (corticotrope) differentiation and maintain undifferentiated progenitors fated for a later, PIT 1-dependent fate. In this way, Notch signaling allows the generation of different endocrine cell types by controlling the time and the context in which they differentiate. The failure of multiple cell types to differentiate in PROP-1 mutants is probably attributed to lack of NOTCH 2 expression.

3.2. The Role of Notch Signaling in the Pathogenesis of Pituitary Adenomas

Notch receptors and their ligands have been demonstrated to be involved in the pathogenesis of numerous neoplasms in humans. Notch 3 affects apoptosis and tumor growth in lung cancer [26, 27] and is able to promote the survival of T-acute lymphoblastic leukemia cells via regulation of the Mitogen Activated Protein Kinase (MAPK) pathway [28].

Abundant evidence suggests that the interaction between Notch 3 and its downstream effector transcription factor Jagged 1 plays a key role in the tumorigenesis of numerous diverse malignancies, including ovarian cancer, colorectal cancer and multiple myeloma cells [29-31]. The majority of these studies revealed that the interaction between Notch 3 and Jagged 1 participates in the growth, proliferation and angiogenesis of these tumors [29, 30, 32, 33].

In the study by Lu et al., the expression of Notch 3 and Jagged 1 protein was significantly elevated in the non-functioning pituitary adenomas compared with normal pituitary tissue [34]. Notch 3 mRNA expression was also increased in prolactinomas by 1.5 to 5.3-fold, while in somatotropinomas there was a significantly reduced expression of Notch 3 [35].

Gene microarrays and proteomic analyses have confirmed increased expression of Notch 3 gene and protein in human clinically non-functioning pituitary adenomas [36, 37] but not in GH- and PRL-secreting adenomas.

At molecular level Notch signaling has been demonstrated to repress MATH 3 expression, which is a PIT 1 target gene and is specifically required for the maturation and proliferation of the GH-producing somatotropes [38]. In addition, Notch3 may promote the maturation and proliferation of gonadotropes, which are the predominant cell type of non-functioning adenomas.

Ligands of the Notch3 receptor and Notch target genes also play a role in the pathogenesis of pituitary adenomas. Previous studies have demonstrated that Delta-like 1 ligand is strongly down-regulated in non-functioning tumors and in PRL-secreting adenomas [35, 36], while Cyclin D1, one of the Notch target genes, was over-expressed in non-functioning pituitary adenomas [39].

Notch signaling may promote tumorigenesis via either the canonical CSL-mediated transcriptional network or through co-operation with other signaling pathways, including the Wnt, MAPK, and EFGR (Endothelial Fibroblast Growth Receptor) pathways. The exact mechanism by which Notch signaling regulates pituitary tumor development and tumorigenesis remains to be elucidated.

As the Notch signaling pathway is involved in the pathogenesis of numerous diverse malignancies, it is hypothesized that inhibition of this pathway may have antitumor effects. Following activation of the Notch receptor, the proteolytic processing of Notch by the γ-secretase protein complex is an essential step that leads to the release of the Notch-IC and transcription of target genes. Therefore, γ-secretase inhibitors are capable of specially blocking Notch signaling pathway activation. It has been demonstrated that γ-secretase inhibitors suppress proliferation and induce apoptosis in T-cell leukemia, and in lung and breast cancer [26, 40, 41]. Furthermore, γ-secretase inhibitors have been used to treat lymphoma in pre-clinical trials [42]. However, the anti-oncogenic potential of γ-secretase inhibitors in non-functioning pituitary adenomas requires further investigation.

4. The Hedgehog Signaling and Its Components

The Hedgehog (Hh) signaling pathway is comprised of a family of evolutionary conserved signaling molecules that play significant role during embryonic development and remain active in adult life regulating a variety of cellular processes in both vertebrates and invertebrates. In adult organisms it is implicated in the maintenance and homeostasis of stem cells and therefore a variety of skin (i.e., basal carcinomas), muscle, and brain cancers develop when this pathway is impaired.

4.1. Ligands

There are three mammalian homologues of the Drosophila Hh gene, Sonic Hh (Shh), Indian Hh (Ihh) and Desert Hh (Dhh). Sonic Hedgehog is coded by the SHH gene, which is located on the long (q) arm of chromosome 7 at position 36 and is the most studied ligand.

The precursor forms of the hedgehog signaling proteins have a molecular weight of 45kDa and they undergo an autocatalytic internal cleavage of the C-terminal leading to a 19-kDa N-terminal domain, which displays the Hedgehog signaling activity and a 25-kD C-terminal domain, which is active in precursor processing. This post-translational auto-processing consists of a simultaneous peptide bond cleavage and attachment of a lipophilic moiety to the newly exposed carboxyl-terminal of the amino-terminal molecule. The lipophilic modification is critical for the spatially restricted localization of the hedgehog proteins on plasma membranes. Further modification to mature forms includes signal peptide cleavage and amino-terminal palmitoylation [43].

This dual lipidation makes mature Hh proteins highly hydrophobic, and thus their release from the plasma membrane is an active process that is mediated by 2 transmembrane proteins, the twelve-pass trans-membrane protein Dispatched (Disp), which is required for release of membrane anchored Hedgehog protein and initiation of signaling to non-adjacent cells and the Tout-velu (Ttv) protein, a homolog of the mammalian EXT tumor suppressor gene family, that regulates the synthesis of proteoglycans enabling the movement of Hedgehog ligands after their release and promoting long range signaling.

Due to their lipophilic nature the majority of secreted Hh are found in soluble multimeric forms reminiscent of intestinal micelle [44, 45].

4.2. Receptors

In vertebrates Hh proteins bind to twelve-pass trans-membrane receptors Patched 1 (Ptch1) and Patched 2 (Ptch2) on responding cells. The trans-membrane loops of patched proteins are divided into two groups. Five loops compose the sterol-sensing domain (SSD) of the receptor, which is important for the internalization of Ptch and the repression of Hh target genes. In the absence of hedgehog proteins, Ptch receptors repress the activity of smoothened (Smo), a seven-pass trans-membrane protein, which is attached to membranes of cytoplasmic microsomes that belong to G-protein-coupled receptors and related to the frizzled class of Wnt receptors. In contrast to frizzled receptors family, however, Smo is not connected to the trimeric complex of G-proteins and does not bind directly to the ligand. Moreover, it is constitutively active and is associated with lipid rafts, biochemically defined fractions of membranes enriched in cholesterol, sphingo-lipids, and certain proteins, which are related with the intracellular trafficking events [46, 47].

Mutant Ptch-SDD leads to inappropriate activation of Smo protein and downstream target genes [48].

Movement of Smo in the cell surface leads to interactions with elements of the plasma membrane.

Loss-of-function mutations in Ptch receptors are associated with the **Gorlin syndrome** that predisposes to basal cell carcinomas, medulloblastomas, and rhabdomyosarcomas [49]. In addition, activating mutations of Smo have been implicated in the development of basal cell carcinomas [50].

4.3. The Intracellular Cascade

In the absence of the Hedgehog ligand, the Ptch receptor represses activity of Smo by preventing its membrane incorporation from endosomes. Downstream of Smo is a multi-protein complex, the hedgehog signaling complex (HSC), which includes the Gli (glioblastoma proteins) family of zinc finger transcription factors in mammals, the serine/threonine kinase Fused (Fu), the kinesin-like molecule, Costal 2 (Cos2) and the Suppressor of fused (Sufu). Cos2 is a docking protein that also binds to protein kinase A (PKA), casein kinase 1 (CK1) and glycogen synthase kinase 3 (GSK3) [51].

The HSC is bound to microtubules/membranes and associates with Smo through Cos 2. There are three Gli genes in mammalian cells, Gli1, Gli2 and Gli3, which have partially overlapping functions. Gli1 and Gli2 are transcriptional activators, while Gli3 functions as a transcriptional repressor. When the Hedgehog signaling is inactive the Sufu and Cos2 allow phosphorylation of the microtubule-bound pool of Gli transcription factors, leading to their degradation through ubiquitination [52-54].

In the unstimulated cells Gli2 and Gli3 are expressed at significant levels, while Gli1 transcription is increased in the presence of hedgehogs and activates expression of Hh target genes. Binding of hedgehog signaling proteins to Ptch receptors promote their internalization and de-represses the activity of Smo. Phosphorylation of the intracellular carboxy-terminal part of Smo [44] promotes its translocation from intracellular vesicles to plasma membrane. In turn activation of Smo inhibits the proteolytic processing of Gli2 and Gli3, and enhances the production of full-length EXPtranscription-activating forms of these proteins that translocate to the nucleus and activate transcription of target genes [55]. (Figure 2) Gli1 acts in conjunction with Gli2 and Gli3, although the loss of Gli1 alone does not cause Hh signaling defects [56]. Hh target genes include several components of the pathway itself including Gli1, which is considered the earliest response of Hh activation, Gli3 which is regulated by a negative manner [57], Ptch1 and hedgehog interacting protein (Hip). Hip is a trans-membrane glycoprotein that functions as putative antagonist of the pathway binding to Hh proteins with similar affinity to Ptch1 and sequester them in a negative feedback loop [58, 59]. Among the Hh target genes the expression of Gli1 particularly, which is not observed in the absence of Hh, is a very useful marker of Hh signaling activation [60, 61].

5. The Hedgehog Signaling and the Pituitary Gland

5.1. The Role of Hedgehog Signaling in the Development of the Pituitary Gland

During embryogenesis, SHH is expressed in the early oral ectoderm and ventral diencephalon at 8 dpc in the mouse embryo. The pituitary placode, which arises from a patch of oral ectoderm by 9 dpc is negative for SHH expression, reflecting the role of Shh signaling as the molecular boundary that defines the area of the developing pituitary [62, 63]. The PTCH 1 gene is expressed in the Rathke's pouch, demonstrating that these cells can receive Hh signaling. Expression of SHH gene, however, is excluded from the pouch as soon as it becomes morphologically visible, allowing the proliferation of the anterior pituitary cells [62].

SHH null mice display pituitary agenesis, but is not clear whether SHH is directly required for pituitary development, since these mice also have disrupted ventral diencephalon [58]. Expression of SHH in ventral diencephalon is necessary for restriction of pituitary expansion to the middle brain and attenuation of the Shh signaling leads to pituitary enlargement [64]. However, it has been shown that increased expression of HIP under the control of the Pitx1 enhancer, which is active in the oral ectoderm and Rathke's pouch, leads to pituitary agenesis but normal ventral diencephalon [63], indicating a direct role of Hh signaling. On the other hand, overexpression of SHH in the pituitary under the control of aGSU promoter leads to pituitary hyperplasia particularly of the ventral pituitary cell types (gonadotropes and thyrotropes) [63]. It has been shown that SHH regulation of ventral pituitary cell specification and proliferation is mediated at least in part, through bone morphogenetic proteins (BMPs). GLI 2 null embryos have reduced expression of BMP 4 and fibroblast growth factor expression 8 (FGF8), demonstrating the essential role of Gli family of transcription factors in proliferation of early progenitors and induction of transforming factors during embryogenesis [65]. In line with the mouse model, inactivating GLI 2 germline mutations in humans are associated with severe pituitary developmental defects and holoprosencephaly [66].

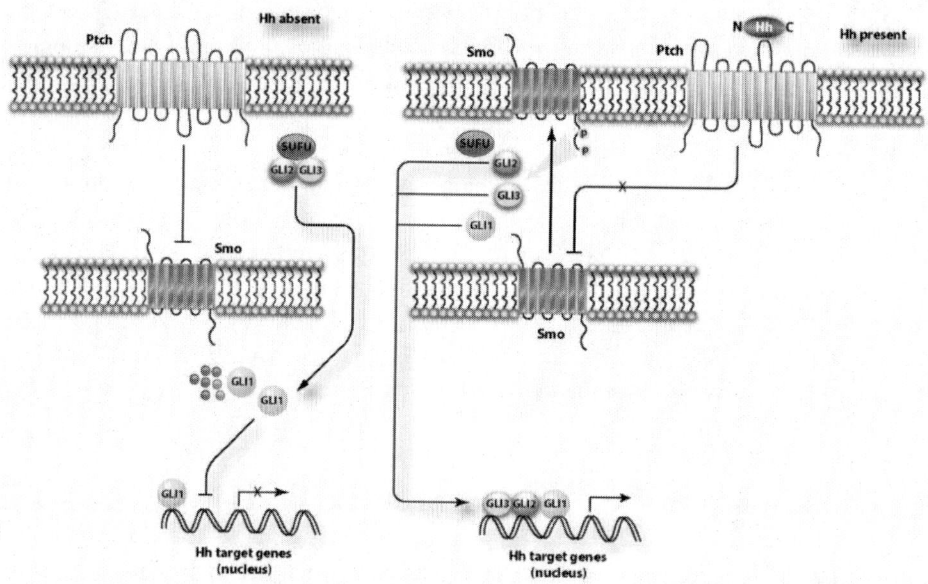

Figure 2. The intracellular cascade of Hedgehog signaling [55].

5.2. The Role of Hedgehog Signaling in the Adult Pituitary and the Pathogenesis of Pituitary Adenomas

Expression of SHH, PTCH2 but not PTCH1, and GLI1 at the level of RNA and protein has been detected in normal anterior pituitary gland in corticotropic cells [67]. Cells that express other pituitary hormones did not show SHH expression. Since GLI1 expression requires activation of Shh signaling, this study demonstrated that Shh/Pth2/Gli1 signaling is active in the corticotropic cells of the adult pituitary [67]. PTCH1 expression was found in thyrotropes and gonadotropes, and PTCH2 was also expressed in somatotropes and in lower percentage in lactotropes [68]. In addition, Shh administration in a rat primary pituitary cell culture and mouse corticotropinoma cell line (AtT20) induced ACTH and pro-opiomelanocortin secretion through a Gli1-dependent transcriptional activity [67]. Co-stimulation of mouse corticotropinoma cells with Shh and CRH showed additive effect on ACTH and POMC secretion. Moreover, Shh increased the expression of CRH receptor, while CRH stimulated Gli1-transcriptional activity, demonstrating a crosstalk between CRH and Shh pathways that converge to Gli-1 transcription factor.

Although Shh was found to be selectively produced by corticotropes, addition of Shh in rat pituitary primary cultures increased secretion of growth hormone (GH) and prolactin (PRL).

In pituitary adenomas PTCH1 and PTCH2 proteins are expressed at variable levels [68]. In conflict with data from normal pituitary, SHH protein is not expressed in corticotropinomas. However, in primary cell cultures established from pituitary adenomas, exogenous Shh increased secretion of GH, PRL and ACTH from somatotropinomas, lactotropinomas and Cushing tumors, respectively [68]. In addition, administration of Shh in pituitary tumor cell lines exerted antiproliferative effects, and thus its significant downregulation in pituitary adenomas could play a pathogenetic role in their development.

Collectively data reported so far are indicative of a functional role of Shh signaling in pituitary tumorigenesis.

6. The Wnt Signaling Pathway and Its Components

Wnt form a family of 19 highly conserved secreted signaling molecules, rich in cysteine, which play an important role in the development and function of multiple tissues. The name derives from the first 2 members of the family: int-1 (mouse) and wingless (Drosophila) [69]. The Wnt1 class (Wnt1 and Wnt3a) activates the canonical Wnt signaling pathway, which involves the formation of a complex between Wnt proteins, Frizzled and LRP5 or LRP6 receptors [70]. These complexes promote the phosphorylation and inactivation of GSK 3b, the inhibition of β-catenin degradation and the subsequent accumulation of β-catenin in the nucleus [71]. The non-canonical Wnt5a class binds to frizzled proteins, activates heterotrimeric G proteins and increases intracellular calcium via protein kinase C-dependent mechanisms or induces Rho- or c-Jun N-terminal kinase (JNK)-dependent changes, mediating the formation of cytoskeleton [72].

6.1. Receptors and Effectors

LRP5/6 receptor family. There are currently at least 13 known members of the LDL receptor family that serve a variety of transport and cell signaling functions in various tissues and cell types [73]. All members of the family are single-pass trans-membrane proteins that contain highly conserved motifs, most notably, all contain copies of a complement-like, cysteine-rich repeat motif (the LDL repeat).

Human low-density lipoprotein (LDL) receptor–related proteins 5 (LRP5) and 6 (LRP6) are unique with respect to other members of the LDL receptor family in that they do not contain the internalization signal sequence for endocytosis.

The extra-cellular portion of LRP5/6 binds several different molecules, principally the Wnt proteins and Wnt antagonists such as DKK and sclerostin, and the co-receptor protein, frizzled (Fz). LRP5/6 functions cooperatively with Fz to stimulate the catenin pathway in response to different Wnt proteins.

The frizzled proteins are seven-trans-membrane serpentine receptors, which consist of an extra-cellular cysteine-rich domain (CRD) that serves as a ligand-binding unit and a seven-trans-membrane signaling portion [74-77]. The extracellular CRD binds Wnt proteins and antagonists of the Wnt signaling. The LRP5/6, co-receptor also binds to the frizzled CRD in a Wnt-dependent manner. Ten members of the frizzled receptors family have been described but little is known about the mechanism of frizzled signaling. Some but not all frizzled proteins stimulate Ca2+ release and protein kinase C (PKC) activity [78].

The key intracellular effector of Wnt signaling is β-catenin a cytoplasmic phosphoprotein, which under resting conditions forms a polyprotein complex with intracellular proteins axin, disheveled (DVL) and adenomatous polyposis coli (APC). Being a part of this complex β-catenin is phosphorylated by specific intracellular kinases glycogen synthase kinase (GSK3b) and casein kinase Ia (CKIa) and is degraded by the proteolytic ubiquitin system.

Upon Wnt activation, β-catenin cannot be phosphorylated, thus it accumulates in the cytoplasm and translocates to the nucleus where it interacts with transcription factors and controls the transcriptional activation of genes [71].

6.2. The Intracellular Cascade

Wnt proteins operate in three different pathways.

6.2.1. The Wnt/β-Catenin or Canonical Pathway

In the absence of Wnt proteins or inhibition of their binding to membrane receptors β-catenin is degraded and the signaling cascade is inactivated. Axin assembles a multi-protein complex with APC, GSK3b and CKIa, permitting GSK3b and CKIa to bind and phosphorylate β-catenin, allowing its degradation by the β-Trcp mediated ubiquitin proteasome pathway [79]. In the nucleus, T cell factor-1 (TCF) and lymphoid enhancing factor-1 (LEF) transcription factors join with transcriptional co-repressor Groucho and histone deacetylases to form a repressive complex and block transcription of Wnt target genes [80]. Activation of Wnt/β-catenin signaling is initiated by binding of Wnt to the seven-trans-membrane domain-spanning frizzled receptor and low-density lipoprotein receptor-related protein 5 and 6 (LRP5/6) co-receptors. DVL, Axin and GSK3b form a ternary complex bridged by Axin that results in the dissociation of GSK3b from Axin. Beta-catenin then accumulates and enters the nucleus where it binds to the TCF/LEF transcription factors, displaces transcriptional co-repressors and recruits transcriptional co-activators, e.g., the histone acetylase p300/CBP and CREB (cAMP response element-binding protein), which act through the remodeling of chromatin surrounding TCF binding sites [81-83]. The formation of the heterodimeric β-catenin-TCF/LEF is crucial for the activation of transcription of target-genes [84]. (Figure 3a)

6.2.2. The Wnt/Ca2+ Pathway

Wnt5a, after binding to receptor frizzled 2, causes the cytosolic G-Protein to break off into its α and β/γ components. The Gα subunit activates phosphodiesterase (PDE), which inhibits cyclic guanosine monophosphate (cGMP) activity in the cell. The Gβ/γ subunits activate phospholipase C (PLC), which in turns hydrolyzes phosphatidylinositol 4,5-bisphosphate (PIP2) into inositol 1,4,5-trisphosphate (IP3) and diacylglycerol (DAG). DAG activates protein kinase C (PKC), while IP3 increases the Ca2+ level in the cell, activating calcineurin and Ca2+-calmodulin-dependent protein kinase II (CamKII). Finally, calcineurin activates the nuclear factor of activated T cells (NFAT), influencing gene expression [84]. (Figure 3b)

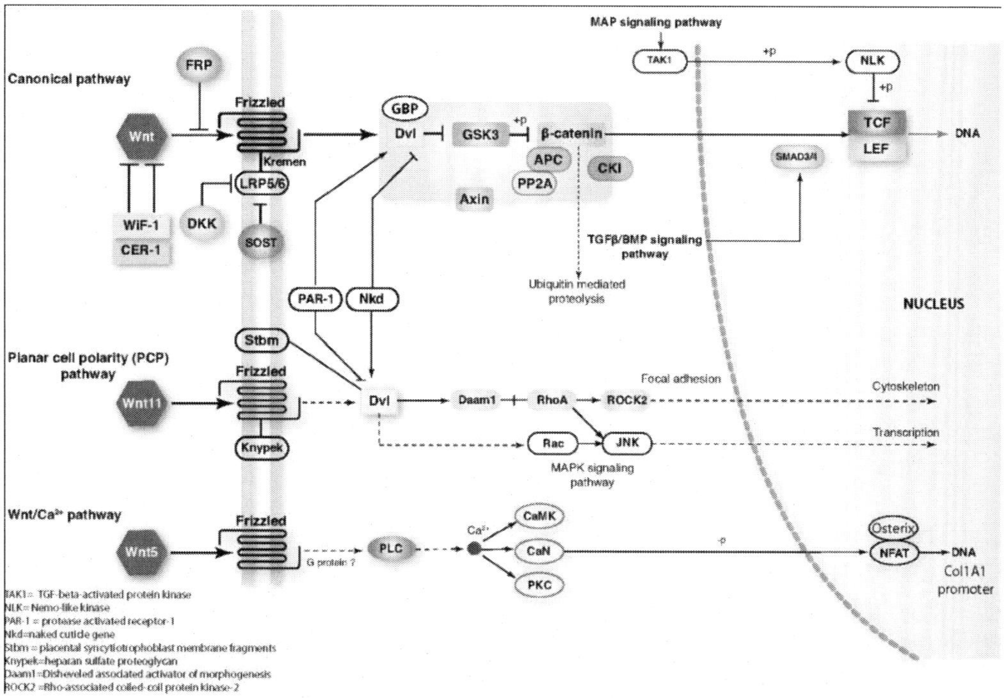

Figure 3. The intracellular cascade of Wntsignaling a) The canonical signaling: Wnt/β-catenin pathway. b) The non-canonical signaling: Wnt/Ca2+ pathway. c) The non-canonical signaling: Planar cell polarity pathway [84].

6.2.3. The Planar Polarity Cell Pathway

In flies, mutant for the frizzled receptor, the normally uniform direction of hair and bristles on the wings and thorax are perturbed, a result of disrupting what is now known as the planar cell polarity (PCP) pathway [85]. This signaling pathway includes frizzled and DVL but not the Axin complex proteins [86]. The non-classical cadherins (a class of trans-membrane proteins that play important roles in cell adhesion and are dependent on calcium ions to function) can apparently modulate frizzled function. Other proteins, including rhoA and rho-kinase act downstream of frizzled and DVL to regulate the cytoskeleton and planar cell polarity. DVL acts in both the PCP pathway and the canonical Wnt signaling pathway [87]. (Figure 3c)

7. THE WNT SIGNALING AND THE PITUITARY GLAND

7.1. The Role of Wnt Signaling in the Development of the Pituitary Gland

Several Wnt proteins have been identified in the developing pituitary [62, 88-90], with Wnt4, expressed in Rathke's pouch and Wnt5a, expressed in the diencephalon [88, 90], capturing most of the attention.

Pituitaries of Wnt4-deficient mice are smaller in size probably due to reduced populations of hormone-expressing cells, such as GH and TSHb, whereas cells expressing POMC were not disturbed [62, 90]. Wnt4 mutant mice also have fewer Pit1-expressing cells, suggesting that there is a general reduction of early precursors of hormone-producing cells. What was interesting in these mice was the intact expression of β-catenin, and intact immune reactivity of TCF 4 and LEF 1 transcription factors in the nucleus of pituitary cells, suggesting a role for non-canonical Wnt pathways [90].

In contrast to Wnt4-deficient mice, Wnt5a-deficient mice develop pituitaries with normal hormone-producing cell types but of altered morphology. The underlying mechanism of this altered morphology is not clear but the researchers proposed that modification of cell to cell adhesion mechanisms it is more likely to be involved [91]. Also in these mice there was no change of β-catenin expression, pointing again towards a role for non-canonical Wnt pathways.

In Rathke's pouch explant studies from e9.5 to 10.5 murine embryos, Wnt5-a was consistently co-expressed with BMP4, and the presence of both induced the development of hormone-producing cells, suggesting that the two signaling pathways may be linked [62, 90].

The generation of the somatotrope, lactotrope and thyrotrope cell lines is dependent on the expression of the transcription factor PIT 1 (also known as Pou1f1) [92]), which is a pituitary-specific transcription factor responsible for pituitary development and hormone expression, as it has been described already above. PIT 1 expression is dependent upon an interaction between PROP 1 and β-catenin. Transgenic mice expressing a mutant β-catenin in pituitary precursors fail to express PIT1 or develop cells expressing GH, TSHb or PRL [89]. This effect, however, is independent of the expression of TCF and LEF transcription factors that are specifically activated by β-catenin.

TCF 4 regulates the recruitment of cells from the ectoderm to Rathke's pouch and the rate of cell proliferation in the developing pituitary. TCF 4-deficient mice develop larger anterior pituitaries that are fully differentiated, demonstrating the intact function of PIT 1 even in the absence of TCF 4 [93].

Thus, despite the critical role of TCF 4 in migration and proliferation of pituitary precursors, the mechanisms responsible for its activation are yet to be clarified [94].

TCF 3 is required in the developing murine forebrain and dorsal aspect of Rathke's pouch.

However, TCF 3 expression is temporally and spatially different from that of PIT1 [89, 94, 95], and therefore the possible effects of TCF 3–PIT 1 interaction remain unproven at present.

In *in vivo* models in which β-catenin was constitutively active in committed PIT 1 lineage cells, development of the differentiated populations was normal [89, 96].

Collectively, results so far show that activation at specific time points of both canonical and non canonical signaling pathways is required for the normal development of the pituitary gland.

7.2. The Role of Wnt Signaling in the Pathogenesis of Pituitary Adenomas

In a mouse model of multiple endocrine neoplasia type 1 (MEN1), wnt proteins (Wnt4, and Wnt9a), and receptors (Fz6 and LRP2) were found significantly down-regulated in all tumors related to this syndrome, tumors from pituitary, pancreas, parathyroids, ovary and testes [97].

In one study, WNT 4 and FZ 6 were over-expressed in human pituitary adenomas, expressing GH, PRL and TSHb, compared with normal pituitary tissue, whereas no difference was noted in ACTH expressing tumors. Interestingly, the researchers did not find any difference in β-catenin distribution, in phosphorylation of CaMK-II, an indicator of calcium signaling, or the c-jun expression, a target of the planar cell polarity pathway.

Thus, the underlying mechanism by which WNT 4 is implicated in the development of some pituitary adenomas remains unknown [98].

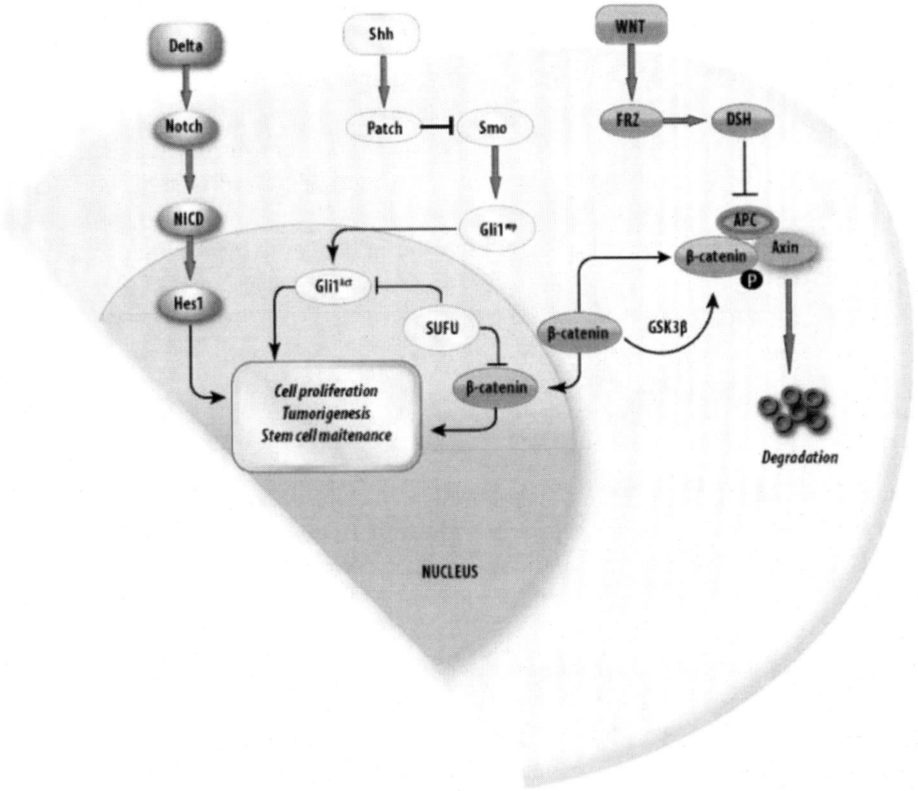

Figure 4. An integrative diagram of Notch, Hedgehog and Wnt signaling crosstalk in the regulation of normal development and tumorigenesis [55].

Studies investigating specifically β-catenin expression in human pituitary adenomas demonstrated inconsistent results. In one study, nuclear accumulation of β-catenin was found in 57% of pituitary tumors. This expression was higher in tumors originated from cells of the PIT 1 lineage [99], but there was no comparison with healthy pituitary tissue, and thus results were not conclusive. In another one, β-catenin expression was not different between pituitary adenomas but the researchers found increased immunostaining for the Wnt target genes cyclin D1 and c-Myc [100]. Used as markers, expression of these genes demonstrated some correlation with the size of the pituitary adenoma, cyclin D1 was associated with a later age of presentation, whereas c-Myc was seen in younger patients [100].

In an *in vitro* study, the aT3-1 gonadotrope tumor cell line was transfected with a dominant-negative PITX 2 and PITX 2 siRNA, which actually resulted in increased apoptosis and significant reduction of cell viability. This effect was replicated in primary cultures from five out of seven human gonadotrope adenomas. Given that PITX 2 is under the control of β-catenin, canonical signaling may be implicated in the pathogenesis of these tumors [101].

Wnt inhibitors were also studied in human pituitary adenomas. Wnt inhibitory factor-1 (WIF 1) is a secreted protein that binds to Wnt proteins and inhibits their activities. This protein has been shown to be significantly down-regulated on a microarray analysis in a series of both functioning and non-functioning pituitary adenomas when compared with healthy pituitary tissue. This finding was associated with the methylation of the CpG island on the promoter of WIF 1, demonstrating the potential epigenetic regulation of Wnt signaling. No changes in β-catenin distribution were observed in this study [102].

In vitro experiments with the GH3 pituitary cell line confirmed reduced expression of WIF-1 in these cells, and when the cells were transfected with WIF 1 there was a significant reduced proliferation.

Collectively, recent studies *in vitro, in vivo* and in human tissue, point to a potential role of Wnt signaling in pituitary oncogenesis, but further work is warranted in order to elucidate the exact molecular mechanisms involved [100].

Conclusion

During embryonic development, the question remains as to how Notch, Wnt and Hh signaling integrate their activity with other cell inputs to control specific developmental events (Figure 4). Another important issue is the mechanisms by which these signaling molecules activate distinct target genes according to cell type and time. Genomic studies will undoubtedly increase the number of target genes and allow development of a systematic approach for understanding these different responses in the future.

Impaired signaling activity of these pathways is implicated in the pathogenesis of cancer and disease, but it remains to be determined whether modulation of such pleiotropic and cross-talking pathways could be a promising target for therapeutic approach.

Notch 3 and Jagged 1 have been implicated in the pathogenesis of human non-functioning pituitary adenomas providing a potential therapeutic target for the medical treatment of these tumors. Several elements of the Notch pathways have also been identified in the transcriptome of prolactinomas and multihormonal pituitary adenomas [103].

Hedgehog signaling exerts differential effects on pituitary cell growth (with stimulating effects on progenitor cells and inhibiting effects in differentiated cells) and is able to modulate hormone secretion and proliferation in pituitary adenomas. Moreover exogenous treatment with Hh proteins in cell cultures has been shown to increase hormone secretion from pituitary tumor cells, reflecting their role as hypophysiotropic factors that regulate pituitary hormone release in normal and tissue cells.

There is accumulating evidence that Wnt signaling plays a significant role in pituitary morphogenesis and tumorigenesis [104]. Beta-catenin appears to exert a differential role in embryonic and mature cells, and most *ex vivo* studies of pituitary tumors fail to identify activation of canonical signaling, suggesting a role for non-canonical pathways in the adult pituitary.

Taken together Hedgehog, Notch and Wnt signaling pathways cross-talk appear to exert significant roles in pituitary development and tumorigenesis establishing novel targets for therapeutic interventions. So far, however, experimental work has focused on mouse models, and therefore transfer of these results in humans needs further investigation.

Ongoing research will definitely increase our understanding on the role of these pathways in the development of pituitary adenomas and pave the way for their potential therapeutic targeting in humans.

REFERENCES

[1] Ezzat, S, Asa, SL, Couldwell, WT, Barr, CE, Dodge WE, Vance ML, McCutcheon IE. The prevalence of pituitary adenomas: a systematic review. *Cancer*, 2004;101:613-619.

[2] Ezzat, S, Asa, SL. Mechanisms of disease: The pathogenesis of pituitary tumors. *Nat Clin Pract Endocrinol Metab*, 2006;2:220-230.

[3] Lewis, J. Notch signalling and the control of cell fate choices in vertebrates. *Semin Cell Dev Biol*, 1998;9:583-589.

[4] Bray, S. Notch signalling in Drosophila: three ways to use a pathway. *Semin Cell Dev Biol*, 1998;9:591-597.

[5] Schweisguth, F. Regulation of notch signaling activity. *Curr Biol*, 2004, 14, R129-138.

[6] Ehebauer, M, Hayward, P, Martinez-Arias, A. Notch Signaling Pathway. *Sci STKE*, 2006;364:cm7-cm7.

[7] Ehebauer, M, Hayward, P, Arias, AM. Notch, a universal arbiter of cell fate decisions. *2 Science.*, 2006;314:1414-1415.

[8] Dahmann, C, Oates, AC, Brand, M. Boundary formation and maintenance in tissue development. *Nat Rev Genet*, 2011;12:43-55.

[9] Tossell, K, Kiecker, C, Wizenmann, A, Lang, E, Irving, C. Notch signalling stabilises boundary formation at the midbrain-hindbrain organiser. *Development*, 2011;138:3745-3757.

[10] Yavropoulou, MP, Yovos, JG. The role of Notch signaling in bone development and disease. *Hormones* (*Athens*), 2014;13:24-37.

[11] Wendorff, AA, Koch, U, Wunderlich, FT, Wirth, S, Dubey, C, Bruning, JC, MacDonald, HR, Radtke, F. Hes1 is a critical but context-dependent mediator of canonical Notch signaling in lymphocyte development and transformation. *Immunity*, 2010;33: 671-684.

[12] Sparrow, DB, Guillen-Navarro, E, Fatkin, D, Dunwoodie, SL. Mutation of Hairy-and-Enhancer-of-Split-7 in humans causes spondylocostal dysostosis. *Hum Mol Genet*, 2008, 17:3761-3766.

[13] Takebe, N, Nguyen, D, Yang, SX. Targeting notch signaling pathway in cancer: clinical development advances and challenges. *Pharmacol Ther*, 2014, 141:140-149.

[14] Azizidoost, S, Shanaki Bavarsad, M, Shanaki Bavarsad, M, Shahrabi, S, Jaseb, K, Rahim, F, Shahjahani, M, Saba, F, Ghorbani, M, Saki, N. The role of notch signaling in bone marrow niche. *Hematology*, 2014;DOI:10.1179/1607845414Y.0000000167.

[15] Zhou, Y, Atkins, JB, Rompani, SB, Bancescu, DL, Petersen, PH, Tang, H, Zou, K, Stewart, SB, Zhong, W. The mammalian Golgi regulates numb signaling in asymmetric cell division by releasing ACBD3 during mitosis. *Cell*, 2007;129:163-178.

[16] Watkins-Chow, DE, Camper, SA. How many homeobox genes does it take to make a pituitary gland? *Trends Genet*, 1998;14:284-290.

[17] Raetzman, LT, Ross, SA, Cook, S, Dunwoodie, SL, Camper, SA, Thomas, PQ. Developmental regulation of Notch signaling genes in the embryonic pituitary: Prop1 deficiency affects Notch2 expression. *Dev Biol*, 2004;265:329-340.

[18] Zhu, X, Zhang, J, Tollkuhn, J, Ohsawa, R, Bresnick, EH, Guillemot, F, Kageyama, R, Rosenfeld, MG. Sustained Notch signaling in progenitors is required for sequential emergence of distinct cell lineages during organogenesis. *Genes Dev*, 2006;20:2739-2753.

[19] Raetzman, LT, Wheeler, BS, Ross, SA, Thomas, PQ, Camper, SA. Persistent expression of Notch2 delays gonadotrope differentiation. *Mol Endocrinol*, 2006;20:2898-2908.

[20] Rainbow, LA, Rees, SA, Shaikh, MG, Shaw, NJ, Cole, T, Barrett, TG, Kirk, JM. Mutation analysis of POUF-1, PROP-1 and HESX-1 show low frequency of mutations in children with sporadic forms of combined pituitary hormone deficiency and septo-optic dysplasia. *Clin Endocrinol* (Oxf), 2005;62:163-168.

[21] Osorio, MG, Kopp, P, Marui, S, Latronico, AC, Mendonca, BB, Arnhold, IJ. Combined pituitary hormone deficiency caused by a novel mutation of a highly conserved residue (F88S) in the homeodomain of PROP-1. *J Clin Endocrinol Metab*, 2000;85:2779-2785.

[22] Raetzman, LT, Wheeler, BS, Ross, SA, Thomas, PQ, Camper, SA. Persistent expression of Notch2 delays gonadotrope differentiation. *Mol Endocrinol*, 2006;20:2898-2908.

[23] Chen, J, Crabbe, A, Van Duppen, V, Vankelecom, H. The notch signaling system is present in the postnatal pituitary: marked expression and regulatory activity in the newly discovered side population. *Mol Endocrinol*, 2006, 20:3293-3307.

[24] Kita, A, Imayoshi, I, Hojo, M, Kitagawa, M, Kokubu, H, Ohsawa, R, Ohtsuka, T, Kageyama, R, Hashimoto, N. Hes1 and Hes5 control the progenitor pool, intermediate lobe specification, and posterior lobe formation in the pituitary development. *Mol Endocrinol*, 2007;21:1458-1466.

[25] Raetzman, LT, Cai, JX, Camper, SA. Hes1 is required for pituitary growth and melanotrope specification *Dev Biol*, 2007;304:455-466.

[26] Konishi, J, Yi, F, Chen, X, Vo, H, Carbone, DP, Dang, TP. Notch3 cooperates with the EGFR pathway to modulate apoptosis through the induction of bim. *Oncogene*, 2010;29:589-596.

[27] Haruki, N, Kawaguchi, KS, Eichenberger, S, Massion, PP, Olson, S, Gonzalez, A, Carbone, DP, Dang, TP. Dominant-negative Notch3 receptor inhibits mitogen-activated protein kinase pathway and the growth of human lung cancers. *Cancer Res*, 2005;65:3555-3561.

[28] Masiero, M, Minuzzo, S, Pusceddu, I, Moserle, L, Persano, L, Agnusdei, V, Tosello, V, Basso, G, Amadori, A, Indraccolo, S. Notch3-mediated regulation of MKP-1 levels

promotes survival of T acute lymphoblastic leukemia cells. *Leukemia*, 2011;25:588-598.

[29] Chen, X, Stoeck, A, Lee, SJ, Shih Ie, M, Wang, MM, Wang, TL. Jagged1 expression regulated by Notch3 and Wnt/beta-catenin signaling pathways in ovarian cancer. *Oncotarget*, 2010;1:210-218.

[30] Rodilla, V, Villanueva, A, Obrador-Hevia, A, Robert-Moreno, A, Fernandez-Majada, V, Grilli, A, Lopez-Bigas, N, Bellora, N, Alba, MM, Torres, F, Dunach, M, Sanjuan, X, Gonzalez, S, Gridley, T, Capella, G, Bigas, A, Espinosa, L. Jagged1 is the pathological link between Wnt and Notch pathways in colorectal cancer. *Proc Natl Acad Sci U S A*, 2009;106:6315-6320.

[31] Jundt, F, Probsting, KS, Anagnostopoulos, I, Muehlinghaus, G, Chatterjee, M, Mathas, S, Bargou, RC, Manz, R, Stein, H, Dorken, B. Jagged1-induced Notch signaling drives proliferation of multiple myeloma cells. *Blood*, 2004;103:3511-3515.

[32] Choi, JH, Park, JT, Davidson, B, Morin, PJ, Shih IE, M, Wang, TL. Jagged-1 and Notch3 juxtacrine loop regulates ovarian tumor growth and adhesion. *Cancer Res*, 2008;68:5716-5723.

[33] Zeng, Q, Li, S, Chepeha, DB, Giordano, TJ, Li, J, Zhang, H, Polverini, PJ, Nor, J, Kitajewski, J, Wang, CY. Crosstalk between tumor and endothelial cells promotes tumor angiogenesis by MAPK activation of Notch signaling. *Cancer Cell*, 2005;8:13-23.

[34] Lu, R, Gao, H, Wang, H, Cao, L, Bai, J, Zhang, Y. Overexpression of the Notch3 receptor and its ligand Jagged1 in human clinically non-functioning pituitary adenomas. *Oncol Lett*, 2013;5:845-851.

[35] Evans, CO, Moreno, CS, Zhan, X, McCabe, MT, Vertino, PM, Desiderio, DM, Oyesiku, NM. Molecular pathogenesis of human prolactinomas identified by gene expression profiling, RT-qPCR, and proteomic analyses. *Pituitary*, 2008;11:231-245.

[36] Moreno, CS, Evans, CO, Zhan, X, Okor, M, Desiderio, DM, Oyesiku, NM. Novel molecular signaling and classification of human clinically nonfunctional pituitary adenomas identified by gene expression profiling and proteomic analyses. *Cancer Res*, 2005;65:10214-10222.

[37] Desiderio, DM, Zhan, X. The human pituitary proteome: the characterization of differentially expressed proteins in an adenoma compared to a control. *Cell Mol Biol (Noisy-le-grand)*, 2003;49:689-712.

[38] Zhu, X, Zhang, J, Tollkuhn, J, Ohsawa, R, Bresnick, EH, Guillemot, F, Kageyama, R, Rosenfeld, MG. Sustained Notch signaling in progenitors is required for sequential emergence of distinct cell lineages during organogenesis. *Genes Dev*, 2006;20:2739-2753.

[39] Jordan, S, Lidhar, K, Korbonits, M, Lowe, DG, Grossman, AB. Cyclin D and cyclin E expression in normal and adenomatous pituitary. *Eur J Endocrinol*, 2000;143:R1-6.

[40] Tammam, J, Ware, C, Efferson, C, O'Neil, J, Rao, S, Qu, X, Gorenstein, J, Angagaw, M, Kim, H, Kenific, C, Kunii, K, Leach, KJ, Nikov, G, Zhao, J, Dai, X, Hardwick, J, Scott, M, Winter, C, Bristow, L, Elbi, C, Reilly, JF, Look, T, Draetta, G, Van der Ploeg, L, Kohl, NE, Strack, PR, Majumder, PK. Down-regulation of the Notch pathway mediated by a gamma-secretase inhibitor induces anti-tumour effects in mouse models of T-cell leukaemia. *Br J Pharmacol*, 2009;158:1183-1195.

[41] Kondratyev, M, Kreso, A, Hallett, RM, Girgis-Gabardo, A, Barcelon, ME, Ilieva, D, Ware, C, Majumder, PK, Hassell, JA. Gamma-secretase inhibitors target tumor-initiating cells in a mouse model of ERBB2 breast cancer. *Oncogene*, 2012;31:93-103.

[42] Ramakrishnan, V, Ansell, S, Haug, J, Grote, D, Kimlinger, T, Stenson, M, Timm, M, Wellik, L, Halling, T, Rajkumar, SV, Kumar, S. MRK003, a gamma-secretase inhibitor exhibits promising *in vitro* pre-clinical activity in multiple myeloma and non-Hodgkin's lymphoma. *Leukemia*, 2012;26:340-348.

[43] Pepinsky, RB, Zeng, C, Wen, D, Rayhorn, P, Baker, DP, Williams, KP, Bixler, SA, Ambrose, CM, Garber, EA, Miatkowski, K, Taylor, FR, Wang, EA, Galdes, A. Identification of a palmitic acid-modified form of human Sonic hedgehog. *J Biol Chem*, 1998;273:14037-14045.

[44] Chen, MH, Li, YJ, Kawakami, T, Xu, SM, Chuang, PT. Palmitoylation is required for the production of a soluble multimeric Hedgehog protein complex and long-range signaling in vertebrates. *Genes Dev*, 2004;18:641-659.

[45] Goetz, JA, Singh, S, Suber, LM, Kull, FJ, Robbins, DJ. A highly conserved amino-terminal region of sonic hedgehog is required for the formation of its freely diffusible multimeric form. *J Biol Chem*, 2006;281:4087-4093.

[46] Denef, N, Neubuser, D, Perez, L, Cohen, SM. Hedgehog induces opposite changes in turnover and subcellular localization of patched and smoothened. *Cell*, 2000;102:521-531.

[47] Karpen, HE, Bukowski, JT, Hughes, T, Gratton, JP, Sessa, WC, Gailani, MR. The sonic hedgehog receptor patched associates with caveolin-1 in cholesterol-rich microdomains of the plasma membrane. *J Biol Chem*, 2001;276, 19503-19511.

[48] Martin, V, Carrillo, G, Torroja, C, Guerrero, I. The sterol-sensing domain of Patched protein seems to control Smoothened activity through Patched vesicular trafficking. *Curr Biol*, 2001;11:601-607.

[49] Gailani, MR, Stahle-Backdahl, M, Leffell, DJ, Glynn, M, Zaphiropoulos, PG, Pressman, C, Unden, AB, Dean, M, Brash, DE, Bale, AE, Toftgard, R. The role of the human homologue of Drosophila patched in sporadic basal cell carcinomas. *Nat Genet*, 1996;14:78-81.

[50] Xie, J, Murone, M, Luoh, SM, Ryan, A, Gu, Q, Zhang, C, Bonifas, JM, Lam, CW, Hynes, M, Goddard, A, Rosenthal, A, Epstein, EH, Jr. de Sauvage, FJ. Activating Smoothened mutations in sporadic basal-cell carcinoma. *Nature*, 1998;391:90-92.

[51] King, PJ, Guasti, L, Laufer, E. Hedgehog signalling in endocrine development and disease. *J Endocrinol*, 2008;198:439-450.

[52] Wang, B, Li, Y. Evidence for the direct involvement of TrCP in Gli3 protein processing. *Proc Natl Acad Sci U S A*, 2006;103:33-38.

[53] Tempe, D, Casas, M, Karaz, S, Blanchet-Tournier, MF, Concordet, JP. Multisite protein kinase A and glycogen synthase kinase 3beta phosphorylation leads to Gli3 ubiquitination by SCFbetaTrCP. *Mol Cell Biol*, 2006;26:4316-4326.

[54] Sheng, T, Chi, S, Zhang, X, Xie, J. Regulation of Gli1 localization by the cAMP/protein kinase A signaling axis through a site near the nuclear localization signal. *J Biol Chem*, 2006;281:9-12.

[55] Yavropoulou, MP, Maladaki, A, Yovos, JG. The role of Notch and Hedgehog signaling pathways in pituitary development and pathogenesis of pituitary adenomas. *Hormones (Athens)*, 2015;14:5-18.

[56] Bai, CB, Stephen, D, Joyner, AL. All mouse ventral spinal cord patterning by hedgehog is Gli dependent and involves an activator function of Gli3. *Dev Cell*, 2004;6:103-115.

[57] Marigo, V, Johnson, RL, Vortkamp, A, Tabin, CJ. Sonic hedgehog differentially regulates expression of GLI and GLI3 during limb development. *Dev Biol*, 1996;180:273-283.

[58] Chuang, PT, McMahon, AP. Vertebrate Hedgehog signalling modulated by induction of a Hedgehog-binding protein. *Nature*, 1999;397:617-621.

[59] Bak, M, Hansen, C, Friis Henriksen, K, Tommerup, N. The human hedgehog-interacting protein gene: structure and chromosome mapping to 4q31.21-->q31.3. *Cytogenet Cell Genet*, 2001;92:300-303.

[60] Ahn, S, Joyner, AL. Dynamic changes in the response of cells to positive hedgehog signaling during mouse limb patterning. *Cell*, 2004;118:505-516.

[61] Vokes, SA, Ji, H, McCuine, S, Tenzen, T, Giles, S, Zhong, S, Longabaugh, WJ, Davidson, EH, Wong, WH, McMahon, AP. Genomic characterization of Gli-activator targets in sonic hedgehog-mediated neural patterning. *Development*, 2007;134:1977-1989.

[62] Treier, M, Gleiberman, AS, O'Connell, SM, Szeto, DP, McMahon, JA, McMahon, AP, Rosenfeld, MG. Multistep signaling requirements for pituitary organogenesis *in vivo*. *Genes Dev*, 1998;12:1691-1704.

[63] Treier, M, O'Connell, S, Gleiberman, A, Price, J, Szeto, DP, Burgess, R, Chuang, PT, McMahon, AP, Rosenfeld, MG. Hedgehog signaling is required for pituitary gland development. *Development*, 2001;128:377-386.

[64] Zhao, L, Zevallos, SE, Rizzoti, K, Jeong, Y, Lovell-Badge, R, Epstein, DJ. Disruption of SoxB1-dependent Sonic hedgehog expression in the hypothalamus causes septo-optic dysplasia. *Dev Cell*, 2012;22:585-596.

[65] Wang, Y, Martin, JF, Bai, CB. Direct and indirect requirements of Shh/Gli signaling in early pituitary development. *Dev Biol*, 2010;348:199-209.

[66] Roessler, E, Du, YZ, Mullor, JL, Casas, E, Allen, WP, Gillessen-Kaesbach, G, Roeder, ER, Ming, JE, Ruiz i Altaba, A, Muenke, M. Loss-of-function mutations in the human GLI2 gene are associated with pituitary anomalies and holoprosencephaly-like features. *Proc Natl Acad Sci U S A*, 2003;100:13424-13429.

[67] Vila, G, Papazoglou, M, Stalla, J, Theodoropoulou, M, Stalla, GK, Holsboer, F, Paez-Pereda, M. Sonic hedgehog regulates CRH signal transduction in the adult pituitary. *FASEB J*, 2005;19:281-283.

[68] Vila, G, Theodoropoulou, M, Stalla, J, Tonn, JC, Losa, M, Renner, U, Stalla, GK, Paez-Pereda, M. Expression and function of sonic hedgehog pathway components in pituitary adenomas: evidence for a direct role in hormone secretion and cell proliferation. *J Clin Endocrinol Metab*, 2005;90:6687-6694.

[69] Dierick, H, Bejsovec, A. Cellular mechanisms of wingless/Wnt signal transduction. *Curr Top Dev Biol*, 1999;43:153-190.

[70] Tamai, K, Semenov, M, Kato, Y, Spokony, R, Liu, C, Katsuyama, Y, Hess, F, Saint-Jeannet, JP, He, X. LDL-receptor-related proteins in Wnt signal transduction. *Nature*, 2000;407:530-535.

[71] Liu, C, Li, Y, Semenov, M, Han, C, Baeg, GH, Tan, Y, Zhang, Z, Lin, X, He, X. Control of beta-catenin phosphorylation/degradation by a dual-kinase mechanism. *Cell*, 2002;108:837-847.

[72] Veeman, MT, Axelrod, JD, Moon, RT. A second canon. Functions and mechanisms of beta-catenin-independent Wnt signaling. *Dev Cell*, 2003;5:367-377.

[73] Kanazawa, A, Tsukada, S, Sekine, A, Tsunoda, T, Takahashi, A, Kashiwagi, A, Tanaka, Y, Babazono, T, Matsuda, M, Kaku, K, Iwamoto, Y, Kawamori, R, Kikkawa, R, Nakamura, Y, Maeda, S. Association of the gene encoding wingless-type mammary tumor virus integration-site family member 5B (WNT5B) with type 2 diabetes. *Am J Hum Genet*, 2004;75:832-843.

[74] Schweizer, L, Varmus, H. Wnt/Wingless signaling through beta-catenin requires the function of both LRP/Arrow and frizzled classes of receptors. *BMC Cell Biol*, 2003;4:4.

[75] Bhanot, P, Brink, M, Samos, CH, Hsieh, JC, Wang, Y, Macke, JP, Andrew, D, Nathans, J, Nusse, R. A new member of the frizzled family from Drosophila functions as a Wingless receptor. *Nature*, 1996;382:225-230.

[76] Moon, RT, Brown, JD, Yang-Snyder, JA, Miller, JR. Structurally related receptors and antagonists compete for secreted Wnt ligands. *Cell*, 1997;88:725-728.

[77] Hsieh, JC, Rattner, A, Smallwood, PM, Nathans, J. Biochemical characterization of Wnt-frizzled interactions using a soluble, biologically active vertebrate Wnt protein. *Proc Natl Acad Sci U S A*, 1999;96:3546-3551.

[78] Dann, CE, Hsieh, JC, Rattner, A, Sharma, D, Nathans, J, Leahy, DJ. Insights into Wnt binding and signalling from the structures of two Frizzled cysteine-rich domains. *Nature*, 2001;412:86-90.

[79] Gordon, MD, Nusse, R. Wnt signaling: multiple pathways, multiple receptors, and multiple transcription factors. *J Biol Chem*, 2006;281:22429-22433.

[80] Chen, G, Fernandez, J, Mische, S, Courey, AJ. A functional interaction between the histone deacetylase Rpd3 and the corepressor groucho in Drosophila development. *Genes Dev*, 1999;13:2218-2230.

[81] Hecht, A, Vleminckx, K, Stemmler, MP, van Roy, F, Kemler, R. The p300/CBP acetyltransferases function as transcriptional coactivators of beta-catenin in vertebrates. *EMBO J*, 2000;19:1839-1850.

[82] Levy, L, Wei, Y, Labalette, C, Wu, Y, Renard, CA, Buendia, MA, Neuveut, C. Acetylation of beta-catenin by p300 regulates beta-catenin-Tcf4 interaction. *Mol Cell Biol*, 2004;24:3404-3414.

[83] Takemaru, KI, Moon, RT. The transcriptional coactivator CBP interacts with beta-catenin to activate gene expression. *J Cell Biol*, 2000;149:249-254.

[84] Yavropoulou, MP, Yovos, JG. The role of the Wnt signaling pathway in osteoblast commitment and differentiation. *Hormones (Athens)*, 2007;6:279-294.

[85] Strutt, D. Frizzled signalling and cell polarisation in Drosophila and vertebrates. *Development*, 2003;130:4501-4513.

[86] Penton, A, Wodarz, A, Nusse, R. A mutational analysis of dishevelled in Drosophila defines novel domains in the dishevelled protein as well as novel suppressing alleles of axin. *Genetics*, 2002;161:747-762.

[87] Axelrod, JD, Miller, JR, Shulman, JM, Moon, RT, Perrimon, N. Differential recruitment of Dishevelled provides signaling specificity in the planar cell polarity and Wingless signaling pathways. *Genes Dev*, 1998;12:2610-2622.

[88] Rosenfeld, MG, Briata, P, Dasen, J, Gleiberman, AS, Kioussi, C, Lin, C, O'Connell, SM, Ryan, A, Szeto, DP, Treier, M. Multistep signaling and transcriptional

requirements for pituitary organogenesis *in vivo*. *Recent Prog Horm Res*, 2000;55:1-13, discussion 13-14.

[89] Olson, LE, Tollkuhn, J, Scafoglio, C, Krones, A, Zhang, J, Ohgi, KA, Wu, W, Taketo, MM, Kemler, R, Grosschedl, R, Rose, D, Li, X, Rosenfeld, MG. Homeodomain-mediated beta-catenin-dependent switching events dictate cell-lineage determination. *Cell*, 2006;125:593-605.

[90] Potok, MA, Cha, KB, Hunt, A, Brinkmeier, ML, Leitges, M, Kispert, A, Camper, SA. WNT signaling affects gene expression in the ventral diencephalon and pituitary gland growth. *Dev Dyn*, 2008;237:1006-1020.

[91] Cha, KB, Douglas, KR, Potok, MA, Liang, H, Jones, SN, Camper, SA. WNT5A signaling affects pituitary gland shape. *Mech Dev*, 2004;121:183-194.

[92] Li, S, Crenshaw, EB, 3rd, Rawson, EJ, Simmons, DM, Swanson, LW, Rosenfeld, MG. Dwarf locus mutants lacking three pituitary cell types result from mutations in the POU-domain gene pit-1. *Nature*, 1990;347:528-533.

[93] Brinkmeier, ML, Potok, MA, Cha, KB, Gridley, T, Stifani, S, Meeldijk, J, Clevers, H, Camper, SA. TCF and Groucho-related genes influence pituitary growth and development. *Mol Endocrinol*, 2003;17:2152-2161.

[94] Brinkmeier, ML, Potok, MA, Davis, SW, Camper, SA. TCF4 deficiency expands ventral diencephalon signaling and increases induction of pituitary progenitors. *Dev Biol*, 2007;311:396-407.

[95] Andoniadou, CL, Signore, M, Young, RM, Gaston-Massuet, C, Wilson, SW, Fuchs, E, Martinez-Barbera, JP. HESX1- and TCF3-mediated repression of Wnt/beta-catenin targets is required for normal development of the anterior forebrain. *Development*, 2011;138:4931-4942.

[96] Gaston-Massuet, C, Andoniadou, CL, Signore, M, Jayakody, SA, Charolidi, N, Kyeyune, R, Vernay, B, Jacques, TS, Taketo, MM, Le Tissier, P, Dattani, MT, Martinez-Barbera, JP. Increased Wingless (Wnt) signaling in pituitary progenitor/stem cells gives rise to pituitary tumors in mice and humans. *Proc Natl Acad Sci U S A*, 2011;108:11482-11487.

[97] Mould, AW, Duncan, R, Serewko-Auret, M, Loffler, KA, Biondi, C, Gartside, M, Kay, GF, Hayward, NK. Global expression profiling of sex cord stromal tumors from Men1 heterozygous mice identifies altered TGF-beta signaling, decreased Gata6 and increased Csf1r expression. *Int J Cancer*, 2009;124:1122-1132.

[98] Miyakoshi, T, Kajiya, H, Miyajima, K, Takei, M, Tobita, M, Takekoshi, S, Osamura, RY. The expression of Wnt4 is regulated by estrogen via an estrogen receptor alpha-dependent pathway in rat pituitary growth hormone-producing cells. *Acta Histochem Cytochem*, 2009;42:205-213.

[99] Semba, S, Han, SY, Ikeda, H, Horii, A. Frequent nuclear accumulation of beta-catenin in pituitary adenoma. *Cancer*, 2001;91:42-48.

[100] Formosa, R, Gruppetta, M, Falzon, S, Santillo, G, DeGaetano, J, Xuereb-Anastasi, A, Vassallo, J. Expression and clinical significance of Wnt players and survivin in pituitary tumours. *Endocr Pathol*, 2012;23:123-131.

[101] Acunzo, J, Roche, C, Defilles, C, Thirion, S, Quentien, MH, Figarella-Branger, D, Graillon, T, Dufour, H, Brue, T, Pellegrini, I, Enjalbert, A, Barlier, A. Inactivation of PITX2 transcription factor induced apoptosis of gonadotroph tumoral cells. *Endocrinology*, 2011;152:3884-3892.

[102] Elston, MS, Gill, AJ, Conaglen, JV, Clarkson, A, Shaw, JM, Law, AJ, Cook, RJ, Little, NS, Clifton-Bligh, RJ, Robinson, BG, McDonald, KL. Wnt pathway inhibitors are strongly down-regulated in pituitary tumors. *Endocrinology*, 2008;149:1235-1242.
[103] Jiang, Z, Gui, S, Zhang, Y. Analysis of differential gene expression in plurihormonal pituitary adenomas using bead-based fiber-optic arrays. *J Neurooncol*, 2012;108:341-348.
[104] Chambers, TJ, Giles, A, Brabant, G, Davis, JR. Wnt signalling in pituitary development and tumorigenesis. *Endocr Relat Cancer*, 2013;20:R101-111.

In: Pituitary Adenoma
Editor: Dimitrios N. Kanakis

ISBN: 978-1-63484-985-2

Chapter 4

CLINICAL SYMPTOMATOLOGY OF PITUITARY ADENOMAS: FROM A NEUROPSYCHIATRIC POINT OF VIEW

Magda Tsolaki**, *MD, PhD
Professor of Neuropsychiatry, 3rd Department of Neurology,
School of Health Sciences, Medical Faculty,
Aristotle University of Thessaloniki, Thessaloniki, Greece

ABSTRACT

Pituitary adenomas have been associated with multiple co-morbidities, including neuropsychiatric disorders. The overall perceived prevalence and severity of *cognitive dysfunction* were the highest among Non-Functional Pituitary Adenomas (NFPA) groups, particularly in the areas of mental agility, verbal recall, and memory recall. The main psychiatric symptom of hypopituitarism is a combination of dementia and delirium. However, the most common neurologic symptoms are *headaches* and *visual changes.* Thirty-three to seventy-two percent of pituitary adenomas, independently of their dimensions, induce headache. Non-functional pituitary adenomas tend to affect *visual acuity* more than adenomas with other pathological diagnoses, which produce either adrenocorticotropic hormone or prolactin. Visual *Field defects* occurred in 95% of patients with non-functioning pituitary macroadenoma. The above neurologic symptoms are more common in nonfunctioning adenomas but also in gonadotroph adenomas because these tumors do not secrete sufficient hormones to cause endocrine-type symptoms. ACTH-secreting adenomas causing Cushing Disease cause significant morbidity. *Carpal tunnel syndrome, obstructive sleeping apnea* and *headache* are typical neurological features in somatotroph adenomas.

Pain appears to be a frequent problem in pituitary disease. The data suggest that pain should be integrated in the diagnostic and therapeutic work-up of patients with pituitary disease in order to treat them appropriately and improve their Quality of Life (QoL).

Meningitis is an unusual complication of untreated invasive pituitary adenomas and represents the initial symptom leading to diagnosis of a macroadenoma in exceptional

* Corresponding author: Magda Tsolaki, MD, PhD, Despere Str. 3, 54621 Thessaloniki, Greece, E-mail: tsolakim1@gmail.com.

cases. If the adenoma expands laterally into the cavernous sinus, it has the potential to affect the cranial nerves housed there, including cranial nerves III (oculomotor), IV (trochlear), VI (abducens), thus causing *diplopia*. Other neurologic presentations, such as *cerebrospinal fluid rhinorrhea, seizures, and pituitary apoplexy,* can occur but are uncommon. Other uncommon symptoms are *hoarse voice, acute respiratory distress* due to unilateral larynx paralysis and *myopathy*.

Prolactin-secreting pituitary adenomas (PRL-omas) are well-differentiated endocrine tumors expressing D2 dopamine receptor (DRD2). DRD2 polymorphisms correlate with psychiatric disorders, in particular *alcoholism* and *schizophrenia.* Compared with healthy controls, acromegalic patients described themselves as distinctly more *harm avoidant and neurotic and presented themselves with high social conformity.* However, specific for patients with GH-producing adenomas was an even more reduced novelty-seeking behavior, especially in terms of *lower impulsiveness*, compared with patients with non-functioning pituitary adenomas. Patients with pituitary adenomas show a distinct pattern of increased *anxiety-related personality traits* compared with the general population, potentially as a result of the pituitary lesion and/or associated hormonal dysregulations and comorbidities. In conclusion many neurological and psychiatric symptoms can accompany pituitary adenomas.

Keywords: functional and non-functional pituitary adenomas, psychiatric and neurological symptoms

1. Introduction

It is widely accepted that there is a close relationship between the endocrine system and the central nervous system (CNS). This connection between the central nervous system and the endocrine system is extremely complex. The hypothalamus serves as a crucial centre for the integration and co-ordination of autonomic functions by neuronal and hormonal pathways. Among hormones closely related to the nervous system, thyroid hormones (THs) are critical for the development and function of the CNS, not only for neuronal cells but also for glial development and differentiation. Pituitary tumors comprise a quarter of the intracranial neoplasms and the adenomas represent the highest percentage of them. They are benign, but they can be invasive and they have an impact in morbidity and mortality.

2. Pituitary Adenomas (PA)

Increasingly, patients with pituitary disease are evaluated and treated at cancer centers. In many ways, these patients resemble patients with other malignant brain tumors. Although the majority of pituitary adenomas are benign, the physical, emotional, and cognitive changes that these patients experience on their well-being is malignant. Also, it is recorded that patients with pituitary adenoma, even when benign, must be carefully followed for signs of malignant transformation, and spinal or distant metastases [1].

Pituitary disease causes a variety of physical illnesses resulting from the alterations in the hypothalamic-pituitary-end organ axis. In addition, patients with pituitary diseases may experience many emotional problems, including *depression, anxiety, behavioral disturbances, and personality changes,* above and beyond the many reactions these patients may have to the myriad of adjustments that they must make in their lives. There is a growing understanding that pituitary patients may experience these emotional problems as a result of long-term effects that the pituitary tumor itself, treatment, and/or hormonal changes have on the hypothalamic-pituitary-end organ axis.

Pituitary adenomas (PAs) represent 15% of all brain tumors. These tumors have been associated with multiple co-morbidities, including neuropsychiatric disorders.

Acromegaly is the result of excessive amounts of growth hormone (GH) and insulin-like growth factor type 1 (IGF-1), almost always caused by a benign adenoma of the pituitary gland.

Several studies reported decreased quality of life (QoL) and *sleep* as well as increased rates of *depression* for patients with pituitary adenomas [2].

The most common neurologic symptoms in patients with pituitary adenomas are *headaches and visual changes*. The most characteristic neurological sign of pituitary adenoma is the *visual field defect*.

It was recorded a high prevalence of *bodily pain* (n = 180, 65%) and *headache* (n = 178, 64%), adrenocorticotropic adenomas were most frequently associated with pain (n = 34, 76%). *Headache* was equally frequent in patients with macro- and microadenomas (68 vs 60%, P = 0.266). According to painDETECT, the majority of the patients had a nociceptive pain component (n = 193, 80%) [3].

Mental alterations are substantially increased in acromegaly being usually present before the diagnosis of acromegaly. Since its first description by Hofmann in 1953, the association of *acromegaly* and *schizophrenia* has been exceptionally reported. Some of these patients were not under Dopamine Agonist (DA) therapy when developed psychiatric symptoms, but they had been treated with antipsychotic drugs, such as haloperidol, olanzapine, and risperidone before acromegaly diagnosis. However, silent, or clinically nonfunctioning, pituitary adenomas can arise from any anterior pituitary cell type. Some are "clinically silent" in that they result in a supranormal serum concentration of the hormonal product of the cell type from which the adenoma arose but do not cause the clinical manifestations typical of excessive levels of that hormone. Others are "totally silent" in that they result in neither hormonal excess nor clinical manifestations. Those that are silent are usually larger and grow more aggressively than those that cause clinical syndromes. Silent adenomas are usually not discovered until they become very large and cause neurologic defects, such as visual impairment, but are also often discovered incidentally when neuro-imaging is performed for another reason. Silent adenomas may become, rarely, clinically apparent over time. The diagnosis of a silent pituitary adenoma begins with the detection of a sellar mass by MRI.

In a retrospective, descriptive analysis of 102 medical records of a total of 191 patients who attended an endocrinology service from 2003 to 2014, the authors found that 63% were women, and 74.4% had age from 25-60 years. About 54% were nonfunctioning adenomas, 28% prolactinomas, 11.8% and 6.2% somatotropinomas and corticotropinomas respectively. In all types, the female group was predominant, except for the nonfunctioning tumors. Of the nonfunctioning adenomas 79% were macroadenomas, of the prolactinomas 52% were microadenomas and surgery was performed in 37% of them. In case of somatotropinomas, 80% were macroadenomas, 40% radiotherapy was operated. In corticotropinomas, both micro and macroadenomas were represented by the same percentage (50%) and all of them underwent surgery [4].

3. Adenomas and Neurologic Symptoms

3.1. Non-Functional Pituitary Adenomas (NFPA) or Gonadotroph Adenomas

Clinically NFPA is currently the preferred term for designating all the pituitary adenomas which are not hormonally active (in other words, not associated with clinical syndromes such as *amenorrhea-galactorrhea* in the context of prolactinomas, *acromegaly, Cushing's disease or hyperthyroidism* secondary to TSH-secreting adenomas). They account for 15-30% of pituitary adenomas. NFPAs may be totally asymptomatic and discovered "incidentally" during radiological examination for some other indication, or else induce tumoral signs with compression of the optic chiasm and pituitary dysfunction. NFPAs are mainly gonadotrophs, but may also be completely "silent." Functioning gonadotroph adenomas (FGAs) are pituitary tumors secreting biologically active gonadotropins. The published literature includes only small case series or individual case reports.

The overall perceived prevalence and severity of *cognitive dysfunction* were the highest among NFPA groups, particularly in the areas of *mental agility, verbal recall, and memory recall*. Patients with *active acromegaly (AA)* reported greater prevalence and severity of dysfunction with respect to *concentration/distractibility and ability to learn* [5]. NFPAs tended to affect *visual acuity* more than adenomas with other pathological diagnoses, which produced adrenocorticotropic hormone and prolactin [6]. *Field defects* occurred in 95% of patients with NFPA macroadenoma. A severe *visual field loss,* involving at least three quadrants in one or both eyes, was the most common. 20% of patients had atypical field defects. Severity of field defects increased with tumor volume [7].

A giant NFPA extending into the third ventricle and thereby causing *obstructive hydrocephalus* with main complaints consisted of *disturbed vision and somnolence* was also described [8].

Neurologic symptoms are most common in NFPAs or gonadotroph adenomas, because these tumors do not secrete sufficient hormones to cause endocrine-type symptoms, and their diagnosis often is delayed until patients present with symptoms of mass effect. Gonadotroph cell adenoma is the most common pituitary adenoma, constituting 35% of the pituitary adenomas. The most common neurological symptoms are *visual symptoms and headache* [9]. *Headaches*, which are believed to result from stretching of the dural sheath, are nonspecific and do not necessarily correlate with tumor size. Gonadotroph and null cell adenomas are the most prevalent types and are typically silent.

When the tumor enlarges, it compresses the optic chiasm superiorly, primarily causing *visual field deficits*, most often *bitemporal hemianopsia*. If the adenoma expands laterally into the cavernous sinus, it has the potential to affect the cranial nerves housed there, including cranial nerves III (oculomotor), IV (trochlear), and VI (abducens), thus causing diplopia. With more severe compression or direct invasion of the optic nerve, *decreased visual acuity* may occur. In contrast to headaches, visual disturbances tend to correlate with tumor size. They also tend to occur insidiously, so that many patients are not aware of them until they are specifically tested. Other neurologic presentations, such as *cerebrospinal fluid rhinorrhea, seizures*, and *pituitary apoplexy*, can occur but are uncommon [10].

Pain appears to be a frequent problem in pituitary disease. *Headache* was equally frequent in patients with macro- and microadenomas. Neuropathic pain and pain-related disability correlated significantly with depression and impaired QoL. Modifiable factors including tumour size, genetic predisposition, previous surgery, irradiation or medical therapy did not have significant impact neither on neuropathic pain components (painDETECT) nor on headache-related disability (MIDAS).

The data suggest that pain should be integrated in the diagnostic and therapeutic work-up of patients with pituitary disease in order to treat them appropriately and improve their QoL [3].

3.2. Somatotroph Adenomas

Somatotroph and corticotroph adenomas typically cause clinical syndromes but occasionally are clinically or totally silent. *Carpal tunnel syndrome, obstructive sleeping apnea and headache* are typical neurological features in somatotroph adenomas [11]. It has been recorded also neuropathic pain.

a. Carpal Tunnel Syndrome (CTS)

The sensory disturbance in the distribution of the median nerve is typical of right *carpal tunnel syndrome* (CTS). CTS typically presents as pain in the medial three fingers radiating into the arm, worsening during the night. CTS often occurs with acromegaly, however, the pathophysiology of CTS in acromegalic patients remains unclear. The median nerves of acromegalic patients with CTS were enlarged and had impaired nerve conduction. This finding represents a predominant intrinsic feature in the pathophysiology of the disease rather than an extrinsic feature such as a thickened transverse carpal ligament [12]. Following adenomectomy, nerve conduction normalized in only six hands (26%). The postoperative persistence of the conduction delay implies that irreversible narrowing of the carpal tunnel rather than reversible soft tissue edema is the principal cause of CTS associated with acromegaly [13].

b. Carpal Tunnel Syndrome (CTS)

Obstructive sleeping apnea. The detection rate of sleep-related breathing disorders (SRBDs) in patients with active acromegaly was 80%, with obstructive disorders being prevalent. There was a positive relationship between SRBD severity and body mass index (BMI), acromegaly duration, IGF-1 level. Compared to the controls, the patients with acromegaly developed SRBDs similar in severity with lower BMI, more severe SRBDs were detected in the patients with active acromegaly with the similar BMI [14].

It has long been known, that irregular, *heavy snoring and daytime sleepiness* are common features of acromegaly. Only recently has the high incidence (30-60%) and clinical relevance of the sleep apnea underlying these symptoms been recognized. Both diseases have a group of common symptoms and prognostic features: *Increased cardiovascular and respiratory mortality, elevated incidence of hypertension, daytime sleepiness, decreased vitality, headaches and depression.* These are very prominent in sleep apnea and often reversible under treatment. In acromegaly their etiology has been widely unexplained and they commonly persist even when human growth hormone (hGH) levels remain normal after operative treatment [15].

3.3. Prolactinomas

Prolactinomas are less frequent, but more invasive in males. Giant ones (≥ 4cm) are extremely rare in literature. Their neurologic, psychiatric and endocrine complications are life threatening.

In a study with a big number of prolactinomas, neurological complications were: *Memory loss and/or unconsciousness* = 18.2%, *epilepsy* = 15.9%, *frontal syndrome* = 9% and *obstructive hydrocephalus* = 6.8% [16].

However giant prolactinomas are rare tumors, representing only 2-3% of all prolactin (PRL)-secreting tumors and raising special diagnostic and therapeutic challenges. Endocrine symptoms are often present but overlooked for a long period of time, and diagnosis is eventually made when neurologic complications arise from massive extension into the surrounding structures, leading to *cranial nerve palsies, hydrocephalus, temporal epilepsy or exophthalmos* [17].

3.4. TSH-Secreting Pituitary Adenomas (TSH-omas)

Thyroid stimulating hormone-secreting pituitary adenomas (TSH-omas) are uncommon tumors of the anterior pituitary gland. They are rare, particularly in childhood. Patients with TSH-omas may present with *hyperthyroidism*, but the incidence of thyroid storm due to TSH-omas has yet to be determined. TSH-omas are rare tumors, and incidence is 1-3% among pituitary adenomas. They are diagnosed in the fifth and sixth decades of life, and the spontaneous occurrence of TSH-omas is more frequent in women. These tumors may lead to the development of *hyperthyroidism* through a condition called syndrome of inappropriate secretion of TSH (SITSH). Approximately 40% of TSH-omas are associated with a concomitant production of other pituitary hormones, such as GH and PRL. In the case of TSH-omas that concomitantly secrete GH, excessive GH causes *acromegalic features, diabetes mellitus, arthropathy, cardiomyopathy and shortened life expectancy.* Surgical removal can be curative for small adenomas, whereas incomplete removal is common for large adenomas [18].

Thyrotoxic periodic paralysis (TPP) is an uncommon disease characterized by episodes of *flaccid paralysis*, usually accompanied by *hypokalemia*. The disorder occurs most frequently in oriental men in their second and third decades. Most reported cases are associated with Graves' disease. Only a few cases have been described in patients with hyperthyroidism due to other diseases. It is thought that pituitary tumors rarely secrete TSH, but this phenomenon has been increasingly recognized as a cause of hyperthyroidism. Kiso and colleagues published a case of *hyperthyroidism* due to a TSH-secreting pituitary tumor complicated by *periodic paralysis*. This association indicates that thyrotoxicosis may induce paralysis in susceptible persons by a mechanism which is not autoimmune [19].

Pituitary apoplexy (manifested through the following symptoms: sudden headache, photophobia, cranial nerve palsies, and collapse due to hypoadrenalism and in some cases hypoglycaemia) is a rare but potentially life-threatening clinical syndrome characterized by ischemic infarction or hemorrhage into a pituitary tumor. The diagnosis of pituitary tumor apoplexy is frequently complicated because of the nonspecific nature of its signs and symptoms, which can mimic different neurological processes, including meningitis.

Meningitis, however, is an unusual complication of untreated invasive pituitary adenomas and represents only the initial symptom, leading to diagnosis of a macroadenoma in exceptional cases. This fact highlights the importance of differential diagnosis when evaluating patients with pituitary adenomas and acute neurological symptoms [20].

3.5. ACTH-Secreting Pituitary Adenomas

Corticotroph adenomas typically cause clinical syndromes but occasionally are clinically or totally silent. ACTH-secreting adenomas causing Cushing Disease are associated with significant morbidity [21].

4. Adenomas and Psychiatric Symptoms

It has been recognized for some time that psychiatric symptoms, such as *depression, anxiety, and behavioral alterations,* may occur in patients who have pituitary disease. From other research focused on endocrine abnormalities, seen in patients with psychiatric illness, it is understood that there is a significant interrelationship between the endocrine system and mental health. More recent research focusing on neural circuits in the brain and the impact of alterations in neurotransmission and neuro-hormonal modulation has shown that the prefrontal cortex can be affected by perturbations in functioning occurring at distant sites. Such is the situation with the hypothalamic-pituitary axis. Through its rich connections with other limbic structures, the hypothalamic-pituitary axis may affect the behavioral control exerted by the prefrontal cortex, *causing mood and personality alterations*. In the more severe cases, an *apathy* syndrome may develop, which must be carefully differentiated from depression and other cognitive disorders [22].

The main psychiatric symptom of hypopituitarism is a combination of dementia and delirium.

4.1. Prolactin-Secreting Pituitary Adenomas (PRL-omas)

Prolactinomas, the most common type of pituitary tumor, can induce hyperprolactinemia and cause some psychiatric symptoms, such as *anxiety, depression and even psychotic symptoms* [23].

They are well-differentiated endocrine tumors expressing D2 dopamine receptor (DRD2). Their actions on DRD2 and the clinical outcome may be affected by polymorphisms. DRD2 polymorphisms correlate with neuropsychiatricdisorders, in particular *alcoholism and schizophrenia* [24].

4.2. Growth Hormone-Producing Pituitary Adenomas (GH-omas)

Compared with healthy controls, acromegalic patients described themselves as distinctly more harm avoidant and neurotic and presented themselves with high social conformity. On harm avoidant subscales, they reported *more anticipatory worries and pessimism, higher fear of uncertainty, higher fatigability and asthenia*. This personality pattern was not specific for acromegaly, but could similarly be observed in patients with NFPA as well. However, specific for patients with GH-producing adenomas was an even more reduced novelty-seeking behavior, especially in terms of *lower impulsiveness*, compared to patients with NFPA. Patients with pituitary adenomas show a distinct pattern of increased *anxiety-related personality traits* compared with the general population, potentially as a result of the pituitary lesion and/or associated hormonal dysregulations and co-morbidities. *Acromegaly* is additionally associated with *reduced impulsivity and novelty-seeking behavior*, which might affect patients' management and their quality of life [25].

The association between *schizophrenia* and *acromegaly* might not be incidental, and it can be speculated that several pathophysiological mechanisms related to alterations in DA neurotransmission due to psychiatric disease itself or its pharmacological treatment could be in relation with the development of GH-secreting PAs [26].

Any impairment of Thyroid Hormone supply to the developing CNS causes severe and irreversible changes in the overall architecture and function of the human brain, leading to various neurological dysfunctions. In the adult brain, impairment of THs, leading to conditions such as *hypothyroidism and hyperthyroidism*, can cause psychiatric disorders such as *schizophrenia, bipolar disorder, anxiety and depression*. Although impact of hypothyroidism on synaptic transmission and plasticity is known, its effect on glial cells and related cellular mechanisms remains enigmatic. THs are transported into the brain, metabolized in astrocytes and affect microglia and oligodendrocytes, demonstrating an example of glioendocrine system. Neuroglial effects may help to understand physiological and/or pathophysiological functions of THs in the CNS and how hypo- and hyperthyroidism may cause mental disorders [27].

4.3. ACTH-Secreting Pituitary Adenomas

The corticotroph-releasing hormone acts as a neurotransmitter, it *has a special role in stress-behavior, anxiety, and depression, and it blocks deep sleeping*.

5. Other Uncommon Neurological Symptoms

Hoarse voice or acute respiratory distress as a result of unilateral larynx paralysis. This is due to submucosal hypertrophy and vocal cord immobility. *Myopathy* remained unchanged after surgery of adenoma.

Aggressive giant invasive pituitary adenomas, refractory to standard surgical or medical treatment, remain a genuine challenge. In addition, *communicating hydrocephalus (CH),* attributed to malabsorption of cerebrospinal fluid (CSF) developing after radiotherapy for pituitary adenomas, has also been previously reported [28].

Pituitary adenoma combined with *intracranial aneurysm* is not rare. Some aneurysms are located inside pituitary adenomas, and most do not rupture. Pituitary apoplexy caused by aneurysm rupture is rare and is easily misdiagnosed as simple pituitary adenoma apoplexy [29].

5.1. Neurologic Symptoms after Surgery or Radiation Therapy of Pituitary Adenomas

Transsphenoidal surgery is the treatment of choice for large non-functioning pituitary adenomas (NFPA) and symptomatic patients. The therapeutic strategies for the management of NFPA after surgery, i.e., watchful waiting, irradiation, or medical therapy have not been compared by randomized controlled trials. Slow re-growth is common, but the natural history of untreated tumors is variable. Conservative follow-up is associated with progression rates of over 40%. Radiation is highly effective in preventing residual tumor growth, but has serious long-term side effects. Finally, no medications are currently approved for the treatment of NFPA [30].

Radiation is a well-known etiology for many CNS tumors, including meningiomas, sarcomas and gliomas.

Single fraction *stereotactic radiosurgery (SRS)* is a common adjuvant therapy for hormonally active pituitary adenomas, when surgical resection fails to control tumor growth or normalize hypersecretory activity. Marginal doses of 20-24 Gy are used at many centers and in other centers patients are treated with a higher marginal dose of 35 Gy. In a recent study thirty-one patients with secretory pituitary adenomas (adrenocorticotropic hormone, n = 15, growth hormone, n = 13, prolactin, n = 2, thyroid-stimulating hormone, n = 1) were treated with 35 Gy to the 50% isodose line, and had a mean follow-up time of 40.2 months (range = 12-96). All patients were evaluated post-SRS for time to hormonal normalization, time to relapse, as well as incidence and time course of radiation-induced hypopituitarism and cranial neuropathies. Initial normalization of hypersecretion was achieved in 22 patients (70%), with a median time to remission of 17.7 months. After initial hormonal remission, 7 patients (32%) experienced an endocrine relapse, with a mean time to relapse of 21 months. New endocrine deficiency within any of the five major hormonal axes occurred in 10 patients (32%). One patient (3%) developed new-onset unilateral optic nerve pallor within the temporal field three years after SRS. Three patients (10%) reported transient new or increasing frontal headaches of unclear etiology following surgical treatment [31].

However, the management of choice of non-functioning pituitary adenomas (NFPAs) remains debulking surgery when symptomatic. However, patient series systematically reporting the NFPAs outcome that were not treated either surgically, medically or with radiotherapy during long follow-up thereby giving an indication of their natural history are limited. Based on the given lack of approved medical treatment and the possible risks of surgical intervention in presence of significant co-morbidities, Karamouzis et al. propose in their study a conservative approach, with a careful follow-up in patients with NFPAs without visual or neurological abnormalities [32].

The most frequent neurological symptoms after surgery or radiation therapy for treating pituitary adenomas are:

5.2. CSF Rhinorrhea

It has been reported in the literature a patient who developed delayed *cerebrospinal fluid (CSF)* rhinorrhea 11 years after gamma knife radiosurgery for a growth hormone (GH)-secreting adenoma. The treatment dose was 18 Gy for the tumor margin (50% isodose). One year later, an MRI of the head revealed that the tumor size had decreased. Perhaps the cause of the CSF rhinorrhea was a secondary empty sella. The other possible causes may be the original invasiveness of the tumor or delayed radiation damage to the mucous membranes of the skull. Long-term follow-up is required to monitor recurrence of CSF rhinorrhea [33].

5.3. Ocular Motor Cranial Nerve Damage

Radiation therapy is often used in the treatment of pituitary tumor. Diplopia due to radiation damage to the ocular motor cranial nerves has been infrequently reported as a complication. Patients with pituitary tumors treated multiple times with various forms of radiation therapy are at risk to sustain ocular motor cranial nerve injury. The prevalence of acromegalic patients in a study, carried out by Vaphiades et al. reflects an aggressive attempt to salvage patients with recalcitrant growth hormone elevation and may place the patient at a greater risk for ocular motor cranial nerve damage. In a recent study of six patients with diplopia after radiation therapy, five patients developed sixth nerve palsies, three unilateral and two bilateral, and in one patient, a sixth nerve palsy was preceded by a fourth cranial nerve palsy. One patient developed third nerve palsy. Five of the six patients had a growth hormone-secreting pituitary tumor with acromegaly [34].

5.4. Neurocognitive Symptoms

In adult patients with operated pituitary adenomas (PA), radiation therapy (RT) was independently associated with impairment in verbal memory and executive function, when compared to non-irradiated patients. Our data suggest that diagnosis of acromegaly or Cushing's disease, and age at the time of RT were able to modulate these long-term radio-induced neurocognitive sequelae [35].

5.5. Hhypopituitarism, Optic Neuropathy, and Radiation-Induced Neoplasms

Gamma Knife surgery (GKS) has become a significant component of neurosurgical treatment for recurrent secretory and non-secretory pituitary adenomas. Although the long-term risks of visual dysfunction following microsurgical resection of pituitary adenomas has been well studied, the comparable risk following radiosurgery is not well defined. Gamma knife surgery is a safe and effective treatment option in patients with primary NFPAs, especially for patients with advanced age or comorbidity. Attention should be paid to late adverse radiation effects such as hypopituitarism, optic neuropathy, and radiation-induced neoplasms. However, stereotactic radiosurgery with a conformal treatment plan sparing the normal pituitary gland will contribute to avoidance of such complications as well as achievement of long-term tumor control [36]. Therefore, neurological and ophthalmological assessments in addition to routine neuro-imaging and endocrinological follow-up are important to perform following GKS. Patients with a history of radiosurgery or radiation therapy are at higher risk of cranial nerve deficits. Also, a reduction in the number of isocenters delivered, along with volume treated, particularly in the patients with secretory tumors, appears to be the most reasonable strategy to minimize the risk to the visual system when treating recurrent pituitary adenomas with stereotactic radiosurgery [37].

5.6. Brain Abnormalities

The extent to which cognitive dysfunction is related to specific brain abnormalities in patients treated for pituitary macroadenoma is unclear. Brain abnormalities on MRI were not observed more frequently in NFPA patients treated with RT compared to patients treated with surgery-alone in study of 86 NFPA patients. Furthermore, RT was not associated with an increased severity of White Matter Lesions (WMLs) and cerebral atrophy ratings in this cohort of NFPA patients [38]. The absence of brain abnormalities on MRI does not exclude impairments in cognition.

5.7. Visual Field Disorder and Oculomotor Palsy

From 35 patients, who followed stereotactic radiosurgery with median follow-up of eight years and a 5-year overall survival, only one new visual field disorder and a new oculomotor palsy occurred in one patient, respectively. Patients with occurrence of visual/neurological impairments had a longer follow up ($p = 0.049$) [39].

5.8. Other Rare Side Effects

a. Sarcoma

Secondary malignancies are infrequent sequelae of pituitary radiotherapy. There is a report of the illustrative case of a 38-year-old man with acromegaly who had transsphenoidal surgery and radiotherapy seven years before presenting with a sellar high-grade sarcoma. Transsphenoidal and transcranial resection, as well as repeated gamma knife radiosurgery, could not prevent tumor progression and development of meningiosis sarcomatosa. A search in medical literature revealed 51 cases of mesenchymal malignancies after sellar radiotherapy. These tumors occur at normal dose schedules with long latencies. Their growth is very aggressive and they may develop meningiosis sarcomatosa. Until now, no treatment modalities have been able to stop the progression of these neoplasms. Radiation-induced sarcoma is a rare sequela of pituitary radiotherapy. It is important for the treating physician to keep in mind the possibility of post-radiation sarcoma development. Additionally, one must include these tumors into the differential diagnosis, in pituitary patients presenting with tumor recurrence more than five years after radiotherapy, in combination with a secondary lack of hormonal activity [40].

b. Stroke

There is a report of a case of ischemic stroke in a 43-year-old woman with no traditional cardiovascular risk factors and a history of cranial surgery and cranial radiation therapy (CRT) for a GH-secreting pituitary macroadenoma. The neurological work-up on this patient disclosed several cerebral ischemic lesions and demonstrated the occlusion of the right middle cerebral artery together with the narrowing of the right carotid artery, post-radiation brain damage was also visible by nuclear magnetic resonance [41].

REFERENCES

[1] Tanaka, T, Kato, N, Aoki, K, Watanabe, M, Arai, T, Hasegawa, Y, et al. Long-term follow-up of growth hormone-producing pituitary carcinoma with multiple spinal metastases following multiple surgeries: case report. *Neurol Med Chir (Tokyo)*, 2013;53:707-711.

[2] Leistner, SM, Klotsche, J, Dimopoulou, C, Athanasoulia, AP, Roemmler-Zehrer, J, Pieper, L, et al. Reduced sleep quality and depression associate with decreased quality of life in patients with pituitaryadenomas. *Eur J Endocrinol*, 2015;172:733-743.

[3] Dimopoulou, C, Athanasoulia, AP, Hanisch, E, Held, S, Sprenger, T, Toelle, TR, et al. Clinical characteristics of pain in patients with pituitaryadenomas. *Eur J Endocrinol*, 2014;171:581-591.

[4] Cecenarro, LA, Rodrigo Fanton, ET, Estario, P, Papalini, RF, Estario, MÉ. Pituitary tumors: 10 years of experience. *Rev Fac Cien Med Univ Nac Cordoba*, 2015;72:32-38.

[5] Yedinak, CG, Fleseriu, M. Self-perception of cognitive function among patients with active acromegaly, controlled acromegaly, and non-functional pituitary adenoma: a pilot study. *Endocrine*, 2014;46:585-593.

[6] Wang, H, Sun, W, Fu, Z, Si, Z, Zhu, Y, Zhai, G, et al. The pattern of visual impairment in patients with pituitary adenoma. *J Int Med Res*, 2008;36:1064-1069.

[7] Thomas, R, Shenoy, K, Seshadri, MS, Muliyil, J, Rao, A, Paul, P. Visual field defects in non-functioning pituitary adenomas. *Indian J Ophthalmol*, 2002;50:127-130.

[8] Verhelst, J, Berwaerts, J, Abs, R, Dua, G, Van Den Weyngaert, D, Mahler, C. Obstructive hydrocephalus as complication of a giant nonfunctioning pituitary adenoma: therapeutical approach. *Acta Clin Belg*, 1998;53:47-52.

[9] Ho, DM, Hsu, CY, Ting, LT, Chiang, H. The clinicopathological characteristics of gonadotroph cell adenoma: a study of 118 cases. *Hum Pathol*, 1997;28:905-911.

[10] Lake, MG, Krook, LS, Cruz, SV. Pituitary adenomas: an overview. *Am Fam Physician*, 2013;88:319-327.

[11] Aszalós, Z. Some neurological and psychiatric complications of the disorders of the hypothalamo-hypophyseal system. *Orv Hetil*, 2007;148:723-730.

[12] Sasagawa, Y, Tachibana, O, Doai, M, Tonami, H, Iizuka, H. Median nerve conduction studies and wrist magnetic resonance imaging in acromegalic patients with carpal tunnel syndrome. *Pituitary*, 2015;18:695-700.
[13] Kameyama, S, Tanaka, R, Hasegawa, A, Tamura, T, Kuroki, M. Subclinical carpal tunnel syndrome in acromegaly. *Neurol Med Chir (Tokyo)*, 1993;33:547-551.
[14] Tsoi, UA, Sviryaev, IuV, Korostovtseva, LS, Semenov, AP, Vaulina, DA, Nepran, VI, Kravchenko, SO, Konradi, AO, Grineva, EN. Clinical features of obstructive sleep apnea syndrome in patients with acromegaly. *Ter Arkh*, 2015;87:47-52.
[15] Rosenow, F, Reuter, S, Szelies, B, Deuss, U, Hildebrandt, G, Schneider, D, et al. Sleepapnoea in acromegaly--prevalence, pathogenesis and therapy. Report on two cases. *Presse Med*, 1994;23:1203-1208.
[16] Chentli, F, Azzoug, S, Daffeur, K, Akkache, L, Zellagui, H, Haddad, M, et al. Neurological, psychiatric, ophthalmological, and endocrine complications in giant male prolactinomas: An observational study in Algerian population. *Indian J Endocrinol Metab*, 2015;19:359-363.
[17] Maiter, D, Delgrange, E. Therapy of endocrine disease: the challenges in managing giant prolactinomas. *Eur J Endocrinol*, 2014;170:R213-227.
[18] Yasuda, A, Seki, T, Oki, M, Takagi, A, Inomoto, C, Nakamura, N, et al. A Case of a TSH-secreting Pituitary Adenoma Associated with Evans' Syndrome. *Tokai J Exp Clin Med*, 2015;40:44-50.
[19] Kiso, Y, Yoshida, K, Kaise, K, Kaise, N, Masuda, T, Ando, N, et al. A case of thyrotropin (TSH)-secreting tumor complicated by periodic paralysis. *Jpn J Med*, 1990; 29:399-404.
[20] Villar-Taibo, R, Ballesteros-Pomar, MD, Vidal-Casariego, A, Alvarez-San Martín, RM, Kyriakos, G, Cano-Rodríguez, I. Spontaneous remission *Arq Bras Endocrinol Metabol*, 2014;58:76-80.
[21] Mehta, GU, Montgomery, BK, Raghavan, P, Sharma, S, Nieman, LK, Patronas, N, et al. Different imaging characteristics of concurrent pituitary adenomas in a patient with Cushing's disease. *J Clin Neurosci*, 2015;22:891-894.
[22] Weitzner, MA. Neuropsychiatry and pituitary disease: an overview. *Psychother Psychosom*, 1998;67:125-132.
[23] Liao, WT, Bai, YM. Major depressive disorder induced by prolactinoma: a case report. *Gen Hosp Psychiatry*, 2014;36:125.
[24] Filopanti, M, Lania, AG, Spada, A. Pharmacogenetics of D2 dopamine receptor gene in prolactin-secreting pituitary adenomas. *Expert Opin Drug Metab Toxicol*, 2010; 6:43-53.
[25] Sievers, C, Ising, M, Pfister, H, Dimopoulou, C, Schneider, HJ, Roemmler, J, et al. Personality in patients with pituitary adenomas is characterized by increased anxiety-related traits: comparison of 70 acromegalic patients with patients with non-functioning pituitary adenomas and age- and gender-matched controls. *Eur J Endocrinol*, 2009;160:367-373.
[26] Iglesias, P, Bernal, C, Díez, JJ. Curious cases: Acromegaly and schizophrenia: an incidental association? *Schizophr Bull*, 2014;40:740-743.
[27] Noda, M. Possible role of glial cells in the relationship between thyroid dysfunction and mental disorders. *Front Cell Neurosci*, 2015;9:194.

[28] Chentli, F, Azzoug, S, Daffeur, K, Akkache, L, Zellagui, H, Haddad, M, et al. Neurological, psychiatric, ophthalmological, and endocrine complications in giant male prolactinomas: An observational study in Algerian population. *Indian J Endocrinol Metab*, 2015;19:359-363.

[29] Xu, K, Yuan, Y, Zhou, J, Yu, J. Pituitary adenoma apoplexy caused by rupture of an anterior communicating artery aneurysm: case report and literature review. *World J Surg Oncol*, 2015;13:228.

[30] Greenman, Y, Stern, N. Optimal management of non-functioning pituitary adenomas. *Endocrine*, 2015;50:51-55.

[31] Grant, RA, Whicker, M, Lleva, R, Knisely, JP, Inzucchi, SE, Chiang, VL. Efficacy and safety of higher dose stereotactic radiosurgery for functional pituitary adenomas: a preliminary report. *World Neurosurg*, 2014;82:195-201.

[32] Karamouzis, I, Berardelli, R, Prencipe, N, Berton, A, Bona, C, Stura, G, et al. Retrospective observational analysis of non-irradiated non-functioning pituitary adenomas. *J Endocrinol Invest*, 2015 Jul 28 [Epub ahead of print].

[33] Hongmei, Y, Zhe, W, Jing, W, Daokui, W, Peicheng, C, Yongjie, L. Delayed cerebrospinal fluid *J Clin Neurosci*, 2012;19:900-902.

[34] Vaphiades, MS, Spencer, SA, Riley, K, Francis, C, Deitz, L, Kline, LB. Radiation-induced ocular motor cranial nerve palsies in patients with pituitary tumor. *J Neuroophthalmol*, 2011;31:210-213.

[35] Lecumberri, B, Estrada, J, García-Uría, J, Millán, I, Pallardo, LF, Caballero, L, Lucas, T. Neurocognitive long-term impact of two-field conventional radiotherapy in adult patients with operated pituitary adenomas. *Pituitary*., 2015 Mar 29 [Epub ahead of print].

[36] Hasegawa, T, Shintai, K, Kato, T, Iizuka, H. Stereotactic Radiosurgery as the Initial Treatment for Patients with Nonfunctioning Pituitary Adenomas. *World Neurosurg*, 2015;83:1173-1179.

[37] Cifarelli, CP, Schlesinger, DJ, Sheehan, JP. Cranial nerve dysfunction following Gamma Knife surgery for pituitary adenomas: long-term incidence and risk factors. *J Neurosurg*, 2012;116:1304-1310.

[38] Sattler, MG, Meiners, LC, Sluiter, WJ, van den Berg, G, Langendijk, JA, Wolffenbuttel, BH, et al. Brain abnormalities on MRI in non-functioning pituitary adenoma patients treated with or without postoperative radiotherapy. *Radiother Oncol*, 2015;114:239-244.

[39] Boström, JP, Kinfe T, Meyer, A, Pintea, B, Gerlach, R, Surber, G, et al. Treatment of acromegaly *Strahlenther Onkol*, 2015;191:477-485.

[40] Berkmann, S, Tolnay, M, Hänggi, D, Ghaffari, A, Gratzl, O. Sarcoma of the sella after radiotherapy for pituitary adenoma. *Acta Neurochir (Wien)*, 2010;152:1725-1735.

[41] Maffei, P, Albano, I, Martini, C, Barban, M, Manara, R, Meneghetti, G, Sicolo, N. Middle cerebral artery occlusion 25 years after cranial radiation therapy in acromegaly: a case report. *J Thromb Thrombolysis*, 2009;28:358-361.

In: Pituitary Adenoma
Editor: Dimitrios N. Kanakis
ISBN: 978-1-63484-985-2

Chapter 5

CLINICAL PICTURE OF PITUITARY ADENOMAS: ENDOCRINE SIGNS AND SYMPTOMS

Olga Karapanou, MD,
and Stylianos Tsagarakis*, MD, PhD, FRCP
Department of Endocrinology, Diabetes and Metabolism,
"Evaggelismos" Hospital, Athens, Greece

ABSTRACT

Pituitary adenomas are rare tumors confined to the sella turcica. Tumorigenesis mainly results from somatic mutations (sporadic tumors), although in few cases pituitary adenomas are associated with several genetic syndromes such as multiple endocrine neoplasia type 1, McCune-Albright syndrome, Carney syndrome or familiar acromegaly. According to tumor size – these are classified into microadenomas (maximum tumor diameter <10mm) and macroadenomas (maximum diameter >10mm), while according to clinical picture they may be either functional or non-functional. Non-functional tumors represent approximately 10% of pituitary adenomas and some of these on histologic examination stain positive for gonadotropins or solely for alpha-subunit. Among the functional pituitary tumors the most common are prolactinomas, comprising about 60% of pituitary tumors, GH-secreting adenomas (approximately 20%), ACTH-tumors (10%) and the unusual TSH- or gonadotropin secreting adenomas. Clinical manifestations reflect hormone hypersecretion, prolactinomas present with amenorrhea or oligomenorrhea with anovulation and/or galactorrhea in women, decreased libido and erectile dysfunction in men. GH-secreting adenomas cause the classic clinical syndrome of acromegaly and gigantism i.e., acral enlargement, soft tissue overgrowth, coarsening of the facial features, excessive sweating and associated metabolic and cardiovascular complications leading to increased mortality. ACTH-secreting tumors cause signs and symptoms of hypercortisolism (Cushing's syndrome) and adrenal androgen excess. Discriminative clinical signs are moon face, buffalo hump, easy bruisability, obesity with central fat distribution and striae. TSHomas are rare cause of hyperthyroidism associated

* Corresponding author: Stylianos Tsagarakis, MD, PhD, FRCP, Department of Endocrinology, Diabetes and Metabolism, "Evaggelismos" Hospital, Ipsilantou Str. 45-47, 10676 Athens, Greece, E-mail: stsagara@otenet.gr.

with elevated TSH, T3 and T4 levels and goiter. So far, few cases of functional gonadotroph adenomas have been reported presenting with precocious puberty in children and ovarian hyperstimulation syndrome in women of reproductive age. Apart from hormone excess, depending on tumor size and invasiveness, pituitary insufficiency and/or neurologic defects due to suprasellar or carvenous sinus extension may be apparent as well. The most common deficiency is gonadotropin deficiency followed by thyrotropin (TSH and rarely adrenocorticotropin-ACTH) deficiency, while posterior hypophysis function loss manifesting as diabetes insipidus is rather unlikely. Clinical picture is a powerful guide to diagnosis especially for acromegaly and Cushing's syndrome. Therefore clinical suspicion and diagnostic awareness should be high.

Keywords: acromegaly, Cushing's syndrome, hyperprolactinemia, TSH-secreting adenomas, gonadotrophinomas, nonfunctioning pituitary adenomas

1. Introduction

Pituitary adenomas are rare tumors confined to the sella turcica. According to their size there are classified into microadenomas (maximum tumor diameter <10mm) and macroadenomas (maximum diameter >10mm), while according to the secretory status they are classified into functional and non-functional. Non-functional tumors represent approximately 10% of pituitary adenomas, and some of these on histological examination stain positive for gonadotropins or solely for alpha-subunit. The former category (functional adenomas) includes GH-secreting, prolactin-secreting, ACTH-secreting and the rare TSH-secreting and gonadotropin secreting adenomas. Hypersecretion of each of the above hormones produces a dinstinct clinical phenotype especially in the case of GH-secreting and ACTH-secreting adenomas, accompanied by tumor mass effects (pituitary insufficiency and/or neurologic defects) in case the tumor is macroadenoma. The most common deficiency is gonadotropin deficiency followed by thyrotropin (TSH) and rarely adrenocorticotropin (ACTH) deficiency, while posterior hypophysis function loss manifesting as diabetes insipidus, is rather unlikely.

In this chapter the clinical picture of pituitary adenomas concerning their endocrinologic manifestations is thoroughly analyzed.

1.1. GH-Secreting Pituitary Adenomas

GH-secreting pituitary adenomas are usually benign surrounded by non-hyperplastic pituitary tissue and they result in the well-known clinical syndrome of acromegaly [1]. A broad spectrum of changes in growth factor levels can induce a cascade of genetic events, ultimately leading to expansion of a population of somatotroph tumor cells and subsequent transformation into a GH-secreting pituitary adenoma [2]. For instance, roughly 40% of GH-secreting adenomas harbor a mutation in the alpha-subunit of the stimulatory G-protein that confers constitutive activation of cyclic AMP (cAMP) [3]. Expression of a pro-apoptotic factor, growth arrest and DNA damage–inducible (GADD) 45γ protein, is lost in growth hormone–secreting adenomas [4]. On the contrary, the pituitary tumor–transforming gene protein (PTTG), a securin molecule that regulates sister chromatid separation, is overexpressed in growth hormone–secreting adenomas and correlates with tumor size [5]. For GH-secreting adenomas there are two main granulation patterns: densely and sparsely granulated adenonas. Densely granulated somatotroph adenomas grow slowly, and patients presenting with these adenomas are usually older than 50 years of age. Younger patients usually present with more rapidly growing, sparsely granulated adenomas composed of GH cells. About 25% of growth hormone adenomas co secrete prolactin, these include dimorphous adenomas composed of GH and prolactin cells, monomorphous mammosomatotroph adenomas (which produce both prolactin and GH), and more primitive acidophil stem-cell adenomas [6]. The third type is more commonly encountered in teenagers, often causing gigantism [7]. Mixed single cellular or multicellular plurihormonal immunoreactivity is commonly reported by the pathologist, especially for the alpha-subunit of the glycoprotein hormones, and rarely for thyrotropin or corticotropin [8]. Plurihormonal hypersecretion is rarely clinically apparent. Silent somatotroph adenomas have been described in patients with elevated levels of prolactin and IGF-1 [9].

Recently, X-linked acrogigantism (X-LAG), a new infant-onset syndrome of pituitary gigantism has been described [10]. This syndrome is caused by microduplications on chromosome Xq26.3, encompassing the gene GPR101, which is highly up regulated in pituitary tumors and results in a severe clinical phenotype. Patients have marked hypersecretion of GH/IGF1 and usually prolactin, due to a pituitary macroadenoma or hyperplasia, and therapy with either transsphenoidal resection or somatostatin analogues is rather unfavorable, despite moderate to high levels of expression of somatostatin receptor subtype-2 in tumor tissue. Aryl hydrocarbon receptor-interacting gene protein (AIP) mutations occur in approximately 15% of families with familiar isolated pituitary adenomas, the vast majority of which are somatotropinomas [11]. Tumors were significantly larger and diagnosed at a younger age in AIP mutation-positive vs. mutation-negative subjects. Finally, hereditary GH-secreting pituitary adenomas can occur in the setting of multiple endocrine neoplasia-1 (MEN1) and Carney complex (CNC), due to mutations in the genes encoding menin (MEN1) and the R1a regulatory subunit of protein kinase A (PRKAR1A), respectively [12-14].

1.2. Clinical Manifestations

The clinical manifestations of acromegaly range from subtle signs of acral overgrowth, soft-tissue swelling, arthralgias, jaw prognathism, fasting hyperglycemia, and hyperhidrosis to florid osteoarthritis, frontal bone bossing, diabetes mellitus, hypertension, and respiratory and cardiac failure [15, 16]. GH–secreting somatotroph adenomas arising in young patients before the closure of epiphyseal bones result in accelerated growth and gigantism. The incidence of acromegaly is approximately 3 to 4 cases per million persons per year, and its prevalence is 40 to 125 per million [17]. Mean age at diagnosis for both sexes is in the early to mid-40s [18-21]. Disease features develop insidiously over decades, often resulting in a delay of 7 to 10 years in diagnosis after the estimated onset of symptoms [22]. Symptoms are described below in detail:

- **Tumor mass consequences**:
  Headache is a common presenting feature and is reported in approximately 55% of patients. Headaches are generally thought to be due to tumor growth with suprasellar extension and stretching of the dura mater, cavernous sinus invasion with trigeminal nerve irritation, or factors associated with GH hypersecretion as well [18, 19, 23, 24]. Suprasellar extension of the tumor causes visual field defects (Figure 1). Hypopituitarism attributable to compression of the normal pituitary gland, particularly in the setting of a macroadenoma is also prevalent. Hypogonadism can be detected in up to 70% of women of childbearing age and may be accompanied by hyperprolactinemia in up to 45% of patients [25, 26], either due to co-secretion of prolactin or due to stalk compression. Less often, adrenal insufficiency and central hypothyroidism have been described in up to 20% and 9% of cases respectively [27-30]. Thyroid gland enlargement frequently occurs in patients with acromegaly, particularly due to multinodular goiter, thyroid nodules in patients with acromegaly should be monitored according to standard guidelines. In a patient with elevated serum thyroxine levels, the presence of an inappropriately normal or elevated serum thyrotropin level may signify co-secretion of thyrotropin by the pituitary adenoma [31, 32].
- **Changes in facial and acral appearance:**
  Clinical findings include signs of soft-tissue swelling and bone overgrowth, coursing of facial features, mandibular prognathism, and enlargement of the nose, tongue and of the supraorbital and nuchal ridges [33, 18]. Hand volume and heel-pad thickness are often increased and patients frequently describe increased ring and glove sizes as well as shoe width. Thickening of the skin, due to edema and deposition in the papillary and upper reticular dermis of hydrophilic glycosaminoglycans, hyaluronic acid, and chondroitin-4, is common in acromegaly [34]. Excessive perspiration and seborrhea occur in 60% to 80% of patients [35]. Symptomatic carpal tunnel syndrome, due to an increase in median nerve edema within the carpal tunnel, has been described in up to 64% of patients and is a frequent source of disability and discomfort [36, 37].
- **Skeletal disorders**:
  Up to 70% of such patients have large-joint and axial arthropathy that includes thickened articular cartilage, peri-articular calcifications, osteophyte overgrowth, and synovitis [38]. Degenerative osteoarthritis [39], scoliosis, kyphosis, and vertebral fractures develop in patients whose disease is not brought under control [40]. Joint pains may be present in up to three-quarters of the patients [41]. Trabecular bone mineral density (BMD) is more consistently influenced by gonadal status because patients with acromegaly who have hypogonadism may have a reduction in trabecular BMD [42, 43]. Hypercalcemia, hypercalciuria, and hyperphosphatemia can uncommonly occur with GH excess and are due to altered vitamin D metabolism [44]. In addition, the presence of hypercalcemia should trigger consideration of measurement of the parathyroid hormone concentration because the presence of primary hyperparathyroidism suggests that an evaluation for MEN 1 is indicated.
- **Cardiovascular complications:**
  By the time of diagnosis, arrhythmias, hypertension, and valvular heart disease are present in up to 60% of patients. With untreated, prolonged disease, concentric

myocardial hypertrophy develops, and diastolic heart failure occurs [45]. The major determinant is disease duration, patients with an estimated disease duration of >10 years had a relative risk to present cardiac complications three times higher than patients with estimated disease duration <5 years [46]. Unlike heart failure, aortic and mitral valve regurgitation [47] and hypertension are not reversible with octreotide treatment.

- **Respiratory disorders:**
  Sleep apnea syndrome is present in approximately 70% of patients with acromegaly and is present in more than 90% of patients with acromegaly who snore [48]. The cause of sleep apnea syndrome is primarily obstruction due to pharyngeal thickening and macroglossia, but a central component has been described as well. Upper airway obstruction can lead to difficulties with airway management during surgical procedures. Respiratory dysfunction may be caused by soft tissue swelling, nasal polyps, macroglossia, and pneumomegaly, with obstructive sleep apnea documented in more than 50% of patients [49]. Soft tissue edema and impaired exercise capacity are reversed once the hypersecretion of growth hormone is controlled. Centrally altered respiratory control may underlie the sleep apnea in acromegaly, which has been attributed to central effects of growth hormone itself [50].

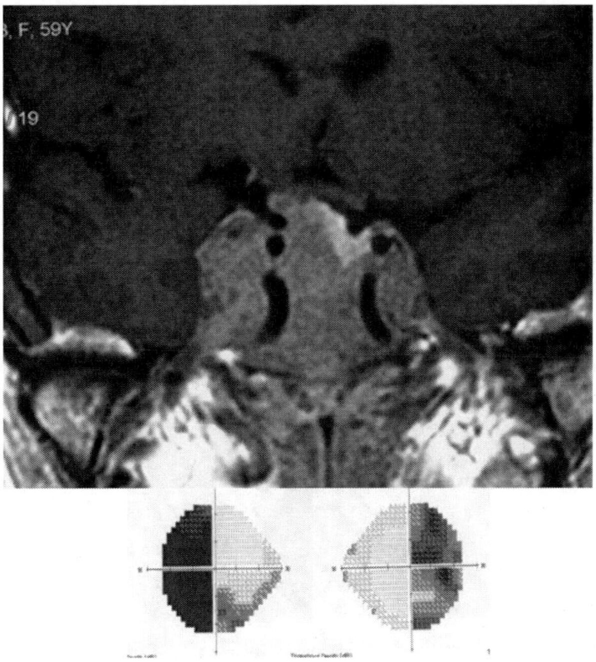

Figure 1. A GH-secreting adenoma with bilateral carvenous sinus invasion (Knosp 4) and suprasellarextension causing bitemporal hemianopsia. Courtesy of Dr. Tsagarakis.

- **Metabolic changes:**
  Insulin resistance is a frequent consequence of acro-megaly. The prevalence of impaired glucose tolerance is up to 46%, and type 2 diabetes mellitus is detected in up to 56% of patients with acromegaly [51-53]. GH has been shown to correlate with

resistance as estimated by clamp [54, 55], oral glucose tolerance test (OGTT) [56], and intravenous glucose tolerance testing [57]. Changes in IGF1- levels also correlated with changes in insulin resistance as assessed by clamp after surgical [58] or octreotide [59] therapy or with the decrease in fasting insulin and glucose values during pegvisomant therapy [60, 61].

- **Colon cancer risk:**
  Standardized mortality ratio for colon cancer risk is estimated 2.47 (95% confidence interval, 1.31 to 4.22) [62]. Furthermore, prospective, controlled studies of colonoscopic screening indicate that the risk of colon cancer in patients with acromegaly is about twice that in the general population [63], which probably reflects a trophic IGF-1 effect on the proliferation of epithelial cells [64]. Screening colonoscopy should be performed when the diagnosis of acromegaly is made, with follow-up according to standard guidelines.
- **Mortality**:
  The overall standardized mortality ratio of patients with acromegaly is 1.48 [65, 66]. Factors contributing to increased mortality among persons with acromegaly include the higher prevalence of hypertension, hyperglycemia or overt diabetes, cardiomyopathy, and sleep apnea in this population. Multivariate analysis of determinants of survival in long-term studies indicates that growth hormone levels of less than 2.5 μg per liter, a younger age, a shorter duration of disease, and the absence of hypertension independently predict longer survival [65, 66]. In some studies, increased IGF-1 levels are associated with higher mortality [67, 21]. However, growth hormone levels seem to be more consistently independent predictors of mortality than are IGF-1 levels [68].
- **Quality of life**:
  Furthermore, the above-mentioned effects of GH excess may affect patients' quality of life. Recently, a disease specific health-related quality of life questionnaire, focusing on physical and psychological quality of life issues in patients with acromegaly, has been developed [69]. Of note, even patients cured after treatment for acromegaly have a persistently decreased quality of life, despite long-term biochemical cure of GH excess. Radiotherapy especially is associated with a reduced quality of life [70].

2. PROLACTINOMAS

Prolactinomas account for 25-30% of functioning pituitary tumors and are the most frequent cause of chronic hyperprolactinemia [71]. Prolactinomas are divided into two groups: (1) microprolactinomas (smaller than 10mm) which are more common in premenopausal women, and (2) macroprolactinomas (10mm or larger) which are more common in men and postmenopausal women. Circulating prolactin (PRL) levels usually parallel tumor size, such that microadenomas rarely result in PRL levels higher than 200mg per l and macroadenomas usually result in PRL levels higher than 200mg per l. On the other hand, if a very large macroadenoma (greater than 3cm) is found in a patient with a normal or only mildly elevated PRL level, "hook effect" must be suspected. The hook effect is an assay artifact caused by an extremely high level of PRL, which saturates the detecting antibody used in the PRL assay, thus resulting in a falsely low reported value [72]. Raised prolactin levels can also be caused by pituitary adenomas co-secreting prolactin. For example many patients with acromegaly have concomitant co-secretion of prolactin. Lesions affecting the hypothalamus and pituitary stalk such as nonfunctioning adenomas, gliomas, and craniopharyngiomas also result in prolactin elevation. Disorders such as hypothyroidism and chronic renal failure must be excluded since 40% patients with primary hypothyroidism, 30% patients with chronic renal failure, and up to 80% patients on hemodialysis have mild elevation of prolactin levels [73]. The predominant physiologic consequence of hyperprolactinemia is hypogonadotropic hypogonadism (HH) due to suppression of pulsatile gonadotropin releasing hormone (GnRH). The clinical manifestations of this condition vary significantly depending on the age and the sex of the patient and the magnitude of the prolactin excess. Clinical presentation in women is more obvious and occurs earlier than in men. Women can present with symptoms of oligomenorrhea, amenorrhea, galactorrhea, decreased libido, infertility, and decreased bone mass. Galactorrhea requires adequate estrogen or progesterone priming of the breast, although it is a common finding in premenopausal women, it is very uncommon in postmenopausal women. Prolonged hypoestrogenism secondary to hyperprolactinemia may result in osteopenia [74]. Spinal bone mineral density (BMD) is decreased by approximately 25% in such women and is not necessarily restored with normalization of prolactin levels [75]. Women with hyperprolactinemia and normal menses have normal BMD [76, 77]. Hyperprolactinemic women may present with signs of chronic hyperandrogenism such as hirsutism and acne, possibly due to increased dehydroepiandrosterone sulfate secretion from the adrenals [78], as well as reduced sex hormone binding globulin leading to high free testosterone levels.

Men with hyperprolactinemia may present with erectile dysfunction, decreased libido, infertility, gynecomastia, decreased bone mass, but rarely galactorrhea. Over time, the patient may have diminished energy, reduced muscle mass, and increased risk of osteopenia [79].

Macroprolactinomas usually present with neurological symptoms caused by mass effects of the tumor. Symptoms include headaches, visual field losses, cranial neuropathies, hypopituitarism, seizures, and cerebrospinal fluid rhinorrhea [79].

3. ACTH-Secreting Pituitary Adenomas

ACTH-secreting pituitary adenomas (usually microadenomas) promote excess cortisol production from the adrenal glands resulting in a clinical phenotype widely known as Cushing's disease (CD). Several population-based studies estimate an incidence of 1.2-2.4 per million persons per year [80, 81], while the prevalence of diagnosed cases is approximately 39 per million population with a female preponderance [80]. However, the prevalence of CD may be underestimated due to unrecognized patients with mild symptoms and/or patients with a cyclic form of CD [82]. On the basis of data from the prospective European Registry on Cushing's syndrome (ERCUSYN) (total number of patients 481, of whom 66% of patients had CD), median delay in diagnosis was 2 years [83]. When compared with the general population, CD patients showed a greater than two-fold increase in hypertension, diabetes, and osteoporosis, and an increase of over five times the rate of major depression and impaired glucose tolerance [84]. Some of the clinical characteristics of CD are described in detail below:

- **Obesity with centripetal fat deposition**:
  (facial plethora, rounded face, buffalo-hump, supraclavicular and dorso-cervical fat pads). The prevalence of overweight (defined as a body mass index (BMI) of 25–30 kg/m^2) ranges from 21 to 48% [85-88]. In addition, these patients also express an unfavorable adipocytokine profile (increased inflammatory markers and reduced adiponectin), which is implicated in increased coronary heart disease risk and has been hypothesized to be a link between adiposity and increased cardiovascular risk [89].
- **Insulin resistance, impaired glucose tolerance and diabetes mellitus:**
  Insulin resistance is a well-known complication of CD and seems to persist after biochemical remission [90, 85]. The high values of homeostatic model assessment (HOMA) [91] and low values of the insulin sensitivity index (ISI) [92] in patients with CD confirm the decrease in insulin sensitivity in this condition without significant differences between obese, overweight and normal weight patients, suggesting that the alteration in insulin sensitivity is due not only to obesity but also to the state of hypercortisolism per se [86]. Epidemiological studies have shown a variable prevalence of abnormalities of glucose metabolism: 20-47% of patients suffer from overt diabetes mellitus, whereas impaired glucose tolerance is present in 21-64% of patients [80-86, 93]. As patients with CD are likely to have impaired glucose tolerance, assessment by an oral glucose tolerance test (OGTT) may have utility in monitoring.
- **Dyslipidemia:**
  The prevalence of dyslipidemia in patients with CD ranges from 38 to 71% [86, 93]. A study by Mancini et al. [86] has shown dyslipidemia to occur less frequently than the other metabolic complications and that it was not correlated to the degree of hypercortisolism or duration of the disease. It is recommended that dyslipidemia should be aggressively treated in patients with Cushing's disease to manage increased cardiovascular morbidity and mortality risk [94].
- **Signs of protein wasting such as thin skin, abdominal purple to red and wide cutaneous striae (abdomen (Figure 2), flanks, breasts, hips, axillae), easy bruising, slow healing, muscle wasting (lower limbs muscle atrophy)**: Myopathy and bruising are discriminatory features of Cushing's disease and involve mainly the proximal muscles of lower limb and shoulder girdle [95]. A sensitive clinical test to demonstrate muscle involvement (or diagnose myopathy) is to ask the patient to rise from a crouching position or to raise upper limbs.
- **Bone wasting leading to osteoporosis:**
  Osteoporosis is a frequent, severe, and often underestimated consequence of long-term hypercortisolism, and fractures can be the presenting manifestation of CD [96, 97]. Pecori Giraldi et al. reported a prevalence of osteoporosis ranging from 31.6 to 46.8% in a gender-comparison study in 280 CD patients [98]. Both overt and subtle endogenous hypercortisolism affect bone, leading to vertebral fractures in up to 70% of patients [96]. Correction of hypercortisolism is able to reverse glucocorticoid-induced osteoporosis [99-101].

- **Hypertension:**
  Hypertension mild to moderate in most cases has been reported in 55-85% of patients with CD [80-86, 93]. Hypertension remits in a subset of patients (44-75%) after successful treatment but persists in approximately 24-56% [80, 85, 86], presumably due to microvessel remodeling or concomitant underlying essential hypertension [102].
- **Coagulation defect:**
  Patients with CD show various abnormalities of hemostatic parameters and those with active CD show an increased thrombotic tendency [103]. Increased cortisol levels stimulate the synthesis of several clotting factors, such as fibrinogen by the liver and von Willebrand factor by endothelial cells. Glucocorticoid also up regulate the synthesis of plasminogen activator inhibitor type 1, the main inhibitor of the fibrinolytic system [104]. This hypercoagulability state is a crucial factor predisposing CD patients to thromboembolic events, mostly after surgery and during inferior petrosal sinus sampling. Before introduction of anticoagulant prophylaxis, 10% of CD patients died due to thromboembolism and 10% had vascular morbidity. Since the introduction of prophylaxis, however, morbidity and mortality due to thromboembolic events were reduced to 6 and 0.4% respectively [104]. However, prophylaxis is not routinely applied in all centers. There is a clear need for guidelines on the dose and duration of thromboprophylaxis in patients with CD, both in the pre- and postoperative phases.
- **Impaired immune defense mechanisms with increased rate of infections:**
  Another complication of Cushing's disease is opportunistic or bacterial infections. Immunosuppression resulting from corticosteroid excess is usually thought of as a cellular immune deficiency [105] that increases the risk of opportunistic infections. Recent studies have also demonstrated the effect of glucocorticoids on the humoral immune system [106, 107]. By inhibiting activation of nuclear factor-κB, glucocorticoids interfere with a number of cytokines including interleukin-6, which plays an integral role in mounting the response to bacterial infections [108].
- **Gonadal dysfunction and hyperandrogenism manifesting with hirsutism (more frequently on the face), menstrual irregularity (oligomenorrhea, amenorrhea) and decreased libido:**
  Hirsutism and acne are commonly found in females because of ACTH-mediated androgen excess. Hypogonadism is the result of a direct inhibitory effect of cortisol upon GnRH pulsatility and LH/FSH secretion and is reversible upon correction of the hypercortisolism [109, 110].
- **Mild to severe psychic disturbances (anxiety, depression, irritability):**
  Studies show that 54-81% of patients with CD meet Diagnostic Statistics Manual (DSM) criteria for major depressive disorder or generalized anxiety disorder [111-113]. Despite remission, many patients exhibit residual symptoms in the first postoperative year or longer [114, 115, 116]. Cognitive deficits were reported in several studies [117, 118] and ranged in severity from mild (29%) to moderate/severe (34%), when English language and other language study results were compared [118]. Mental disturbances can be associated with structural modification of the brain, namely, atrophy of specific cerebral areas. The normalization of cortisol secretion following remission has been demonstrated to reverse cerebral atrophy, at

least partially [119]. Forget et al. found persistent cognitive impairment among CD patients in remission, which suggests that prolonged exposure to high levels of glucocorticoids can cause chronic deleterious effects to the cognitive function [120].

- **Other non-specific biological characteristics include hypokalemia, increased hemoglobin, increased numbers of neutrophils and decreased numbers of lymphocytes or eosinophils** [121]:
  Especially eosinopenia serves as biochemical co-marker for the diagnosis of Cushing's disease. Hypokalemia is not as common in CD as in case of ectopic Cushing's syndrome or adrenal carcinomas, where excess cortisol binds to both glucocorticoid and mineralcorticoid receptors, despite its lower affinity for the latter.
- **Mortality:**
  Overall mortality rates in patients with Cushing's disease reported as standardized mortality ratio range from 1.7 to 4.8 [122-124]. Among all systemic consequences of hypercortisolism, cardiovascular complications are the most deleterious ones, as these are among the leading causes of death in patients with CD [80, 122]. Cardiovascular risk is increased in CD due to complications such as hypertension, atherosclerosis, hypercoagulability, obesity, diabetes, and dyslipidemia, which are all consequences of chronic cortisol hypersecretion [104, 125]. In addition, CD is associated with left ventricular hypertrophy and diastolic dysfunction [126]. Elevated cardiovascular risk may persist even after remission [86, 127], suggesting that hypercortisolism and the length of exposure to hypercortisolism is associated with increased mortality. As a result there is a significant impact on HRQoL in patients with CD mediated through physical and psychological features and social and role-functioning impairments [128, 129].

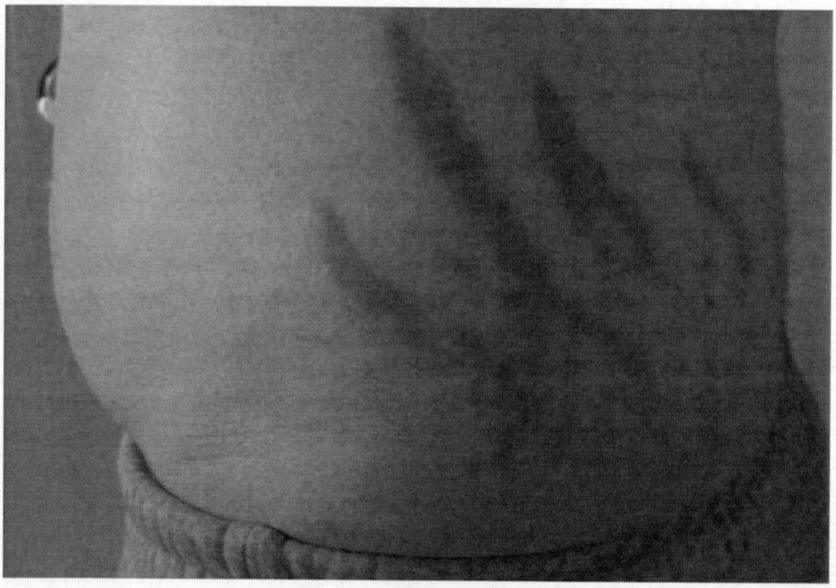

Figure 2. Abdominal purple striae in a male patient with Cushing's disease. Courtesy of Dr. Tsagarakis.

4. Cyclic Cushing's Syndrome (CS)

Cyclic CS is a disorder in which rhythmic fluctuations in ACTH secretion result in a more or less predictable cyclic variation in adrenal steroid production and a clinical course of intermittent, cyclic or periodic symptoms of hypercortisolism. The most frequent causes of cyclic CS are associated with ACTH-secreting pituitary adenoma [130-133], but it has also been reported in association with a well-differentiated neuroendocrine tumor (typical bronchial carcinoid) and malignant carcinoid tumor of the lung [134, 135], oncocytic carcinoid of the kidney [136], bronchial adenoma [137], ectopic ACTH secretion by a pheochromocytoma [138], adrenal adenoma [139] and rare forms of the pigmented variant of micronodular adrenocortical hyperplasia (primary pigmented nodular adrenocortical disease (PPNAD) [140-142]. Patients usually present with episodes of biochemical and clinical remission alternating with periods of frank Cushing's disease, characterized by circadian hyper-pulsatile ACTH and cortisol secretion. The cycles can also vary, lasting from a few hours to 85 days [130], sometimes with long disease-free intervals [143]. Evaluation during such intervals may indicate a normal pituitary function, so the syndrome may be suspected particularly in patients with signs of CS but normal cortisol levels, or with paradoxical responses to dexamethasone suppression tests [144, 145]. It has been suggested that rhythmic fluctuations in ACTH secretion may also be due to a cyclic change in central dopaminergic tone, which is partially responsible for triggering periodic ACTH secretion [146, 147], resulting in temporary damage to actively secreting cells, or the synchronous growth and death of ACTH-secreting tumor cells. Finally, it has been suggested that a serotoninergic influence may somehow be involved in the pathogenesis of cyclic CS, but this hypothesis needs to be confirmed [148].

5. Silent Corticotroph Adenomas (SCAS)

This term refers to pituitary adenomas showing positive staining for adrenocorticotrophic hormone (ACTH) in immunohistochemical studies, but lacking either clinical or laboratory features of hypercortisolemia [149]. They account for 1.1-6% of surgically removed pituitary adenomas and for 17-22% of ACTH immunoreactive tumours [150-152]. Currently, two distinct pathologic subtypes of SCAs are recognized [153]. Macroscopically, both type 1 and type 2 SCAs are generally macroadenomas with variable invasion or compression of parasellar structures. This distinguishes them from typical Cushing's adenomas, which are mostly microadenomas at clinical presentation. Type 1 is densely granulated, basophilic on haematoxylin and eosin staining, periodic acid-Schiff (PAS)-positive, and shows strong ACTH expression by the majority of tumor cells. By contrast, the type 2 adenoma is generally chromophobic or weakly basophilic with scattered PAS-staining and reveals only patchy or faint ACTH-positivity by immunohistochemistry. In both SCA subtypes, ACTH is usually the only immunohistochemically detectable anterior pituitary hormone, although scant co-expression of prolactin has been reported [153]. As expected, Crooke's hyaline change in non-neoplastic corticotrophs, which is a reliable indicator of recent hypercortisolemia, is absent. The lack of manifestations of cortisol excess (despite the occasionally found elevated serum ACTH levels) has not been, as yet, conclusively elucidated, proposed scenarios include defective packaging of ACTH into secretary granules due to an inadequately developed Golgi complex, secretion of biologically inactive hormones, increased intracellular degradation of hormones and the presence of morphologically similar, but functionally different parent cell type, deriving from the pars intermedia that processes preopiomelanocortin (POMC) differently [154-156]. Notably, it has been shown that, in contrast to adenomas obtained from patients with Cushing's disease, which demonstrate strong positive pro-hormone convertase 1/3 immunoreactivity (the enzyme involved in the post-translational processing of POMC into ACTH), silent corticotroph adenomas exhibit very weak expression [157].

As it has been already mentioned above, these tumors are usually macroadenomas with suprasellar extension present in 87-100% of the cases [152, 153, 158, 159] and carvenous sinus invasion in 30-52% [153, 158, 159]. Thus, SCAs present with local mass effects such as headaches (98.3-70.4%), visual field defects (41.7-86.7%), cranial nerve palsies (7-18.5%) and hypopituitarism (26-33.3%), mainly manifesting as hypogonadism [152, 153, 159, 160]. Acute or subacute pituitary apoplexy has been described in 9-41.7% [152, 158, 159].

6. Nonfunctioning Pituitary Adenomas (NFPAS)

Nonfunctioning pituitary adenomas do not secrete biologically active pituitary hormones and represent approximately 30% of all pituitary tumors [161]. Besides glucoprotein hormones and/or their free α- and β- subunits, this group of tumors includes the null cell adenomas and oncocytomas [162]. According to Kovacs et al. due to the lack of hypersecretory endocrine signs and symptoms, the diagnosis of NFPA is often delayed and usually presented as a macroadenoma [163]. Clinical picture is often insidious and represented by endocrinological symptoms, such as hypopituitarism and prolactin hypersecretion, but also neurological symptoms due to mass effects, at initial diagnosis 5% of patients have visual field defects and 15% have some degree of pituitary dysfunction [164]. In specific, the most frequent clinical manifestations are amenorrhea or menstrual irregularities, erectile dysfunction/decreased libido, headaches, visual field defects, dizziness and fatigue or indisposition [166, 167]. Diagnosis is usually made during the fifth decade of life [165-167].

Because of the increased availability and use of magnetic resonance image (MRI) an increasing number of patients have been incidentally diagnosed as harboring a pituitary adenoma [168, 169]. One third of them shows significant tumor growth on serial imaging, thus regular clinical and radiological follow-up is mandatory [170, 171].

7. TSH-Secreting Adenomas

TSH-secreting pituitary adenomas account for less than 2% of pituitary tumors with an incidence of one case per million [172]. The vast majority of these tumors secrete TSH alone, though it is often accompanied by imbalanced hypersecretion of a-GSU. Mixed adenomas are found in about one-fourth of TSH-omas and they are characterized by concomitant hypersecretion of other anterior pituitary hormones, mainly growth hormone (GH) or prolactin (PRL), which are known to share common transcription factors, such as PROP-1,

Pit-1 and HESX-1 [173, 174]. Indeed, hypersecretion of TSH and GH is the most frequent association (16%), followed by hypersecretion of TSH and PRL (10.4%) and seldom TSH and gonadotropins. The molecular mechanisms leading to the formation of TSHomas are presently unknown, it has been suggested that TSH-secreting adenomas derive from the clonal expansion of a single initially transformed cell followed by secondary mutations or alterations favouring tumor progression [175]. Similarly to other pituitary adenomas, no mutations in oncogenes commonly activated in human cancer, particularly *Ras*, have been reported in TSHomas. In contrast to GH-secreting adenomas, in which the oncogene *gsp* is present in about 40% of cases, none of the screened TSHomas has been shown to express activating mutations of genes encoding for G-protein alpha subunits, such as alpha s, alpha q, alpha 11, or for TRH receptor [176]. Recent data suggest that somatic mutations of TRb may be responsible for the defect in negative regulation of TSH secretion in some TSHomas [177]. Finally, it has recently been demonstrated that knock-in mutant mice harboring a mutation in the TRb gene spontaneously develop TSHomas and that aberrant pituitary growth is due to the activation of phosphatidylinositol 3-kinase signaling [178]. This entity is characterized by autonomous, inappropriate TSH-secretion refractory to the negative feedback mechanism of thyroid hormones i.e., "central hyperthyroidism" [179-182]. The presence of goitre is the rule even in previously thyroidectomised patients, since thyroid residue may re-grow as a consequence of TSH hyperstimulation. Occurrence of uni- or multi-nodular goitre is frequent (about 70% of reported cases), whereas differentiated thyroid carcinomas were documented in a few cases [183, 184]. Progression towards toxic goitre is very infrequent [185]. In contrast to Graves' disease, the occurrence of circulating anti-thyroid auto-antibodies is similar to that found in the general population, being about 8%. Bilateral exophthalmos occurred in a few patients, who subsequently developed autoimmune thyroiditis, while unilateral exophthalmos due to orbital invasion by pituitary tumor has rarely been reported [179, 186]. Disorders of the gonadal axis are frequent, menstrual disorders are present in all females with mixed TSH/PRL tumors and in one-third of those with pure TSHoma. Central hypogonadism, delayed puberty and decreased libido were also found in a number of males with TSHomas and/or mixed TSH/FSH adenomas. Most patients have a long history of thyroid dysfunction, frequently misdiagnosed as Graves' disease, and about 30% of them had inappropriate thyroidectomy or radio-iodine thyroid ablation [172, 173]. As a result, the clinical appearance of hyperthyroidism may be sometimes overshadowed by neurological symptoms (headaches, visual field defects) due to compression on the surrounding anatomical structures by the pituitary tumor. Diagnostic evaluation reveals high levels of free thyroid hormones in the presence of measurable (normal or high) TSH levels [179]. TSH-secreting pituitary adenomas share the same biochemical profile with resistance to thyroid hormone action (RTH), although the main difference is the presence of signs and symptoms of hyperthyroidism in patients with TSHoma, while RTH patients are in general euthyroid (the so-called generalised RTH, GRTH). However, in a minority of RTH patients, features of hyperthyroidism may be present involving some organs and not others, for example, heart (tachycardia) and brain (nervousness, insomnia, attention deficit, hyperactivity). T3 suppression test and TRH test are useful in the differential diagnosis between TSHomas and syndromes of thyroid hormone resistance [172].

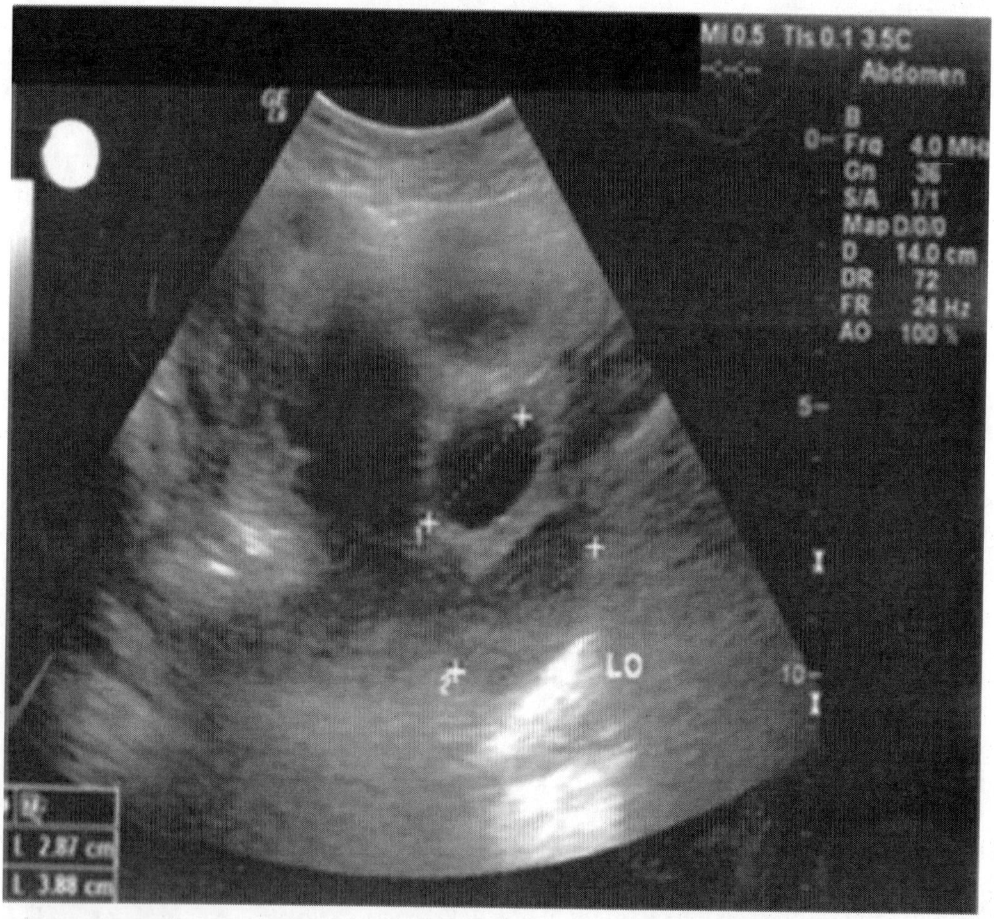

Figure 3. Pelvic ultrasound: ovarian hyperstimulation syndrome due to functional gonadotroph adenoma. Courtesy of Dr. Tsagarakis.

8. Functioning Gonadotroph Adenomas (FGAS)

Although, most immunohistochemically positive gonadotroph adenomas are hormonally silent, very few have been reported to express and secrete biologically active gonadotropins, causing distinct clinical manifestations (mainly menstrual irregularity and ovarian hyperstimulation syndrome in premenopausal females and adolescent girls, testicular enlargement in males, and isosexual precocious puberty in children) [187]. Several mechanisms for excess production and secretion of gonadotropins leading to a distinct clinical syndrome have been proposed, among them the prevailing theory is that functioning gonadotroph adenomas produce intact and biologically active FSH with an increased bioactivity to immunoreactivity ratio [188-190]. Another possible explanation is that the degree of glycosylation of the gonadotropins affects their biological activity, and the secretion of glycosylated variants with increased biological activity cannot be excluded. Presenting clinical features vary according to sex and age at diagnosis.

Many reports involve premenopausal women presenting with menstrual irregularities (oligo-/amenorrhea, spotting-menorrhagia), infertility, galactorrhea, mass effects (headaches, visual deterioration) and ovarian hyperstimulation syndrome. This latter syndrome is usually mild, with the enlarged ovaries increasing abdominal girth and causing pain and discomfort of varying severity due to irritation of the peritoneum [191-214]. Acute abdomen attributed to multiple ovarian cysts causing bilateral adnexal torsion has also been reported [215]. Hyper-estrogenism is a characteristic biochemical finding, although in a few cases estrogen levels have been found normal or fluctuating. Serum FSH is within reference range or mildly elevated, serum LH is suppressed or within reference range and serum α-subunit and inhibin normal or elevated [187]. Pelvic imaging demonstrates multiseptated cysts of variable size (often larger than 5cm) (Figure 3) [216]. Most of the reported FGAs in premenopausal women are macroadenomas, often showing a suprasellar extension, invading into the cavernous sinus, and abutting the optic chiasm, although few cases of microadenomas have been also described [202, 206, 211, 217, 218]. In postmenopausal women no clinical syndrome has been demonstrated because the ovaries are depleted of pre-antral follicles and are insensitive to FSH stimulation [219]. FSH hypersecretion by a FGA in males can lead to testicular enlargement due to the trophic effect to the testicles, leading to increased length of the seminiferous tubules [220]. FSH levels have been found elevated in all cases [189, 220-222]. whereas LH and testosterone have been reported as slightly below the reference range, normal, or elevated [189-222]. All published cases in adult males involve macroadenomas, some of which had significant suprasellar and parasellar extension [189, 220-223]. A microadenoma has been described only in an adolescent male [224]. Gonadotroph-secreting pituitary adenomas are quite rare in childhood and present with isosexual precocious puberty and mass effects [225-228]. Serum FSH is usually elevated, serum LH low or elevated, and estradiol/testosterone elevated.

REFERENCES

[1] Sanno, N, Teramoto, A, Osamura, RY, Horvath, E, Kovacs, K, Lloyd, RV, et al. Pathology of pituitary tumors. *Neurosurg Clin N Am*, 2003;14:25-39.

[2] Asa, SL, Ezzat, S. Genetics and proteomics of pituitary tumors. *Endocrine*, 2005;28: 43-7.

[3] Landis, CA, Masters, SB, Spada, A, Pace, AM, Bourne, HR, Vallar, L. GTPase inhibiting mutations activate the alpha chain of Gs and stimulate adenylyl cyclase in human pituitary tumours. *Nature*, 1989;340:692-696.

[4] Zhang, X, Sun, H, Danila, DC, Johnson, SR, Zhou, Y, Swearingen, B, et al. Loss of expression of GADD45 gamma, a growth inhibitory gene, in human pituitary adenomas: implications for tumorigenesis. *J Clin Endocrinol Metab*, 2002;87:1262-1267.

[5] Heaney, AP, Horwitz, GA, Wang, Z, Singson, R, Melmed, S. Early involvement of estrogen-induced pituitary tumor transforming gene and fibroblast growth factor expression in prolactinoma pathogenesis. *Nat Med*, 1999;5:1317-1321.

[6] Al-Shraim, M, Asa, SL. The 2004 World Health Organization classification of pituitary tumors: what is new? *Acta Neuropathol* (Berl), 2006;111:1-7.

[7] Maheshwari, HG, Prezant, TR, Herman-Bonert, V, Shahinian, H, Kovacs, K, Melmed, S. Long-acting peptidomimergic control of gigantism caused by pituitary acidophilic stem cell adenoma. *J Clin Endocrinol Metab*, 2000;85:3409-3416.

[8] Tahara, S, Kurotani, R, Ishii, Y, Sanno, N, Teramoto, A, Osamura, RY. A case of Cushing's disease caused by pituitary adenoma producing adrenocorticotropic hormone and growth hormone concomitantly: aberrant expression of transcription factors Neuro-D1 and pit-1 as proposed mechanism. *Mol Pathol*, 2002;15:1102-1105.

[9] Sakharova, AA, Dimaraki, EV, Chandler, WF, Barkan, AL. Clinically silent somatotropinomas may be biochemically active. *J Clin Endocrinol Metab*, 2005;90:2117-2121.

[10] Beckers, A, Lodish, MB, Trivellin, G, Rostomyan, L, Lee, M, Faucz, FR, et al. X-linked acrogigantism syndrome: clinical profile and therapeutic responses. *Endocr Relat Cancer*, 2015;22:353-367.

[11] Dady, AF, Vanbellinghen, JF, Khoo, SK, Jaffrain-Rea, ML, Naves, LA, Guitelman, MA, et al. Aryl Hydrocarbon Receptor-Interacting Protein Gene Mutations in Familial Isolated Pituitary Adenomas: Analysis in 73 Families. *J Clin Endocrinol Metab*, 2007;92:1891-1896.

[12] Agarwal, SK, Lee Burns, A, Sukhodolets, KE, Kennedy, PA, Obungu, VH, Hickman, AB, et al. Molecular pathology of the MEN1 gene. *Ann NY Acad Sci*, 2004;1014:189-198.

[13] Verges, B, Boureille, F, Goudet, P, Murat, A, Beckers, A, Sassolas, G, et al. Pituitary disease in MEN type 1 (MEN1), data from the France-Belgium MEN1 multicenter study. *J Clin Endocrinol Metab*, 2002;87:457-465.

[14] Stratakis, CA, Matyakhina, L, Courkoutsakis, N, Patronas, N, Voutetakis, A, Stergiopoulos, S, et al. Pathology and molecular genetics of the pituitary gland in patients with the "complex of spotty skin pigmentation, myxomas, endocrine overactivity and schwannomas" (Carney complex). *Front Horm Res*, 2004;32:253-264.

[15] Clayton, RN. Cardiovascular function in acromegaly. *Endocr Rev*, 2003;24:272-277.

[16] Colao, A, Ferone, D, Marzullo, P, Lombardi, G. Systemic complications of acromegaly: epidemiology, pathogenesis, and management. *Endocr Rev*, 2004;25:102-152.

[17] Holdaway, IM, Rajasoorya, C. Epidemiology of acromegaly. *Pituitary*, 1999;2:29-41.

[18] Ezzat, S, Forster, MJ, Berchtold, P, Redelmeier, DA, Boerlin, V, Harris, AG. Acromegaly: clinical and biochemical features in 500 patients. *Medicine* (Baltimore), 1994;73:233-240.

[19] Molitch, ME. Clinical manifestations of acromegaly. *Endocrinol Metab Clin North Am*, 1992;21:597-614.

[20] Nabarro, JD. Acromegaly. *Clin Endocrinol* (Oxf), 1987;26:481-512.

[21] Swearingen, B, Barker, FG, 2nd, Katznelson, L, Biller, BM, Grinspoon, S, Klibanski, A, et al. Long-term mortality after transsphenoidal surgery and adjunctive therapy for acromegaly. *J Clin Endocrinol Metab*, 1998;83:3419-3426.

[22] Rajasoorya, C, Holdaway, IM, *Wrightson*, P, Scott, DJ, Ibbertson, HK. Determinants of clinical outcome and survival in acromegaly. *Clin Endocrinol* (Oxf), 1994;41:95-102.

[23] Levy, MJ, Matharu, M, Goadsby, PJ. Chronic headache and pituitary tumors. *Curr Pain Headache Rep*, 2008;12:74-78.

[24] Melmed, S. Medical progress: acromegaly. *N Engl J Med*, 2006;355:2558-2573.

[25] Katznelson, L, Kleinberg, D, Vance, ML, Stavrou, S, Pulaski, KJ, Schoenfeld, DA, et al. Hypogonadism in patients with acromegaly: data from the multi-centre acromegaly registry pilot study. *Clin Endocrinol* (Oxf), 2001;54:183-188.

[26] Grynberg, M, Salenave, S, Young, J, Chanson, P. Female gonadal function before and after treatment of acromegaly. *J Clin Endocrinol Metab*, 2010;95:4518-4525.

[27] Corrigan, DF, Wartofsky, L, Dimond, RC, Schaaf, M, Earll, JM, Rogers, JE, et al. Parameters of thyroid function in patients with active acromegaly. *Metabolism*, 1978;27:209-216.

[28] Geelhoed-Duijvestijn, PH, Bussemaker, JK, Roelfsema, F. Changes in basal and stimulated TSH and other parameters of thyroid function in acromegaly after transsphenoidal surgery. *Acta Endocrinol* (Copenh), 1989;121:207-215.

[29] Gordon, DA, Hill, FM, Ezrin, C. Acromegaly: a review of 100 cases. *Can Med Assoc J*, 1962;87:1106-1109.

[30] Kanis, JA, Gillingham, FJ, Harris, P, Horn, DB, Hunter, WM, Redpath, AT, et al. Clinical and laboratory study of acromegaly: assessment before and one year after treatment. *Q J Med*, 1974;43:409-431.

[31] Skorić, T, Korsić, M, Zarković, K, Plavsić, V, Besenski, N, Breskovac, L, et al. Clinical and mor-phological features of undifferentiated monomorphous GH/TSH-secreting pituitary adenoma. *Eur J Endocrinol*, 1999;140:528-537.

[32] Wémeau, JL, Dewailly, D, Leroy, R, D'Herbomez, M, Mazzuca, M, Decoulx, M, et al. Long term treatment with the somatostatin analog SMS 201-995 in a patient with a thyrotropin- and growth hormone-secreting pituitary adenoma. *J Clin Endocrinol Metab*, 1988;66:636-639.

[33] Nabarro, JD. Acromegaly. *Clin Endocrinol* (Oxf), 1987;26:481-512.

[34] Matsuoka, LY, Wortsman, J, Kupchella, CE, Eng, A, Dietrich, JE. Histochemical characterization of the cutaneous involvement of acromegaly. *Arch Intern Med*, 1982;142:1820-1823.

[35] Jadresic, A, Banks, LM, Child, DF, Diamant, L, Doyle, FH, Fraser, Tr, et al. The acromegaly syndrome: relation between clinical features, growth hormone values and radiological characteristics of the pituitary tumours. *Q J Med*, 1982;51:189-204.

[36] Jenkins, PJ, Sohaib, SA, Akker, S, Phillips, RR, Spillane, K, Wass, JA, et al. The pathology of median neuropathy in acromegaly. *Ann Intern Med*, 2000;133:197-201.

[37] Baum, H, Lüdecke, DK, Herrmann, HD. Carpal tunnel syndrome and acromegaly. *Acta Neurochir* (Wien), 1986;83:54-55.

[38] Lieberman, SA, Bjorkengren, AG, Hoffman, AR. Rheumatologic and skeletal changes in acromegaly. *Endocrinol Metab Clin North Am*, 1992;21:615-631.

[39] Colao, A, Cannavo, S, Marzullo, P, Pivonello, R, Squadrito, S, Vallone, G, et al. Twelve months of treatment with octreotide- LAR reduces joint thickness in acromegaly. *Eur J Endocrinol*, 2003;148:31-38.

[40] Bonadonna, S, Mazziotti, G, Nuzzo, M, Bianchi, A, Fusco, A, De Marinis, L, et al., Increased prevalence of radiological spinal deformities in active acromegaly: a cross-sectional study in postmenopausal women. *J Bone Miner Res*, 2005;20:1837-1844.

[41] Biermasz, NR, Pereira, AM, Smit, JW, Romijn, JA, Roelfsema, F. Morbidity after long-term remission for acromegaly: persisting joint-related complaints cause reduced quality of life. *J Clin Endocrinol Metab*, 2005;90:2731-2739.

[42] Lesse, GP, Fraser, WD, Farquharson, R, Hipkin, L, Vora, JP. Gonadal status is an important determinant of bone density in acromegaly. *Clin Endocrinol* (Oxf), 1998;48:59-65.

[43] Scillitani, A, Battista, C, Chiodini, I, Salcuni, AS, Eller-Vainicher, C, Viti, R, et al. Bone mineral density in acromegaly: the effect of gender, disease activity and gonadal status. *Clin Endocrinol* (Oxf), 2003;58:725-731.

[44] Lund, B, Eskildsen, PC, Lund, B, Norman, AW, Sørensen, OH. Calcium and vitamin D metabolism in acromegaly. *Acta Endocrinol* (Copenh), 1981;96:444-450.

[45] Giustina, A, Boni, E, Romanelli, G, Grassi, V, Giustina, G. Cardiopulmonary performance during exercise in acromegaly, and the effects of acute suppression of growth hormone hypersecretion with octreotide. *Am J Cardiol*, 1995;75:1042-1047.

[46] Colao, A, Pivonello, R, Grasso, LF, Auriemma, F, Galdiero, M, Savastano, S, et al. Determinants of cardiac disease in newly diagnosed patients with acromegaly. *Eur J Endocrinol*, 2011;165:713-721.

[47] Pereira, AM, van Thiel, SW, Lindner, JR, Roelsema, F, van der Wall, EE, Morreau, H, et al., Increased prevalence of regurgitant valvular heart disease in acromegaly. *J Clin Endocrinol Metab*, 2004;89:71-75.

[48] Attal, P, Chanson, P. Endocrine aspects of obstructive sleep apnea. *J Clin Endocrinol Metab*, 2010;95:483-495.

[49] Mestron, A, Webb, SM, Astorga, R, Benito, P, Catala, M, Gaztambide, S, et al. Epidemiology, clinical characteristics, outcome, morbidity and mortality in acromegaly based on the Spanish Acromegaly Registry (Registro Espanol de Acromegalia, REA). *Eur J Endocrinol*, 2004;151:439-446.

[50] Biering, H, Knappe, G, Gerl, H, Lochs, H. Prevalence of diabetes in acromegaly and Cushing syndrome [in German]. *Acta Med Austriaca*, 2000;27:27-31.

[51] Kasayama, S, Otsuki, M, Takagi, M, Saito, H, Sumitani, S, Kouhara, H, et al. Impaired beta-cell function in the presence of reduced insulin sensitivity determines glucose tolerance status in acromegalic patients. *Clin Endocrinol* (Oxf), 2000;52:549-555.

[52] Luger, A, Prager, R, Gaube, S, Graf, H, Klauser, R, Schernthaner, G. Decreased peripheral insulin sensitivity in acromegalic patients. *Exp Clin Endocrinol*, 1990;95:339-343.

[53] Ho, KK, Jenkins, AB, Furler, SM, Borkman, M, Chisholm, DJ. Impact of octreotide, a long-acting somatostatin analogue, on glucose tolerance and insulin sensitivity in acromegaly. *Clin Endocrinol* (Oxf), 1992;36:271-279.

[54] Rieu, M, Girard, F, Bricaire, H, Binoux, M. The importance of insulin-like growth factor (somatomedin) measurements in the diagnosis and surveillance of acromegaly. *J Clin Endocrinol Metab*, 1982;55:147-153.

[55] Sonksen, PH, Greenwood, FC, Ellis, JP, Lowy, C, Rutherford, A, Nabarro, JD. Changes of carbohydrate tolerance in acromegaly with progress of the disease and in response to treatment. *J Clin Endocrinol Metab*, 1967;27:1418-1430.

[56] Wasada, T, Aoki, K, Sato, A, Katsumori, K, Muto, K, Tomonaga, O, Yokoyama, H, Iwasaki, N, Babazono, T, Takahashi, C, Iwamoto, Y, Omori, Y, Hizuka, N. Assessment of insulin resistance in acromegaly associated with diabetes mellitus before and after transsphenoidal adenomectomy. *Endocr J*, 1997;44:617-620.

[57] Breidert, M, Pinzer, T, Wildbrett, J, Bornstein, SR, Hanefeld, M. Long-term effect of octreotide in acromegaly on insulin resistance. *Horm Metab Res*, 1995;27:226-230.

[58] van der Lely, AJ, Hutson, RK, Trainer, PJ, Besser, GM, Barkan, AL, Katznelson, L, Klibanski, A, Herman-Bonert, V, Melmed, S, Vance, ML, Freda, PU, Stewart, PM, Friend, KE, Clemmons, DR, Johannsson, G, Stavrou, S, Cook, DM, Phillips, LS, Strasburger, CJ, Hackett, S, Zib, KA, Davis, RJ, Scarlett, JA, Thorner, MO. Long-term treatment of acromegaly with pegvisomant, a growth hormone receptor antagonist. *Lancet*, 2001;358:1754-1759.

[59] Rose, DR, Clemmons, DR. Growth hormone receptor antagonist improves insulin resistance in acromegaly. *Growth Horm IGF Res*, 2002;12:418-424.

[60] Rosenow, F, Reuter, S, Deuss, U, Szelies, B, Hilgers, RD, Winkelmann, W, et al. Sleep apnoea in treated acromegaly: relative frequency and predisposing factors. *Clin Endocrinol* (Oxf), 1996;45:563-569.

[61] Grunstein, RR, Ho, KK, Sullivan, CE. Effect of octreotide, a somatostatin analog, on sleep apnea in patients with acromegaly. *Ann Intern Med*, 1994;121:478-483.

[62] Orme, S, McNally, RJ, Cartwright, RA, Belchetz, PE. Mortality and cancer incidence in acromegaly: a retrospective cohort study. *J Clin Endocrinol Metab*, 1998;83:2730-2734.

[63] Renehan, AG, Shalet, SM. Acromegaly and colorectal cancer: risk assessment should be based on population-based studies. *J Clin Endocrinol Metab*, 2002;87:1909.

[64] Cats, A, Dullaart, RP, Kleibeuker, JH, Kuipers, F, Sluiter, WJ, Hardonk, MJ, et al. Increased epithelial cell proliferation in the colon of patients with acromegaly. *Cancer Res*, 1996;56:523-526.

[65] Holdaway, IM, Rajasoorya, RC, Gamble, GD. Factors influencing mortality in acromegaly. *J Clin Endocrinol Metab*, 2004;89:667-674.

[66] Kauppinen-Makelin, R, Sane, T, Reunanen, A, Välimäki, MJ, Niskanen, L, Markkanen, H, et al., A nationwide survey of mortality in acromegaly. *J Clin Endocrinol Metab*, 2005;90:4081-4086.

[67] Biermasz, NR, Dekker, FW, Pereira, AM, van Thiel, Sw, Schutte, PJ, van Dulken, H, et al., Determinants of survival in treated acromegaly in a single center: predictive value of serial insulin-like growth factor I measurements. *J Clin Endocrinol Metab*, 2004;89:2789-2796.

[68] Ayuk, J, Clayton, RN, Holder, G, Sheppard, MC, Stewart, PM, Bates, AS. Growth hormone and pituitary radiotherapy, but not serum insulin-like growth factor-I concentrations, predict excess mortality in patients with acromegaly. *J Clin Endocrinol Metab*, 2004;89:1613-1617.

[69] Webb, SM, Prieto, L, Badia, X, Albareda, M, Catala, M, Gaztambide, S, et al. Acromegaly Quality of Life Questionnaire (ACROQOL) a new health-related quality of life questionnaire for patients with acromegaly: development and psychometric properties. *Clin Endocrinol* (Oxf), 2002;57:251-258.

[70] Biermasz, NR, van Thiel, SW, Pereira, AM, Hoftijzer, HC, van Hemert, AM, Smit, JW, Romijn, JA, Roelfsema, F. Decreased Quality of Life in Patients with Acromegaly Despite Long-Term Cure of Growth Hormone Excess. *J Clin Endocrinol Metab*, 2004;89:5369-5376.

[71] Webster, J, Scanlon, MF. Prolactinomas. In Sheaves R, Jenkins PJ, Wass JA, (editors): Clinical Endocrine Oncology. Blackwell Science, Oxford, 1997;189-194.

[72] Barkan, AL, Chandler, WF. Giant pituitary prolactinoma with falsely low serum prolactin: the pitfall of the "high-dose hook effect": case report. *Neurosurgery*, 1998;42:913-916.

[73] Bevan, JS, Webster, J, Burke, CW, Scanlon, MF. Dopamine agonists and pituitary tumor shrinkage. *Endocr Rev*, 1992;13:220-240.

[74] Klibanski, A, Neer, RM, Beitins, IZ, Ridgway, EC, Zervas, NT, McArthur, JW. Decreased bone density in hyperprolactinemic women. *N Engl J Med*, 1980;303:1511-1514.

[75] Schlechte, J, el-Khoury, G, Kathol, M, Walkner, L. Forearm and vertebral bone mineral in treated and untreated hyperprolactinemic amenorrhea. *J Clin Endocrinol Metab*, 1987;64:1021-1026.

[76] Biller, BM, Baum, HB, Rosenthal, DI, Saxe, VC, Charpie, PM, Klibanski, A. Progressive trabecular osteopenia in women with hyperprolactinemic amenorrhea. *J Clin Endocrinol Metab*, 1992;75:692-697.

[77] Klibanski, A, Biller, BM, Rosenthal, DI, Schoenfeld, DA, Saxe, V. Effects of prolactin and estrogen deficiency in amenorrheic bone loss. *J Clin Endocrinol Metab*, 1988;67:124-130.

[78] Biller, BM. Hyperprolactinemia. *Int J Fertil Womens Med*, 1999;44:74-77.

[79] Luciano, AA. Clinical presentation of hyperprolactinemia. *J Reprod Med*, 1999;44(Suppl 12):1085-1090.

[80] Etxabe, J, Vazquez, JA. Morbidity and mortality in Cushing's disease: an epidemiological approach. *Clin Endocrinol* (Oxf), 1994;40:479-484.

[81] Lindholm, J, Juul, S, Jorgensen, JO, Astrup, J, Bjerre, P, Feldt-Rasmussen, U, et al. Incidence and late prognosis of Cushing's syndrome: a population-based study. *J Clin Endocrinol Metab*, 2001;86:117-123.

[82] Meinardi, JR, Wolffenbuttel, BH, Dullaart, RP. Cyclic Cushing's syndrome: a clinical challenge. *Eur J Endocrinol*, 2007;157:245-254.

[83] Valassi, E, Santos, A, Yaneva, M, Toth, M, Strasburger, CJ, Chanson, P, et al. The European Registry on Cushing's syndrome: 2-year experience. Baseline demographic and clinical characteristics. *Eur J Endocrinol*, 2011;165:383-392.

[84] Feelders, RA, Pulgar, SJ, Kempel, A. Significant burden of illness in patients with Cushing's disease. 12th International Pituitary Congress. Boston, MA, USA, 1-3 June, 2011 abst 41. Data from CDC statistics and NHANES III (2005-2006). 2011. Available at: http://www.cdc.gov/nchs/nhanes.htm.

[85] Faggiano, A, Pivonello, R, Spiezia, S, De Martino, MC, Filippella, M, di Somma, C, et al. Cardiovascular risk factors and common carotid artery caliber and stiffness in patients with Cushing's disease during active disease and 1 year after disease remission. *J Clin Endocrinol Metab*, 2003;88:2527-2533.

[86] Mancini, T, Kola, B, Mantero, F, Boscaro, M, Arnaldi, G. High cardiovascular risk in patients with Cushing's syndrome according to 1999 WHO/ISH guidelines. *Clin Endocrinol* (Oxf), 2004;61:768-777.

[87] Tauchmanova, L, Rossi, R, Biondi, B, Pulcrano, M, Nuzzo, V, Palmieri, EA, et al. Patients with subclinical Cushing's syndrome due to adrenal adenoma have increased cardiovascular risk. *J Clin Endocrinol Metab*, 2002;87:4872-4878.

[88] Colao, A, Pivonello, R, Spiezia, S, Faggiano, A, Ferone, D, Filippella, M, et al. Persistence of increased cardiovascular risk in patients with Cushing's disease after five years of successful cure. *J Clin Endocrinol Metab*, 1999;84:2664-2672.
[89] Barahona, MJ, Sucunza, N, Resmini, E, Fernandez-Real, JM, Ricart, W, Moreno-Navarrete, JM, et al. Deleterious effects of glucocorticoid replacement on bone in women after long-term remission of Cushing's syndrome. *J Bone Min Res*, 2009;24: 1841-1846.
[90] Colao, A, Pivonello, R, Spiezia, S, Faggiano, A, Ferone, D, Filippella, M, et al. Persistence of increased cardiovascular risk in patients with Cushing's disease after five years of successful cure. *J Clin Endocrinol Metab*, 1999;84:2664-2672.
[91] Barahona, MJ, Sucunza, N, Resmini, E, Fernandez-Real, JM, Ricart, W, Moreno-Navarrete, JM, et al. Persistent body fat mass and inflammatory marker increases after long-term cure of Cushing's syndrome. *J Clin Endocrinol Metab*, 2009;94:3365-3371.
[92] Terzolo, M, Pia, A, Ali, A, Osella, G, Reimondo, G, Bovio, S, et al. Adrenal incidentaloma: a new cause of the metabolic syndrome? *J Clin Endocrinol Metab*, 2002;87:998-1003.
[93] Tauchmanova, L, Rossi, R, Biondi, B, Pulcrano, M, Nuzzo, V, Palmieri, EA, et al. Patients with subclinical Cushing's syndrome due to adrenal adenoma have increased cardiovascular risk. *J Clin Endocrinol Metab*, 2002;87:4872-4878.
[94] Greenman, Y. Management of dyslipidemia in Cushing's syndrome. *Neuroendocrinology*, 2010;92(Suppl 1):91-95.
[95] Pleasure, DE, Engel, WK. Atrophy of skeletal muscle in patients with Cushing's syndrome. *Arch Neurol*, 1970; 22:118-125.
[96] Kaltsas, G, Manetti, L, Grossman, AB. Osteoporosis in Cushing's syndrome. *Front Horm Res*, 2002;30:60-72.
[97] di Somma, C, Pivonello, R, Loche, S, Faggiano, A, Klain, M, Salvatore, M, et al. Effect of 2 years of cortisol normalization on the impaired bone mass and turnover in adolescent and adult patients with Cushing's disease, a prospective study. *Clin Endocrinol* (Oxf), 2003;58:302-308.
[98] Pecori Giraldi, F, Moro, M, Cavagnini, F. Gender-related differences in the presentation and course of Cushing's disease. *J Clin Endocrinol Metab*, 2003;88:1554-1558.
[99] Hermus, AR, Smals, AG, Swinkels, LM, Huysmans, DA, Pieters, GF, Sweep, CF, et al., Bone mineral density and bone turnover before and after surgical cure of Cushing's syndrome. *J Clin Endocrinol Metab*, 1995;80:2859-2865.
[100] Gennari, L, Bilezikian, JP. Glucocorticoid-induced osteoporosis: hope on the HORIZON. *Lancet*, 2009;373:1225-1226.
[101] di Somma, C, Colao, A, Pivonello, R, Klain, M, Faggiano, A, Tripodi, FS, et al. Effectiveness of chronic treatment with alendronate in the osteoporosis of Cushing's disease. *Clin Endocrinol* (Oxf), 1998;48:655-662.
[102] Fallo, F, Sonino, N, Barzon, L, Pistorello, M, Pagotto, U, Paoletta, A, et al. Effect of surgical treatment on hypertension in Cushing's syndrome. *Am J. Hypertension*, 1996;9:77-80.
[103] Fatti, LM, Bottasso, B, Invitti, C, Coppola, R, Cavagnini, F, Mannucci, PM. Markers of activation of coagulation and fibrinolysis in patients with Cushing's syndrome. *J Endocrinol Invest*, 2000;23:145-150.

[104] Boscaro, M, Sonino, N, Scarda, A, Barzon, L, Fallo, F, Sartori, MT, et al. Anticoagulant prophylaxis markedly reduces thromboembolic complications in Cushing's syndrome. *J Clin Endocrinol Metab*, 2002;87:3662-3666.

[105] Boumpas, DT, Paliogianni, F, Anastassiou, ED, Balow, JE. Glucocorticoid action on the immune system: molecular and cellular aspects. *Clin Exp Rheumatol*, 1991;9:413-423.

[106] Auphan, N, DiDonato, JA, Rosette, C, Helmberg, A, Karin, M. Immunosuppression by glucocorticoids: inhibition of NF-κβ activity through of induction of I kβ synthesis. *Science*, 1995;270:286-290.

[107] Scheinmen, RI, Cogswell, PC, Lofquist, AK, Baldwin, AS. Role of transcriptional activation of I k β alpha in mediation of immunosuppression by glucocorticoids. *Science*, 1995;270:283-286.

[108] Papanicolaou, DA, Wilder, RL, Manolagas, SC, Chrousos, GP. The pathophysiologic roles of interleukin-6 in human disease. *Ann Intern Med*, 1998;128:127-137.

[109] Luton, JP, Thieblot, P, Valcke, JC, Mahoudeau, JA, Bricaire, H. Reversible gonadotropin deficiency in male Cushing's disease. *J Clin Endocrinol Metab*, 1977;45:488-495.

[110] Lado Abeal, J, Rodriguez-Arnao, J, Newell-Price, JD, Perry, LA, Grossman, AB, Besser, GM, et al. Menstrual abnormalities in women with Cushing's disease are correlated with hypercortisolemia rather than raised circulating androgen levels. *J Clin Endocrinol Metab*, 1998;83:3083-3088.

[111] Sonino, N, Fava, GA, Raffi, AR, Boscaro, M, Fallo, F. Clinical correlates of major depression in Cushing's disease. *Psychopathol*, 1998, 31, 302-306.

[112] Hudson, JI, Hudson, MS, Griffing, GT, Melby, JC, Pope, HG. Jr. Phenomenology and family history of affective disorder in Cushing's disease. *Am J Psychiatry*, 1987;144:951-953.

[113] Loosen, PT, Chambliss, B, DeBold, CR, Shelton, R, Orth, DN. Psychiatric phenomenology in Cushing's disease. *Pharmacopsychiatry*, 1992;25:192-198.

[114] Sonino, N, Fava, GA, Boscaro, M. A role for life events in the pathogenesis of Cushing's disease. *Clin Endocrinol* (Oxf), 1993;38:261-264.

[115] Sonino, N, Fava, GA, Belluardo, P, Girelli, ME, Boscaro, M. Course of depression in Cushing's syndrome: response to treatment and comparison with Graves' disease. *Horm Res*, 1993;39:202-206.

[116] Starkman, MN, Schteingart, DE, Schork, MA. Cushing's syndrome after treatment: changes in cortisol and ACTH levels, and amelioration of the depressive syndrome. *Psychiatry Res*, 1986;19:177-188.

[117] Starkman, MN, Giordani, B, Berent, S, Schork, MA, Schteingart, DE. Elevated cortisol levels in Cushing's disease are associated with cognitive decrements. *Psychosom Med*, 2001;63:985-993.

[118] Whelan, TB, Schteingart, DE, Starkman, MN, Smith, A. Neuropsychological deficits in Cushing's syndrome. *J Nerv Mental Dis*, 1980;168:753-757.

[119] Bourdeau, I, Bard, C, Noel, B, Leclerc, I, Cordeau, MP, Belair, M, et al. Loss of brain volume in endogenous Cushing's syndrome and its reversibility after correction of hypercortisolism. *J Clin Endocrinol Metab*, 2002;87:1949-1954.

[120] Forget, H, Lacroix, A, Cohen, H. Persistent cognitive impairment following surgical treatment of Cushing's syndrome. *Psychoneuroendocrinology*, 2002;27:367-383.

[121] Castinetti, F, Morange, I, Conte-Devolx, B, Brue, T. Cushing's disease. *Orph J Rare Dis*, 2012, 7, 41-49.

[122] Dekkers, OM, Biermasz, NR, Pereira, AM, Roelfsema, F, van Aken, MO, Voormolen, JH, et al. Mortality in patients treated for Cushing's disease is increased, compared with patients treated for nonfunctioning pituitary macroadenoma. *J Clin Endocrinol Metab*, 2007;92: 976-981.

[123] Pikkarainen, L, Sane, T, Reunanen, A. The survival and wellbeing of patients treated for Cushing's syndrome. *J Int Med*, 1999;245:463-468.

[124] Lindholm, J, Juul, S, Jorgensen, JO, Astrup, J, Bjerre, P, Feldt-Rasmussen, U, et al., Incidence and late prognosis of Cushing's syndrome: a population-based study. *J Clin Endocrinol Metab*, 2001;86:117-123.

[125] Arnaldi, G, Angeli, A, Atkinson, AB, Bertagna, X, Cavagnini, F, Chrousos, GP, et al. Diagnosis and complications of Cushing's syndrome: a consensus statement. *J Clinical Endocrinol Metab*, 2003;88:5593-5602.

[126] Pereira, AM, Delgado, V, Romijn, JA, Smit, JW, Bax, JJ, Feelders, RA. Cardiac dysfunction is reversed upon successful treatment of Cushing's syndrome. *Eur J Endocrinol*, 2010;162:331-340.

[127] Colao, A, Pivonello, R, Spiezia, S, Faggiano, A, Ferone, D, Filippella, M, et al. Persistence of increased cardiovascular risk in patients with Cushing's disease after five years of successful cure. *J Clin Endocrinol Metab*, 1999;84:2664-2672.

[128] Webb, SM, Badia, X, Barahona, MJ, Colao, A, Strasburger, CJ, Tabarin, A, et al. Evaluation of health-related quality of life in patients with Cushing's syndrome with a new questionnaire. *Eur J Endocrinol*, 2008;158:623-630.

[129] Pikkarainen, L, Sane, T, Reunanen, A. The survival and wellbeing of patients treated for Cushing's syndrome. *J Int Med*, 1999;245:463-468.

[130] Shapiro, MS, Shenkman, L. Variable hormonogenesis in Cushing's syndrome. *Q J Med*, 1991;79:351-363.

[131] Bailey, RE. Periodic hormonogenesis: a new phenomenon. Periodicity in function of a hormone-producing tumor in man. *J Clin Endocrinol Metab*, 1971;32:317-327.

[132] Brown, RD, Van Loon, GR, Orth, DN, Liddle, GW. Cushing's disease with periodic hormonogenesis: one explanation for paradoxical response to dexamethasone. *J Clin Endocrinol Metab*, 1973;36:445-451.

[133] Liberman, B, Wajchenberg, BL, Tambascia, MA, Mesquita, CH. Periodic remission in Cushing's disease with paradoxical dexamethasone response: an expression of periodic hormonogenesis. *J Clin Endocrinol Metab*, 1976;43:913-918.

[134] Arnaldi, G, Mancini, T, Kola, B, Appolloni, G, Freddi, S, Concettoni, C, et al., Cyclical Cushing's syndrome in a patient with a bronchial neuroendocrine tumor (typical carcinoid) expressing ghrelin and growth hormone secretagogue receptors. *J Clin Endocrinol Metab*, 2003;88:5834-5840.

[135] Chajek, T, Romanoff, H. Cushing syndrome with cyclical edema and periodic secretion of corticosteroids. *Arch Intern Med*, 1976;136:441-443.

[136] Hannah, J, Lippe, B, Lai-Goldman, M, Bhuta, S. Oncocytic carcinoid of the kidney associated with periodic Cushing's syndrome. *Cancer*, 1988;61:2136-2140.

[137] Shapiro, MS, Gutman, A, Bruderman, I, Myers, B, Griffel, WB. Cushing's syndrome associated with a bronchial adenoma. Possible periodic hormonogenesis. *Isr J Med Sci*, 1975;11:919-924.

[138] Terzolo, M, Ali, A, Pia, A, Bollito, E, Reimondo, G, Paccotti, P, et al. Cyclic Cushing's syndrome due to ectopic ACTH secretion by an adrenal pheochromocytoma. *J Endocrinol Invest*, 1994;17:869-874.

[139] Blau, N, Miller, WE, Miller, ER, Jr. Cervi-Skinner, SJ. Spontaneous remission of Cushing's syndrome in a patient with an adrenal adenoma. *J Clin Endocrinol Metab*, 1975;40:659-663.

[140] Gomez Muguruza, MT, Chrousos, GP. Periodic Cushing syndrome in a short boy: usefulness of the ovine corticotrophin releasing hormone test. *J Pediatr*, 1989;115:270-273.

[141] Carson, DJ, Sloan, JM, Cleland, J, Russell, CF, Atkinson, AB, Sheridan, B. Cyclical Cushing's syndrome presenting as short stature in a boy with recurrent atrial myxomas and freckled skin pigmentation. *Clin Endocrinol* (Oxf), 1988;28:173-180.

[142] Oelkers, W, Bahr, V, Hensen, J, Pickartz, H. Primary adrenocortical micronodular adenomatosis causing Cushing's syndrome. Effects of ketoconazole on steroid production and *in vitro* performance of adrenal cells. *Acta Endocrinol* (Copenh), 1986;113:370-377.

[143] Peri, A, Bemporad, D, Parenti, G, Luciani, P, Serio, M, Mannelli, M. Cushing's syndrome due to intermittent ectopic ACTH production showing a temporary remission during a pulmonary infection. *Eur J Endocrinol*, 2001;145:605-611.

[144] Brown, RD, Van Loon, GR, Orth, DN, Liddle, GW. Cushing's disease with periodic hormonogenesis: one explanation for paradoxical response to dexamethasone. *J Clin Endocrinol Metab*, 1973;36:445-451.

[145] Liberman, B, Wajchenberg, BL, Tambascia, MA, Mesquita, CH. Periodic remission in Cushing's disease with paradoxical dexamethasone response: an expression of periodic hormonogenesis. *J Clin Endocrinol Metab*, 1976;43:913-918.

[146] Watanobe, H, Aoki, R, Takebe, K, Nakazono, M, Kudo, M. *In vivo* and *in vitro* studies in a patient with cyclical Cushing's disease showing some responsiveness to bromocriptine. *Horm Res*, 1991;36:227-234.

[147] Thorner, MO, Martin, WH, Ragan, GE, MacLeod, RM, Feldman, PS, Bruni, C, et al. A case of ectopic ACTH syndrome: diagnostic difficulties caused by intermittent hormone secretion. *Acta Endocrinol* (Copenh), 1982;99:364-370.

[148] Jordan, RM, Ramos-Gabatin, A, Kendall, JW, Gaudette, D, Walls, RC. Dynamics of adrenocorticotropin (ACTH) secretion in cyclic Cushing's syndrome: evidence for more than one abnormal ACTH biorhythm. *J Clin Endocrinol Metab*, 1982;55:531-537.

[149] Horvath, E, Kovacs, K, Killinger, DW, Smyth, HS, Platts, ME, Singer, W. Silent corticotropic adenomas of the human pituitary gland: a histologic, immunocytologic, and ultrastructural study. *Am J Pathol*, 1980;98:617-638.

[150] Sahli, R, Christ, ER, Seiler, R, Kappeler, A, Vajtai, I. Clinicopathologic correlations of silent corticotroph adenomas of the pituitary: report of four cases and literature review. *Pathol Res Pract*, 2006;202:457-464.

[151] Baldeweg, SE, Pollock, JR, Powell, M, Ahlquist, J. A spectrum of behaviour in silent corticotroph pituitary adenomas. *Br J Neurosurg*, 2005;19:38-42.

[152] Lopez, JA, Kleinschmidt-Demasters, BkB, Sze, CI, Woodmansee, WW, Lillehei, KO. Silent corticotroph adenomas: further clinical and pathological observations. *Hum Pathol*, 2004;35:1137-1147.

[153] Scheithauer, BW, Jaap, AJ, Horvath, E, Kovacs, K, Lloyd, RV, Meyer, FB, et al. Clinically silent corticotroph tumors of the pituitary gland. *Neurosurgery*, 2000;47:723-729.

[154] Reincke, M, Allolio, B, Saeger, W, Kaulen, D, Winkelmann, W. A pituitary adenoma secreting high molecular weight adrenocorticotropin without evidence of Cushing's disease. *J Clin Endocrinol Metab*, 1987;65:1296-1300.

[155] Nagaya, T, Seo, H, Kuwayama, A, Sakurai, T, Tsukamoto, N, Nakane, T, et al. Pro-opiomelanocortin gene expression in silent corticotroph- cell adenoma and Cushing's disease. *J Neurosurg*, 1990;72:262-267.

[156] Braithwaite, SS, Clasen, RA, D'Angelo, CM. Silent corticotroph adenoma: case report and literature review. *Endocr Pract*, 1997;3:297-301.

[157] Ohta, S, Nishizawa, S, Oki, Y, Yokoyama, T, Namba, H. Significance of absent prohormone convertase 1/3 in inducing clinically silent corticotroph pituitary adenoma of subtype I - immunohistochemical study. *Pituitary*, 2002;5:221-223.

[158] Baldeweg, SE, Pollock, JR, Powell, M, Ahlquist, J. A spectrum of behaviour in silent corticotroph pituitary adenomas. *Br J Neurosurg*, 2005;19:38-42.

[159] Webb, MK, Laurent, JJ, Okonkwo, DO, Lopes, MB, Vance, ML, Laws, ER. Clinical characteristics of silent corticotrophic adenomas and creation of an internet-accessible database to facilitate their multi-institutional study. *Neurosurgery*, 2003;53:1076-1084.

[160] Sahli, R, Christ, ER, Seiler, R, Kappeler, A, Vajtai, I. Clinicopathologic correlations of silent corticotroph adenomas of the pituitary: report of four cases and literature review. *Pathol Res Pract*, 2006;202:457-464.

[161] Milker-Zabel, S, Debus, J, Thilmann, C, Schlegel, W, Wannenmacher, M. Fractionated stereotactically guided radiotherapy and radiosurgery in the treatment of functional and nonfunctional adenomas of the pituitary gland. *Int J Radiat Oncol Biol Phys*, 2001;50:1279-1286.

[162] Laws, ER, Ebersold, MJ, Piepgras, DG. The results of transsphenoidal surgery in specific clinical entities. In Laws ER, Randall RV, Kern EB, Abboud CF. Management of Pituitary Adenomas and Related Lesions with Emphasis on Transsphenoidal Microsurgery. Appleton-Century-Crofts, New York 1982, pp 277-305.

[163] Kovacs, K, Scheithauer, BW, Horvath, E, Lloyd, RV. The World Health Organization classification of adenohypophysial neoplasms. A proposed five-tier scheme. *Cancer*, 1996;78:502-510.

[164] Feldkamp, J, Santen, R, Harms, E, Aulich, A, Modder, UM, Scherbaum WA. Incidentally discovered pituitary lesions: high frequency of macroadenomas and hormone-secreting adenomas - results of a prospective study. *Clin Endocrinol* (Oxf), 1999;51:109-113.

[165] Drange, MR, Fram, NR, Herman-Bonert, V, Melmed, S. Pituitary tumour registry: a novel clinical resource. *J Clin Endocrinol Metab*, 2000;85:168-174.

[166] Cury, ML, Fernandes, JC, Machado, HR, Elias, LL, Moreira, AC. Castro Md. Non functioning pituitary adenomas: clinical feature: *Laboratorial and imaging assessment, therapeutic management and outcome Arq Bras Endocrinol Metab*, 2009;53:31-39.

[167] Dekkers, OM, Hammer, S, de Keizer, RJW, Roelfsema, F, Schutte, PJ, Smitt, JWA, et al., The natural course of non-functioning pituitary macroadenomas. *Eur J Endocrinol*, 2007;156:217-224.

[168] Ebersold, MJ, Quast, LM, Laws, ER, Scheithauer, B, Randall, RV. Long-term results in transsphenoidal removal of nonfunctioning pituitary adenomas. *J Neurosurg*, 1986;64: 713-719.

[169] Scheithauer, BW, Kovacs, KT, Laws, ER, Jr. Randall, RV. Pathology of invasive pituitary tumors with special reference to functional classification. *J Neurosurg*, 1986; 65:733-744.

[170] Molitch, ME, Russell, EJ. The pituitary "incidentaloma." *Ann Intern Med*, 1990;112: 925-931.

[171] Feldkamp, J, Santen, R, Harms, E, Aulich, A, Modder, UM, Scherbaum, WA. Incidentally discovered pituitary lesions: high frequency of macroadenomas and hormone-secreting adenomas - results of a prospective study. *Clin Endocrinol* (Oxf), 1999;51:109-113.

[172] Beck-Peccoz, P, Brucker-Davis, F, Persani, L, Smallridge, RC, Weintraub, BD. Thyrotropin-secreting pituitary tumors. *Endocr Rev*, 1996;17:610-638.

[173] Cohen, LE, Radovick, S. Molecular bases of pituitary hormone deficiencies. *Endocr Rev*, 2002;23:431-442.

[174] Mantovani, G, Asteria, C, Pellegrini, C, Bosari, S, Alberti, L, Bondioni, S, et al. HESX1 expression in human normal pituitaries and pituitary adenomas. *Mol Cell Endocrinol*, 2006;247:135-139.

[175] Ma, W, Ikeda, H, Watabe, N, Kanno, M, Yoshimoto, T. A plurihormonal TSH-producing pituitary tumor of monoclonal origin in a patient with hypothyroidism. *Horm Res*, 2003;59:257-261.

[176] Dong, Q, Brucker-Davis, F, Weintraub, BD, Smallridge, RC, Carr, FE, Battey, J, et al., Screening of candidate oncogenes in human thyrotroph tumors: absence of activating mutations of the Gaq, Ga11, Gas, or thyrotropin-releasing hormone receptor genes. *J Clin Endocrinol Metab*, 1996;81:1134-1140.

[177] Ando, S, Sarlis, NJ, Oldfield, EH, Yen, PM. Somatic mutation of TRbeta can cause a defect in negative regulation of TSH in a TSH-secreting pituitary tumor. *J Clin Endocrinol Metab*, 2001;86:5572-5576.

[178] Lu, C, Willingham, MC, Furuya, F, Cheng, SY. Activation of phosphatidylinositol 3-kinase signaling promotes aberrant pituitary growth in a mouse model of thyroid-stimulating hormone-secreting pituitary tumors. *Endocrinology*, 2008;149:3339-3345.

[179] Refetoff, S, Weiss, RE, Usala, SJ. The syndromes of resistance to thyroid hormone. *Endocr Rev*, 1993;14:348-399.

[180] Kienitz, T, Quinkler, M, Strasburger, CJ, Ventz, M. Long-term management in five cases of TSH-secreting pituitary adenomas: a single center study and review of the literature. *Eur J Endocrinol*, 2007;157:39-46.

[181] Ness-Abramof, R, Ishay, A, Harel, G, Sylvetzky, N, Baron, E, Greenman, Y, et al. TSH-secreting pituitary adenomas. *Pituitary*, 2007;10:307-310.

[182] Foppiani, L, Del Monte, P, Ruelle, A, Bandelloni, R, Quilici, P, Bernasconi, D. TSH-secreting adenomas: rare pituitary tumors with multifaceted clinical and biological features. *J Endocrinol Invest*, 2007;30:603-609.

[183] Gasparoni, P, Rubello, D, Persani, L, Beck-Peccoz, P. Unusual association between a thyrotropin-secreting pituitary adenoma and a papillary thyroid carcinoma. *Thyroid*, 1998;8:181-183.

[184] Ohta, S, Nishizawa, S, Oki, Y, Namba, H. Coexistence of thyrotropin-producing pituitary adenoma with papillary adenocarcinoma of the thyroid: a case report and surgical strategy. *Pituitary*, 2001;4:271-274.

[185] Abs, R, Stevenaert, A, Beckers, A. Autonomously functioning thyroid nodules in a patient with a thyrotropin-secreting pituitary adenoma: possible cause-effect relationship. *Eur J Endocrinol*, 1994;131:355-358.

[186] Kourides, IA, Pekonen, F, Weintraub, BD. Absence of thyroid-binding immunoglobulins in patients with thyrotropinmediated hyperthyroidism. *J Clin Endocrinol Metab*, 1980, 51, 272-274.

[187] Ntali, G, Capatine, C, Grossman, A, Karavitaki, N. Functioning gonadotroph adenomas. *J Clin Endocrinol Metab*, 2014;99:423-433.

[188] Galway, AB, Hsueh, AJ, Daneshdoost, L, Zhou, MH, Pavlou, SN, Snyder, PJ. Gonadotroph adenomas in men produce biologically active follicle-stimulating hormone. *J Clin Endocrinol Metab*, 1990;71:907-912.

[189] Pigny, P, Henric, B, Lahlou, N, Christin, S, Mazzuca, M, Dewailly, D, et al. A gonadotroph adenoma with a high proportion of basic FSH isohormones by chromatofocusing. *J Clin Endocrinol Metab*, 1996;81:2407-2408.

[190] Borgato, S, Persani, L, Romoli, R, Cortelazzi, D, Spada, A, Beck-Peccoz, P. Serum FSH bioactivity and inhibin levels in patients with gonadotropin secreting and nonfunctioning pituitary adenomas. *J Endocrinol Invest*, 1998;21:372-379.

[191] Sugita, T, Seki, K, Nagai, Y, Saeki, N, Yamaura, A, Ohigashi, S, et al. Successful pregnancy and delivery after removal of gonadotrope adenoma secreting follicle-stimulating hormone in a 29-year-old amenorrheic woman. *Gynecol Obstet Invest*, 2005;59:138-143.

[192] Karapanou, O, Tzanela, M, Tamouridis, N, Tsagarakis, S. Gonadotroph pituitary macroadenoma inducing ovarian hyperstimulation syndrome: successful response to octreotide therapy. *Hormones (Athens)*, 2012;11:199-202.

[193] Garmes, HM, Grassiotto, OR, Fernandes, YB, Queiroz Lde, S, Vassalo, J, de Oliveira, DM, et al. A pituitary adenoma secreting follicle-stimulating hormone with ovarian hyperstimulation: treatment using a gonadotropin-releasing hormone antagonist. *Fertil Steril*, 2012;97:231-234.

[194] Shimon, I, Rubinek, T, Bar-Hava, I, Nass, D, Hadani, M, Amsterdam, A, et al. Ovarian hyperstimulation without elevated serum estradiol associated with pure follicle-stimulating hormone-secreting pituitary adenoma. *J Clin Endocrinol Metab*, 2001;86: 3635-3640.

[195] Christin-Maitre, S, Rongières-Bertrand, C, Kottler, ML, Lahlou, N, Frydman, R, Touraine, P, et al. A spontaneous and severe hyperstimulation of the ovaries revealing a gonadotroph adenoma. *J Clin Endocrinol Metab*, 1998;83:3450-3453.

[196] Castelo-Branco, C, del Pino, M, Valladares, E. Ovarian hyperstimulation, hyperprolactinaemia and LH gonadotroph adenoma. *Reprod Biomed Online*, 2009;19: 153-155.

[197] Ghayuri, M, Liu, JH. Ovarian hyperstimulation syndrome caused by pituitary gonadotroph adenoma secreting follicle-stimulating hormone. *Obstet Gynecol*, 2007;109:547-549.

[198] Roberts, JE, Spandorfer, S, Fasouliotis, SJ, Lin, K, Rosenwaks, Z. Spontaneous ovarian hyperstimulation caused by a follicle-stimulating hormone-secreting pituitary adenoma. *Fertil Steril*, 2005;83:208–210.

[199] Paoletti, AM, Depau, GF, Mais, V, Guerriero, S, Ajossa, S, Melis, GB. Effectiveness of cabergoline in reducing follicle-stimulating hormone and prolactin hypersecretion from pituitary macroadenoma in an infertile woman. *Fertil Steril*, 1994;62: 882-885.

[200] Djerassi, A, Coutifaris, C, West, VA, Asa, SL, Kapoor, SC, Pavlou, SN, et al. Gonadotroph adenoma in a premenopausalwomansecreting follicle-stimulating hormone and causing ovarian hyperstimulation. *J Clin Endocrinol Metab*, 1995;80: 591-594.

[201] Castelbaum, AJ, Bigdeli, H, Post, KD, Freedman, MF, Snyder, PJ. Exacerbation of ovarian hyperstimulation by leuprolide reveals a gonadotroph adenoma. *Fertil Steril*, 2002;78:1311-1313.

[202] Murakami, T, Higashitsuji, H, Yoshinaga, K, Terada, Y, Ito, K, Ikeda, H. Management of ovarian hyperstimulation due to follicle-stimulating hormone-secreting gonadotroph adenoma. *BJOG*, 2004;111:1297-1300.

[203] Benito, M, Asa, SL, Livolsi, VA, West, VA, Snyder, PJ. Gonadotroph tumor associated with multiple endocrine neoplasia type 1. *J Clin Endocrinol Metab*, 2005;90:570-574.

[204] Välimäki, MJ, Tiitinen, A, Alfthan, H, Paetau, A, Poranen, A, Sane, T, et al. Ovarian hyperstimulation caused by gonadotroph adenoma secreting follicle-stimulating hormone in 28-year-old woman. *J Clin Endocrinol Metab*, 1999;84:4204-4208.

[205] Pentz-Vidovíc, I, Skoric, T, Grubisic, G, Korsic, M, Ivicevic-Bakulic, T, Basenski, N, et al., Evolution of clinical symptoms in a young woman with a recurrent gonadotroph adenoma causing ovarian hyperstimulation. *Eur J Endocrinol*, 2000;143:607-614.

[206] Murata, Y, Ando, H, Nagasaka, T, Takahashi, I, Saito, K, Fukugaki, H, et al. Successful pregnancy after bromocriptine therapy in an anovulatory woman complicated with ovarian hyperstimulation caused by follicle-stimulating hormoneproducing plurihormonal pituitary microadenoma. *J Clin Endocrinol Metab*, 2003;88:1988-1993.

[207] Kihara, M, Sugita, T, Nagai, Y, Saeki, N, Tatsuno, I, Seki, K. Ovarian hyperstimulation caused by gonadotroph cell adenoma: a case report and review of the literature. *Gynecol Endocrinol*, 2006;22:110-113.

[208] Sommergruber, M, Yaman, C, Ebner, T, Hartl, J, Moser, M, Tews, G. A case of ovarian hyperstimulation during pituitary down-regulation caused by plurihormonal macroadenoma. *Fertil Steril*, 2000;73:1059-1060.

[209] Macchia, E, Simoncini, T, Raffaelli, V, Lombardi, M, Iannelli, A, Martino, E. A functioning FSH-secreting pituitary macroadenoma causing an ovarian hyperstimulation syndrome with multiple cysts resected and relapsed after leuprolide in a reproductive-aged woman. *Gynecol Endocrinol*, 2012;28:56-59.

[210] Catargi, B, Felicie-Dellan, E, Tabarin, A. Comment on gonadotroph adenoma causing ovarian hyperstimulation. *J Clin Endocrinol Metab*, 1999;84:3404.

[211] Mor, E, Rodi, IA, Bayrak, A, Paulson, RJ, Sokol, RZ. Diagnosis of pituitary gonadotroph adenomas in reproductive-aged women. *Fertil Steril*, 2005;84:757.

[212] Cooper, O, Geller, JL, Melmed, S. Ovarian hyperstimulation syndrome caused by an FSH-secreting pituitary adenoma. *Nat Clin Pract Endocrinol Metab*, 2008;4:234-238.

[213] Kanaya, M, Baba, T, Kitajima, Y, Ikeda, K, Shimizu, A, Morishita, M, et al. Continuous follicle-stimulating hormone exposure from pituitary adenoma causes

periodic follicle recruitment and atresia, which mimics ovarian hyperstimulation syndrome. *Int J Womens Health.*, 2012;4:427-431.
[214] Knoepfelmacher, M, Danilovic, DL, Rosa Nasser, RH, Mendonça, BB. Effectiveness of treating ovarian hyperstimulation syndrome with cabergoline in two patients with gonadotropin-producing pituitary adenomas. *Fertil Steril*, 2006;86:719.e15-e18.
[215] Sicilia, V, Earle, J, Mezitis, SG. Multiple ovarian cysts and oligomenorrhea as the initial manifestations of a gonadotropin-secreting pituitary macroadenoma. *Endocr Pract*, 2006;12:417-421.
[216] van Wijk, JP, ter Braak, EW. Images in clinical medicine: amenorrhea, abdominal pain, and weight gain. *N Engl J Med*, 2011;365:e39.
[217] Davis, JR, McNeilly, JR, Norris, AJ, Pope, C, Wilding, M, McDowell, G, et al. Fetal gonadotrope cell origin of FSH-secreting pituitary adenoma - insight into human pituitary. *Clin Endocrinol* (Oxf), 2006;65:648-54.
[218] Kajitani, T, Liu, S, Maruyama, T, Uchida, H, Sakurai, R, Masuda, H, et al. Analysis of serum FSH bioactivity in a patient with an FSH-secreting pituitary microadenoma and multicystic ovaries: a case report. *Hum Reprod*, 2008;23:435-439.
[219] Hall, JE. Neuroendocrine changes with reproductive aging in women. *Semin Reprod Med*, 2007;25:344-351.
[220] Heseltine, D, White, MC, Kendall-Taylor, P, DeKretser, DM, Kelly, W. Testicular enlargement and elevated serum inhibin concentrations occur in patients with pituitary macroadenomas secreting follicle stimulating hormone. *Clin Endocrinol* (Oxf), 1989;31:411-423.
[221] Snyder, PJ. Gonadotroph cell adenomas of the pituitary. *Endocr Rev*, 1985;6:552-563.
[222] Dahlqvist, P, Koskinen, LO, Brännström, T, Hägg, E. Testicular enlargement in a patient with a FSH-secreting pituitary adenoma. *Endocrine*, 2010;37:289-293.
[223] Zárate, A, Fonseca, ME, Mason, M, Tapia, R, Miranda, R, Kovacs, K, et al. Gonadotropin-secreting pituitary adenoma with concomitant hypersecretion of testosterone and elevated sperm count. Treatment with LRH agonist. *Acta Endocrinol* (Copenh), 1986;113:29-34.
[224] Clemente, M, Caracseghi, F, Gussinyer, M, Yeste, D, Albisu, M, Vasquez, E, et al., Macroorchidism and panhypopituitarism: two different forms of presentation of FSH secreting pituitary adenomas in adolescence. *Horm Res Paediatr*, 201175:225-230.
[225] Tashiro, H, Katabuchi, H, Ohtake, H, Kaku, T, Ushio, Y, Okamura, H. A follicle-stimulating hormone-secreting gonadotroph adenoma with ovarian enlargement in a 10-year-old girl. *Fertil Steril*, 1999;72:158-160.
[226] Di Rocco, C, Maira, G, Borrelli, P. Pituitary microadenomas in children. *Childs Brain*, 1982;9:165-178.
[227] Faggiano, M, Criscuolo, T, Perrone, L, Quarto, C, Sinisi, AA. Sexual precocity in a boy due to hypersecretion of LH and prolactin by a pituitary adenoma. *Acta Endocrinol* (Copenh), 1983;102:167-172.
[228] Ambrosi, B, Bassetti, M, Ferrario, R, Medri, G, Giannattasio, G, Faglia, G. Precocious puberty in a boy with a PRL-, LH- and FSH-secreting pituitary tumour: hormonal and immunocytochemical studies. *Acta Endocrinol* (Copenh), 1990;122:569-576.

In: Pituitary Adenoma
Editor: Dimitrios N. Kanakis

ISBN: 978-1-63484-985-2

Chapter 6

GENDER DIFFERENCE IN PROLACTINOMAS: A COMPARATIVE CLINICOPATHOLOGIC STUDY

Daizo Yoshida**, MD, PhD, Akira Teramoto Akio, MD, PhD, and Akio Morita, MD, PhD

Department of Neurosurgery, Nippon Medical School, Tokyo, Japan

ABSTRACT

Prolactinoma occurrance in males is not a rare event. In general, the occurance is higher in females than in males, clinical manifestation in the form of galactorrhea or gynecomastia is uncommon in males, and the male patients initially complain of bitemporal hemianopia or hypogonadism, such as erectile dysfunction. To the best of our knowledge, in the 21st century, gender-related clinical features have been little discussed with statistical analysis because the number of male patients with prolactinoma were ten cases at the most in each article. From January 2001 to December 2014, we treated 384 cases with clinically and histologicaly proven prolactinomas, which met strict immunohistological criterion. All these patients were surgically treated as they were found to be resistant to dopaminergic agonists. Sixty-two patients (16.1%) were male and 322 patients were female, the female-to-male ratio was 5.19:1. Males were significantly older (male: 49.3 years old, female: 33.4 years old, $p < 0.01$) at surgery. The most common presenting symptom in females was menstrual abonormalities (84%), whereas general fatigue predominated in males (78%, including 8% impotence). Sudden onset of severe headache, indicating pituitary apoplexy, or gradually progressing headache was observed more in males (56%) than in females (32%). Frequency of psychological symptoms, typically depressive state, werenot different between gender (male: 4.2%, female: 5.7%). There was no significant difference between gender for complete or incomplete bitemporal hemianopsia (male: 28.2%, female: 24.5%). Males had a significantly shorter pre-operative duration of symptoms (mean: 93.5 days vs. 189.0 days). Progression free to survival analysis showed that there was no difference between males and females ($p = 0.0510$). Difference between male and female cases of prolactinoma was fewer than that in 1990s, because pre-operative diagnosis with

* Corresponding author: Daizo Yoshida, MD, PhD, Department of Neurosurgery, Nippon Medical School, 1-1-5, Sendagi, Bunkyo-ku, Tokyo,113-8603 Japan, Phone: +81338222131, Fax: +81357050981, E-mail:dyoshida@nms.ac.jp.

progressing neuroimaging system to find early stage in prolactinoma enabling the doctor to find male prolactinomas especially in subclinical stage.

Keywords: comparative study, endocrinology, gender, surgical treatment, pituitary adenoma, prolactinoma

1. INTRODUCTION

A prolactinoma is a benign tumor (adenoma) of the pituitary gland that produces a hormone called prolactin [1]. It is the most common type of pituitary tumor. Symptoms of prolactinoma are hyperprolactinemia, it is induced by compression of the tumor on surrounding tissues [2]. Prolactin stimulates the breast to produce milk and has many other functions such as the regulation of mood and inhibition of the activity of osteoclast in the bone [3]. Prolactin level is usually higher during pregnancy and after childbirth [2]. In males, it is responsible for the sexual refractory period after orgasm and excess levels can lead to erectile dysfunction [3]. Autopsy studies indicate that <10% of the population has small pituitary tumors [4]. Approximately 40% of these pituitary tumors immunohistochemically produce prolactin, however, a vast majority of them are not considered to be clinically manifested. Clinically significant pituitary tumors affect the health of approximately 10 per 100,000 people [1]. On the selective surgical series, this tumor accounts for approximately 25%-30% of all pituitary adenomas [5, 6]. Some growth hormone (GH)-producing tumors also co-secrete prolactin with much lower level [7, 8]. The goal of the treatment is to restore prolactin secretion to normal, reduce tumor size, correct any visual abnormalities, and restore normal pituitary function.

Prolactinomas have a wide variety of symptoms *because of the influence of the elevated serum* prolactin *levels on the reproductive system and/or the size of the tumor* [9, 10]. A very large tumor may produce pressure on the optic nerves or nearby brain tissue, leading to headaches and/or vision problems [11, 12].

In females, high levels of prolactin secreted by the tumor hinders the production of estrogen [13]. When estrogen levels decrease, women have absent or irregular menstrual periods, vaginal dryness, and difficulty conceiving. In addition, because of elevated prolactin levels in the breast, women who are not pregnant experience a milky breast discharge [14]. This symptom is called galactorrhea. Patients rarely have headaches, visual symptoms, or other complaints that are closely related to tumor size. Prolactinomas in women are generally considered relatively small and often do not progressively increase in size [15].

In males, even slight elevations in prolactin levels from very small pituitary tumors can lead to a decrease in sex drive and cause erectile dysfunction because prolactin inhibits testosterone production in the testis, which can infrequently cause infertility [16, 17]. Generally, larger tumors in men are associated with higher levels of prolactin. Breast discharge (galactorrhea) is very uncommon in men as compared to in women [18], simply because the breast is not developed in males. In other words, many authors consider that clinical manifestation of prolactinoma in the early stage is rarely observed [1, 14, 17, 19-23]. Males with prolactinomas are often provided medical attention because of headaches or vision problems due to large tumors that can produce pressure on the optic nerves. Because of the low estrogen and testosterone levels that may occur with elevated prolactin, some men and women also develop low bone density, however, fractures and osteoporosis due to this fact have not been reported well [20, 24].

Recent drammatical progression and development in the field of medical science has accomplished early diagnosis of a number of diseases and also pituitary adenomas [25-28]. Simultaneously, health care insurance system can provide help for the early diagnosis before its clinical manifestation. Therefore, we consider that strategy to treat pituitary tumor should be discussed again in the 21st century. Until 1990, prolactinoma in males tended to be found when it became much larger and invasive to the neighboring cavernous sinus, comparing to these occurred in females. Smaller prolactinoma in males is usually clinically silent. In other words, they did not have a chance to consult a doctor to examine brain CT or MRI [11, 12, 18, 29]. In this chapter, we analyzed operative cases of prolactinoma after 2001 in our institute aiming to discuss the gender related clinical approach in males and to provide a new horizon for treatment strategy.

2. Materials and Methods

From January 2001 to December 2014, we operated 384 cases, which were histologically proven prolactinomas and strictly met the immunohistological criteria. We analyzed their medical records. Sixty-two patients (16.1%) were males and 322 cases were females, the female-to-male ratio was 5.19:1. Age, Knosp grading just prior to the surgery, present symptoms, pre-operative duration after the first diagonosis, pre-and post-operative serum prolactin levels, labeling index of MIB-1 in the tumor tissue, and Progression free to survival was compared.

For statistical analysis, Mann-Whitney test,Kaplan-Meier curve, and log-rank test were mainly employed (GraphPad Prism, ver. 6.0, GraphPad Software, Inc., La Jolla, CA 92037, USA). Statistically significant difference was evaluated when p-value was <0.05.

3. Results

Males were significantly older (male: 49.3 years old, female: 33.4 years old, $p < 0.01$) at surgery. In pre-operative imagings, distribution of tumor invasion in the male cases on Knosp grading was shifted to grade 4, meanwhile plateau distribution in the cases in females showed around grade 2 and 3 (Figure 1).

The most common presenting symptom in females was menstrual abonormalities (84%), whereas general fatigue was predominant in males (78%, including 8% impotence). Sudden onset of severe headache, indicating pituitary apoplexy, or gradually progressing headache tended to be frequently observed in males (56%) than in females (32%). Psychological symptoms, typically depressive state, were not frequently complaint (male 4.2%, female 5.7%). There was no significant difference between gender for complete or incomplete bitemporal hemianopsia (male: 28.2%, female: 24.5%). Males had a significantly shorter pre-operative duration of symptoms (mean: 93.5 days vs. 189.0 days) (Figure 2).

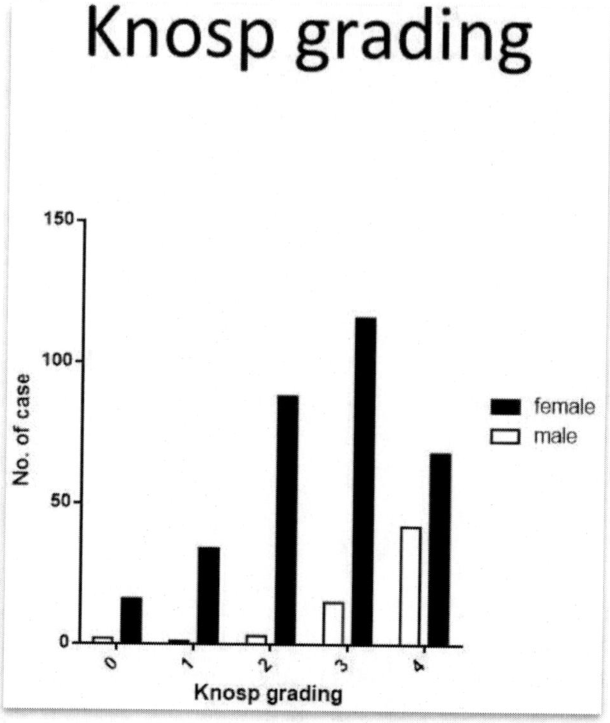

Figure 1. *Distribution of Knosp grading of male or female cases with prolactinoma at surgery.* Distribution of Knosp grading is shifted to grade 4 in male cases, but the peak in the cases in females showed around grade 2 and 3.

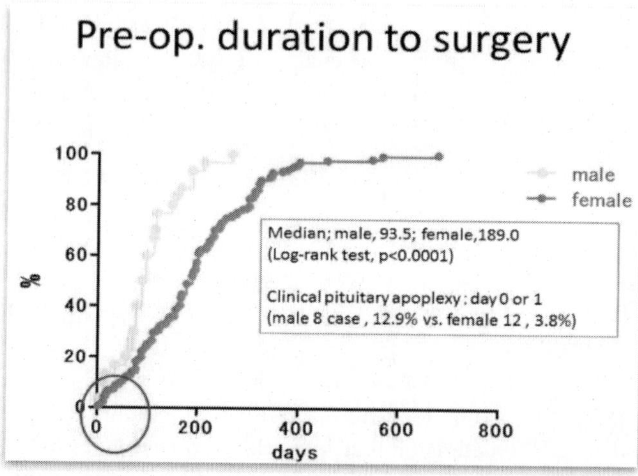

Figure 2. *Pre-operative interval to surgical treatment after diagnosis.* Male cases reveal a significantly shorter pre-operative duration of symptoms (mean: 93.5 days vs. 189.0 days), (Log-rank test, $p < 0.0001$). These involve clinical manifestation as a sudden onset of pituitary apoplexy, those operated at day 0 or 1 (male: 8 cases, female: 12 cases).

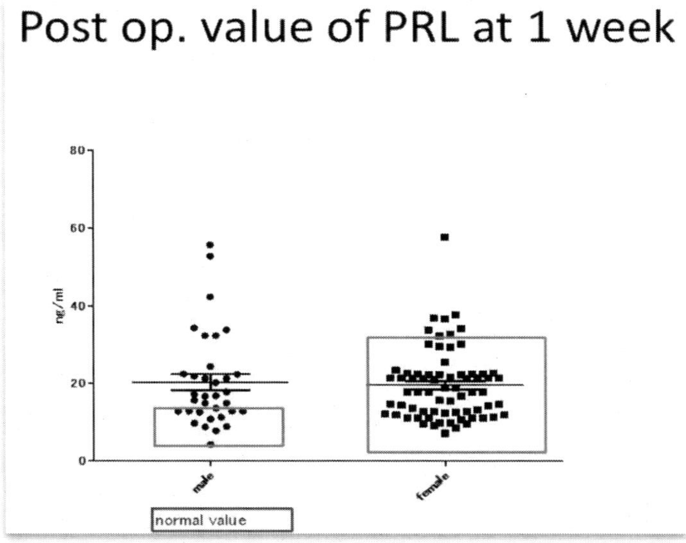

Figure 3. *Post-operative serum prolactin level at 1 week.* Forty-two percent of male cases was still higher than the normal value, compared with female cases, which are much lesser (3.4%).

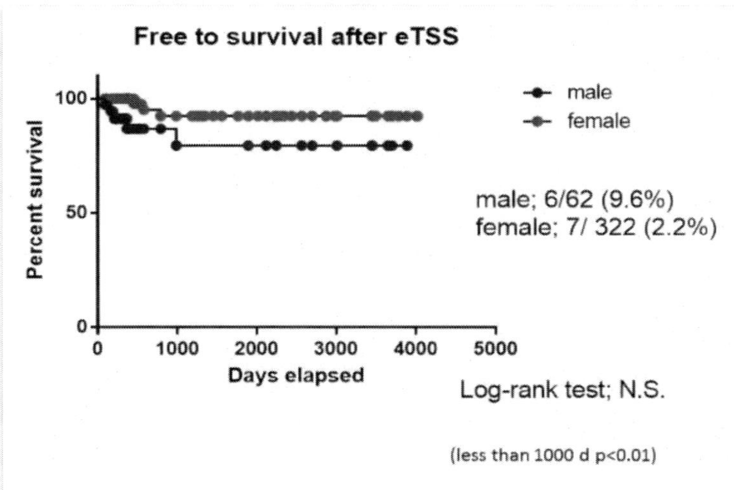

Figure 4. *Progression free to survival period after eTSS surgery.* Six out of 62 male cases (9.6%) recur, whereas 7 out of 322 (2.2%) female cases recur within 100 days. But 4000 days Log-rank test show no siginificant difference between both genders.

They all were operated surgically because their serum prolactin level could not be controlled by dopaminergic agonist therapy, and further the visual field deficit was not recovered. Just prior to surgical operation, serum prolactin level was significantly higher in males (male: 2822.2 g/ml, female: 782.5 g/ml, Mann-Whitney test: $p < 0.001$). Labeling index of MIB-1 showed no difference between genders in operative samples (male: 1.89, female: 2.14%, not significant in the Mann-Whitney test). Post-operative serum level of prolactin at 1 week disclosed that 42% of male cases was still higher than the normal value as compared with females (3.4%) (Figure 3).

Progression free to survival analysis showed there was no difference between male and female cases (p = 0.0510, log-rank test, Figure 4).

4. Discussion

In our series, prolactinoma in male patients were much fewer than in female patients (female-to-male ratio, 5.19:1) and older (male: 49.3 years old, female: 33.4 years old) at surgery. At the operation, distribution of tumor invasion in the male cases on Knosp grading was shifted to grade 4. The result clearly showed that male patients with prolactinoma tended to be found when they were bigger and invaded into the surrounding normal tissue more than in female case. In male prolactinomas, clinical manifestation can be hardly noticed when it is in a small size.

However, we hereby stress that Knosp grading in male cases has gradually shifted to the lower grade at surgery every year. In this century, asymptomatic and small pituitary tumors have been more easily found as so called incidentalomas because of development of neuroimaging system, such as dynamic MRI or targeted *MRI* examination of the *pituitary* egion with contrast enhancement [30, 31]. The diagnosis of smaller tumor within the sella turcica, at the earliest stage in adenoma growth could attribute to the better prognosis. The most common presenting symptom in females was menstrual abnormalities (84%) [20, 21, 32] whereas general fatigue predominated in males (78%, including 8% impotence [5, 24]. Female patients with menstrual abnormality may usually consult a gynecologist and then a sociological examination focusing on hormones can easily disclose that it is caused by hypersecretion of prolactin, sometimes associated with pituitary dysfunction. We strongly wonder whether male patients, complaining only of general fatigue without headache or visual symptom, would consult any neurosurgeon or endocrinologist for evaluation of any possible disease in the brain. The majority of them must rest for a while when the fatigue had temporarily occurred. In this series, we could not find any significant difference between gender for complete or incomplete bitemporal hemianopsia. They could easily notice in the daily life when they felt loss of visual acuity or visual field deficit, and then they immediately visited the department of ophthalmology. It is indeed easy to detect the visual field deficit, typically seen in the case with pituitary tumor.

In comparison with several summaries published in the 20th century [18, 31, 33-36], our experience in a single institute for the treatment of prolactinoma in males highlighted on gender-related analysis and disclosed that the male patients complaining hypogonadism (impotence or decreased sexual libido) was clearly fewer (8%) than the report by Arasho et al. (57%) [35]. Sudden onset of severe headache, plausibly indicating pituitary apoplexy, or gradually progressing headache tended to be frequently observed in males (56%) than in females (32%), in the present study. Psychological symptoms, typically depressive state, were not a frequent complaint (male: 4.2%, female: 5.7%), compared with past studies (Glezer and Bronstein, 48.2%, Loyo-Varela et al., 54.2%, Mindermann and Wilson, 39.8%, Popovic et al., 54.3%) [14, 15, 34, 36]. There was no significant difference between gender for complete or incomplete bitemporal hemianopsia (male: 28.2%, female: 24.5%), which differed from our general impression before starting this statistical analysis. This fact may also be contributed by the tumor size not to the gender, because prolactinoma found in males has decreased year by year. So far, psychological symptoms, like depressive state, were also dramatically fewer in our institute (5.7% vs. 58%) [35]. There may be a difference in the cultural background. At least, males may usually believe that depressive state and erectile dysfunction must be because of general fatigue that is caused by numerous diseases arising in the various organs or blood, otherwise some males hesitate to consult a psychologist or urologist. They may not be willing to consult the department of endocrinology or neurosurgery. Meanwhile, just prior to surgical operation, serum prolactin level and Knosp grading, criteria for invasion into the cavernous sinus, were significantly still higher in male patients in our series but gradually the difference has been also reduced.

Methods for neuroimaging aiming to find small pituitary adenoma has been dramatically improved in this decade. Dynamic MRI helps finding the presence of very small pituitary adenoma that was impossible to detect previously [30, 31]. Progression of high-resolution image of peri- or pre-operative monitoring system suggest the correct location and size of pituitary adenoma and can eliminate any tumor tissue from being uncaptured [31, 39, 40] Concomitantly in our institute, peri-operative enhancement by fluorescence after intravenous can provide a blood vessel observation system capable of observing blood running of the internal carotid arteries and cavernous sinus, thus, the system helps to reduce bleeding during endoscopic surgery. These new techniques must decrease the recurrence from the residual pituitary tumor tissue.

Several reviews insisted that in the male cases, MIB-1 or Ki-67 index, hallmark of cell proliferation, was siginificantly higher than in female cases and consequently, male prolactioma is more aggressive than female [41-45]. But in our series, we could not find any significant differences. As usual, positive cells for such labeling are not diffused but biased distributed. Furthermore, we strongly wonder if tumor of 2.2% MIB-1 index can be really invasive and proliferative than 1.4% index tumor. It appears to be exaggerative.

We started endoscopic transsphenoidal surgery (eTSS) since 1999, and all surgery for pituitary tumors have been performed using eTSS from 2007. For these three years, we employed extra-capsular approach in eTSS along with progression of peri-operative monitoring system, i.e., peri-operative monitoring with 3-D imaging and fluorescence image guidance to reveal the position of the intracarotid arteries. For the past 4 years, we have been eager to employ the extra-capsular approach. When we can find the border of pseudo-membrane between the tumor parenchyma and adjacent normal pituitary, tumor removal is much easier along with pseudo-membrane. Even in the case with Knosp grading 3 or 4, highly invading into the cavernous sinus or in some others extending above the optic chiasm bulging into the third ventricle, this method potentiates better removal. But we should bear in mind the limitation of this method. We often experience the part of pseudo-membrane being too soft to be detached, or incompletely formed all around the tumor mass, sometimes in the case with invading into the cavernous sinus that has obscure border with the cerebral nerves in the sinus. In such a case, we can no longer accomplish the way to remove, even though we undertake before the surgery.

Both in pre- and post-operative follow-up, we should remember that hyperprolactinemia yields osteoporosis risk as mentioned above [24]. Consequently, it is rational to consider that male cases with prolactinoma are exposed to higher serum level of prolactin, hence, they have a risk for complication of osteoporosis. Hyperprolactinemia can cause reduced estrogen production in women and reduced testosterone production in men. Testosterone is chemically changed to estrogen resulting in inhibition of osteoclast activity [46, 47] and therefore, reduction of testosterone by hyperprolactinemia causes osteoporosis in the future. Although estrogen/testosterone production may be restored after treatment of hyperprolactinemia, even a year or two without estrogen/testosterone can compromise bone strength [46], and patients should prevent themselves from osteoporosis by increasing exercise and calcium intake through diet or supplementation and by avoiding smoking. We encourage the patients for bone density measurements to assess the effect of testosterone deficiency on the density. They may also need testosterone replacement therapy by their physician.

On the basis of the previous discussion and our series, in pituitary prolactinomas, serum prolactin levels usually parallel to the tumor size. Osteoporosis induced by post-operative prolactinema is one of critical factors for aged generation post-operatively. We should consider that general symptoms such as depressive state, general fatigue, or impotence are able to be sometimes raised also by prolactinoma. Brain MRI is strongly recommended for these cases.

In conclusion, also in male cases, small prolactinoma can be detected by high-resolutional neuro-imagings and then removed surgically. Early diagnosis before growing over the surrounding organs can be a key factor for the treatment.

REFERENCES

[1] Casanueva FF, Molitch ME, Schlechte JA, Abs R, Bonert V, Bronstein MD, et al. Guidelines of the Pituitary Society for the diagnosis and management of prolactinomas. *Clin Endocrinol* (Oxf) 2006;65:265-273.

[2] Shakir KM. Impotence as a presenting symptom of presumed prolactinoma in a patient with diabetes mellitus. *Diabetes Care* 1983;6:510-511.

[3] Donangelo I, Melmed S. Implication of Pituitary Tropic Status on Tumor Development. *Front Horm Res* 2006;35:1-8.

[4] Eglash A. Treatment of maternal hypergalactia. *Breastfeed Med* 2014;9: 423-425.

[5] Sansone A, Romanelli F, Gianfrilli D, Lenzi A. Endocrine evaluation of erectile dysfunction. *Endocrine* 2014;46:423-430.

[6] Buurman H, Saeger W. Subclinical adenomas in postmortem pituitaries: classification and correlations to clinical data. *Eur J Endocrinol* 2006;154:753-758.

[7] Li J, Stefaneanu L, Kovacs K, Horvath E, Smyth HS. Growth hormone (GH) and prolactin (PRL) gene expression and immunoreactivity in GH- and PRL-producing human pituitary adenomas. *Virchows Arch A Pathol Anat Histopathol* 1993;422:193-201.

[8] Tomita T, Watanabe I, Rengachary SS. Immunoelectron microscopy for growth hormone and prolactin in pituitary adenomas. *Hum Pathol* 1987;18:367-374.

[9] Devi YS, Halperin J. Reproductive actions of prolactin mediated through short and long receptor isoforms. *Mol Cell Endocrinol* 2014;382:400-410.

[10] Gettler LT, McDade TW, Feranil AB, Kuzawa CW. Prolactin, fatherhood, and reproductive behavior in human males. *Am J Phys Anthropol* 2012;148:362-370.

[11] Fong LP, Fabinyi GC. Ophthalmic manifestations of pituitary apoplexy. *Med J Aust* 1985;142:142-143.

[12] Woodhouse NJ, Khouqueer F, Sieck JO. Prolactinomas and optic nerve compression: disappearance of suprasellar extension and visual recovery after two weeks bromocriptine treatment. *Horm Res* 1981;14:141-147.

[13] Tong Y, Zhou J, Mizutani J, Fukuoka H, Ren SG, Gutierrez-Hartmann A, et al. CEBPD suppresses prolactin expression and prolactinoma cell proliferation. *Mol Endocrinol* 2011;25:1880-1891.

[14] Glezer A, Bronstein MD. Prolactinomas, cabergoline, and pregnancy. *Endocrine* 2014;47:64-69.

[15] Loyo-Varela M, Herrada-Pineda T, Revilla-Pacheco F, Manrique-Guzman S. Pituitary tumor surgery: review of 3004 cases. *World Neurosurg* 2013;79:331-336.

[16] Rupp K. You're the flight surgeon: hypogonadism. *Aviat Space Environ Med* 2014;85:1235-1237.

[17] Shimon I, Benbassat C. Male prolactinomas presenting with normal testosterone levels. *Pituitary* 2014;17:246-250.

[18] Gooren LJ, Harmsen-Louman W, van Kessel H. Follow-up of prolactin levels in long-term oestrogen-treated male-to-female transsexuals with regard to prolactinoma induction. *Clin Endocrinol* (Oxf) 1985;22:201-207.

[19] Somma M, Beauregard H, Rasio E. Prolactinoma in the male. Preoperative evaluation of 40 patients. *Neurochirurgie* 1981;27(Suppl 1):S37-S39.

[20] Dorkkam N, Wongdee K, Suntornsaratoon P, Krishnamra N, Charoenphandhu N. Prolactin stimulates the L-type calcium channel-mediated transepithelial calcium transport in the duodenum of male rats. *Biochem Biophys Res Commun* 2013;430:711-716.

[21] Coburger J, Konig R, Seitz K, Bazner U, Wirtz CR, Hlavac M. Determining the utility of intraoperative magnetic resonance imaging for transsphenoidal surgery: a retrospective study. *J Neurosurg* 2014;120:346-356.

[22] Giustina A, Mazziotti G, Fontanella M. Commentary: Postsurgical monitoring of acromegaly. *Neurosurgery* 2013;73:E746-8.

[23] Kuge A, Kikuchi Z, Sato S, Sakurada K, Takemura S, Kayama T. Practical use of a simple technique, insertion of wet cotton pledgets into the tumor resection cavity in transsphenoidal surgery of pituitary tumors, for a better comparison between pre- and intraoperative high-field magnetic resonance images. J Neurol Surg A Cent Eur Neurosurg 2013;74:366-372.

[24] Masopust V, Netuka D, Benes V, Bradac O, Marek J, Hana V. Endonasal endoscopic pituitary adenoma resection: preservation of neurohypophyseal function. *J Neurol Surg A Cent Eur Neurosurg* 2014;75:336-342.

[25] Guo Q, Young WF, Erickson D, Erickson B. Usefulness of dynamic MRI enhancement measures for the diagnosis of ACTH-producing pituitary adenomas. *Clin Endocrinol* (Oxf) 2015;82:267-273.

[26] Sun Y, Sun Q, Fan C, Shen J, Zhao W, Guo Y, et al., Diagnosis and therapy for Cushing's disease with negative dynamic MRI finding: a single-centre experience. *Clin Endocrinol* (Oxf) 2012;76:868-876.

[27] Godinjak Z, Idrizbegovic E, Rama A. Correlation between hyperprolactinemia, MRI of hypophysis and clinical presentation in infertile patients. *Med Arch* 2013;67:22-24.

[28] Lee DY, Oh YK, Yoon BK, Choi D. Prevalence of hyperprolactinemia in adolescents and young women with menstruation-related problems. *Am J Obstet Gynecol* 2012;206:213 e1-5.

[29] Shao S, Li X. Clinical features and analysis in 1385 Chinese patients with pituitary adenomas. *J Neurosurg Sci* 2013;57:267-275.

[30] Drange MR, Fram NR, Herman-Bonert V, Melmed S. Pituitary tumor registry: a novel clinical resource. *J Clin Endocrinol Metab* 2000;85:168-174.

[31] Calle-Rodrigue RD, Giannini C, Scheithauer BW, Lloyd RV, Wollan PC, Kovacs KT, et al., Prolactinomas in male and female patients: a comparative clinicopathologic study. *Mayo Clin Proc* 1998;73:1046-1052.

[32] Delgrange E, Maiter D, Donckier J, Tourniaire J. Influence of age on the clinical presentation of prolactinomas in male patients. *Gerontology* 1999; 45:160-164.

[33] Jaffrain-Rea ML, Petrangeli E, Lubrano C, Minniti G, Di Stefano D, Sciarra F, et al., Epidermal growth factor binding sites in human pituitary macroadenomas. *J Endocrinol* 1998;158:425-433.

[34] Mindermann T, Wilson CB. Age-related and gender-related occurrence of pituitary adenomas. *Clin Endocrinol* (Oxf) 1994;41:359-364.

[35] Arasho BD, Schaller B, Sandu N, Zenebe G. Gender-related differences in pituitary adenomas. *Exp Clin Endocrinol Diabetes* 2009;117:567-572.

[36] Popovic V, Damjanovic S, Micic D, Nesovic M, Djurovic M, Petakov M, et al., Increased incidence of neoplasia in patients with pituitary adenomas. *The Pituitary Study Group. Clin Endocrinol* (Oxf) 1998;49:441-445.

[37] Chittiboina P, Montgomery BK, Millo C, Herscovitch P, Lonser RR. High-resolution(18)F-fluorodeoxyglucose positron emission tomography and magnetic resonance imaging for pituitary adenoma detection in Cushing disease. *J Neurosurg* 2015;122:791-797.

[38] Linn J, Peters F, Lummel N, Schankin C, Rachinger W, Brueckmann H, et al., Detailed imaging of the normal anatomy and pathologic conditions of the cavernous region at 3 Tesla using a contrast-enhanced MR angiography. *Neuroradiology* 2011,53:947-954.

[39] Chacko G, Chacko AG, Kovacs K, Scheithauer BW, Mani S, Muliyil JP, et al. The clinical significance of MIB-1 labeling index in pituitary adenomas. *Pituitary* 2010;13:337-344.

[40] Chiloiro S, Bianchi A, Doglietto F, de Waure C, Giampietro A, Fusco A, et al. Radically resected pituitary adenomas: prognostic role of Ki 67 labeling index in a monocentric retrospective series and literature review. *Pituitary* 2014;17:267-276.

[41] de Aguiar PH, Aires R, Laws ER, Isolan GR, Logullo A, Patil C, et al. Labeling index in pituitary adenomas evaluated by means of MIB-1: is there a prognostic role? A critical review. *Neurol Res* 2010;32:1060-1071.

[42] Hsu CY, Guo WY, Chien CP, Ho DM. MIB-1 labeling index correlated with magnetic resonance imaging detected tumor volume doubling time in pituitary adenoma. *Eur J Endocrinol* 2010;162:1027-1033.

[43] Lath R, Chacko G, Chandy MJ. Determination of Ki-67 labeling index in pituitary adenomas using MIB-1 monoclonal antibody. *Neurol India* 2001;49:144-147.

[44] Ogawa Y, Ikeda H, Tominaga T. Clinicopathological study of prognostic factors in patients with pituitary adenomas and Ki-67 labeling index of more than 3%. *J Endocrinol Invest* 2009;32:581-584.

[45] Widhalm G, Wolfsberger S, Preusser M, Fischer I, Woehrer A, Wunderer J, et al. Residual nonfunctioning pituitary adenomas: prognostic value of MIB-1 labeling index for tumor progression. *J Neurosurg* 2009;111:563-571.

[46] Chen Q, Kaji H, Sugimoto T, Chihara K. Testosterone inhibits osteoclast formation stimulated by parathyroid hormone through androgen receptor. *FEBS Lett* 2001;491:91-93.

[47] Jakob F, Siggelkow H, Homann D, Kohrle J, Adamski J, Schutze N. Local estradiol metabolism in osteoblast- and osteoclast-like cells. *J Steroid Biochem Mol Biol* 1997;61:167-174.

In: Pituitary Adenoma
Editor: Dimitrios N. Kanakis
ISBN: 978-1-63484-985-2

Chapter 7

PATHOLOGY OF PITUITARY ADENOMAS

Wolfgang Saeger*[*], *MD
Professor Emeritus of Neuropathology,
Institute of Pathology and Neuropathology of the University of Hamburg,
UKE, Hamburg, Germany

ABSTRACT

Most pituitary tumors are typical adenomas. Nearly half of them are invasive, by growing into surrounding tissues. If invasive adenomas show mitoses, with a Ki-67 index of more than 3% and a significant number of p53-positive nuclei, they are designated as atypical adenomas (3 to 15% of all adenomas). The very rare (less than 1%) pituitary carcinoma is defined by demonstration of metastases. In endocrine active adenomas, the over-produced hormone has to be demonstrated in the surgical specimens by immunocytochemistry. Pituitary adenomas are called clinically silent, if hormones - with exception of FSH-or LH-positive adenomas - are found in clinically inactive adenomas. According to the WHO classification of 2004, all adenomas have to be classified in the following types: densely and sparsely granulated GH cell adenomas, mixed GH- and Prolactin secreting adenomas, mammosomatotroph adenomas, acidophil stem cell adenomas, densely and sparsely granulated Prolactin cell adenomas, densely and sparsely ACTH cell adenomas, Crooke's cell adenomas, TSH cell adenomas, FSH/LH cell adenomas, null cell adenomas and plurihormonal adenomas. Sparsely granulated GH cell adenomas, densely granulated Prolactin cell adenomas, acidophil stem cell adenomas, Crooke's cell adenomas, null cell adenomas and some plurihormonal adenomas are for aggressive adenomas. Craniopharyngiomas are the second most frequent pituitary tumors. They have to be differentiated into the adamantinomatous type, which is more frequent and present often strong regressive changes and into the papillary type being less frequent and always free of regressive changes. Third most frequent tumors of the pituitary are the group of TTF-1 positive spindle cell tumors which are classified into spindle cell oncoytomas, pituicytomas and granular cell tumors.

[*] Corresponding author: Wolfgang Saeger, MD, Institutes of Pathology and Neuropathology of the University of Hamburg, UKE, Martinistraße 52, D-20246 Hamburg, Germany, E-mail: w.saeger@uke.de.

Keywords: pituitary, adenoma, WHO classification, spindle cell tumors, craniopharyngioma, immunocytochemistry

1. Definition

By definition, pituitary adenomas are benign neuroendocrine glandular tumors of the pituitary, originating from glandular cells of the anterior pituitary gland. Depending on their grade of differentiation the different adenoma cells are very similar or less similar to the corresponding cell types of the normal pituitary.

2. Epidemiology

Pituitary adenomas are not rare. Examinations of unselected series of post-mortem pituitaries account for proportions of 8 to 26% [1, 2, 3]. These are mostly microadenomas of Prolactin cell type or FSH-LH cell adenomas.

Clinically significant pituitary adenomas are much less frequent. In clinics of neurosurgery they comprehend 5 to 14% of all patients with intracranial tumors [1, 2, 3]. Each age can be involved, but before the age of 8 years they are very rare. The frequency of distribution shows a peak between 40 and 50 years. The sex distribution is very similar, but in higher ages men are over-represented, whereas women are more frequent before the age of 45 [4].

3. Pathogenesis

The etiology of pituitary adenomas is not yet known. For only very few tumors increased releasing factors were demonstrated and accepted as co-factors for the pathogenesis [5]. Experiments with GHRH-transgenic mice revealed hyperplasias of GH cells that were transformed to GH cell adenomas [6]. Deletions of 11q13 locus are characteristic for MEN 1 tumors, which can also be found in some sporadic adenomas [5]. For the development of far most (the majority of) adenomas, a defect in the cellular level of the pituitary is supposed. Activating mutations of the Gs-alpha-gene could be found in about 40% of GH secreting adenomas. Pituitary tumor transforming gene (PTTG) and fibroblastic growth factor (FGF) are overexpressed in most adenomas [7]. The fibroblastic growth factor receptor-4-gene was demonstrated in adenomas in its truncated form [7]. Transgenic mice with this mutation develop Prolactin secreting adenomas. Monoclonality after somatic mutation was supposed for the adenomas and was demonstrated in many of them [8, 9].

Concerning the pathogenesis, a development of microadenomas from nodular hyperplasias is also a possible mechanism, since transition from hyperplasia to adenoma was demonstrated in many unselected postmortem pituitaries [10].

4. Classification

The main principle of classification of pituitary adenomas is the similarity of the different adenoma types with the structural and immunohistochemical features of the special cell types of the normal anterior pituitary (GH cells, Prolactin cells, ACTH cells, TSH cells, FSH cells, and LH cells) [11-15]. For GH-, Prolactin- and ACTH-cell adenomas the density of secretory granules is also important for classification, although in the normal pituitary only Prolactin cells can be densely or sparsely granulated, the latter especially during pregnancy and lactation [16]. Pathologists are requested to use the WHO classification in the current version [17].

5. Adenoma Subtypes

5.1. GH Secreting Adenomas

Pituitary adenomas secreting GH only comprehend 15.1% of ordinary pituitary adenomas (Table 1). Common feature of GH secreting adenomas is an acidophilic granulation, which is weak in sparsely granulated GH cell adenomas and strong in densely granulated GH cell adenomas.

Table 1. Pituitary Adenomas in surgical specimens 1996 - 2014 (German Pituitary Tumor Registry)

Adenoma type	**N**	**%**
Densely granulated GH cell adenoma	708	9.1%
Sparsely granulated GH cell adenoma	467	6.0%
Mixed GH-Prolactin cell adenoma	472	6.1%
Mammosomatotropic adenoma	77	1.0%
Acidophil stem cell adenoma	8	0.1%
Densely granulated Prolactin cell adenoma	16	0.2%
Sparsely granulated Prolactin cell adenoma	631	8.1%
Densely granulated ACTH cell adenoma	628	8.1%
Sparsely granulated ACTH cell adenoma	594	7.7%
Crooke's cell adenoma	2	0.0%
TSH cell adenoma	109	1.4%
FSH/LH cell adenoma	2322	30.0%
Null cell adenoma	1,509	19.5%
Plurihormonal adenoma	78	1.0%
Adenomas, not classified	129	1.7%
All adenomas	**7,750**	**100.0%**

a. Densely granulated GH cell adenomas show a diffuse pattern, slightly pleomorphic, medium-sized or large, partly angular cells. The cytoplasm is strongly acidophilic and PAS-negative. The nuclei may be monomorphic, oval and poor in chromatin or slightly pleomorphic and rich in chromatin. The nuclei are small to medium-sized. Mitoses are very rare or lacking. Immunostaining for GH is mostly very strong. The Ki-67 index does not exceed 3%.

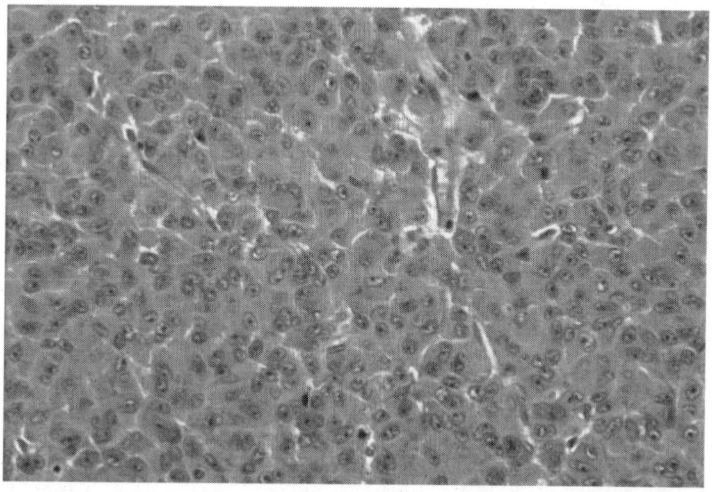

Figure 1. Densely granulated GH cell adenoma: diffusely arranged medium-sized cell with eosinophilic cytoplasm and monomorphic nuclei. Hematoxylin-eosin stain, Magnification: X440.

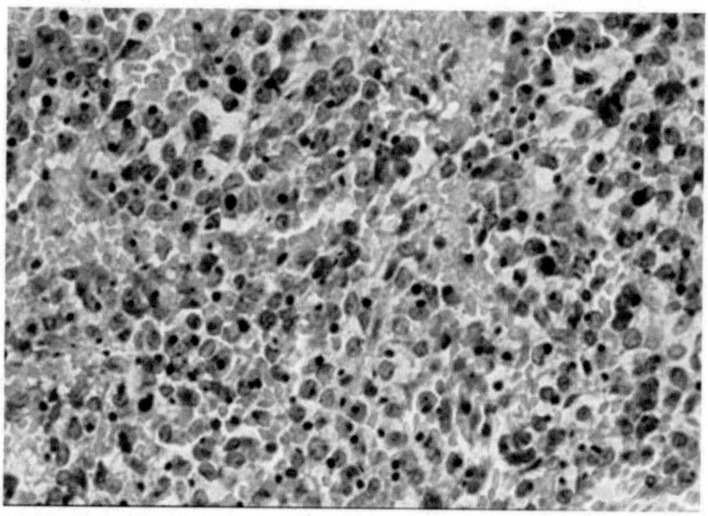

Figure 2. Sparsely granulated GH cell adenoma: medium-sized cells with strongly Keratin-positive globular fibrous bodies in the cytoplasm. Keratin Kl-1 immunostaining-hematoxylin, Magnification: X250.

b. Sparsely granulated GH cell adenomas are composed of slightly acidophilic or chromophobe and PAS-negative cells in a diffuse pattern. Besides the nuclei many cells show globular chromophobe bodies that correspond to ultrastructural fibrous bodies composed of densely arranged cytofilament. These can be demonstrated by immunostaining for Pan-Keratin. The nuclei can be pleomorphic and rich in chromatin. Mitoses are rarely found. The immunostaining for GH is often weak and in rare cases negative. For those adenomas, not only a monoclonal antibody for GH but also a polyclonal antibody for GH should be used.

5.2. Prolactin Secreting Adenomas

Two types of solely Prolactin producing adenomas have to be subclassified (Table 1). They have a proportion of 8.3% of all adenomas.

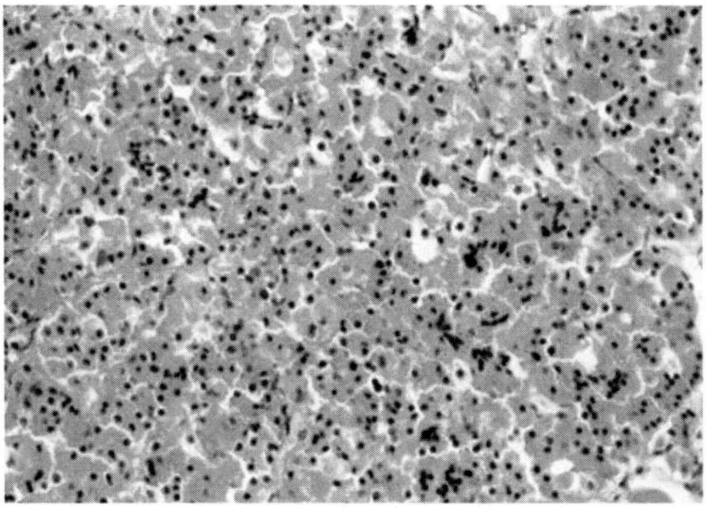

Figure 3. Densely granulated Prolactin cell adenoma: diffusely arranged large cells with eosinophilic cytoplasm. Hematoxylin-eosin stain, Magnification: X250.

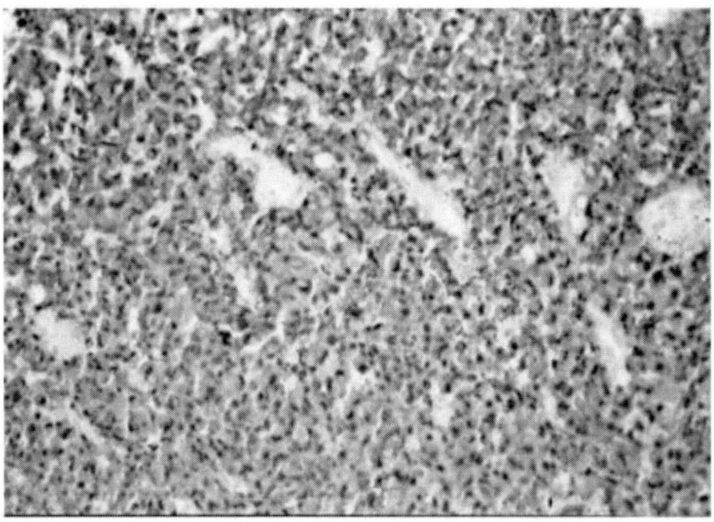

Figure 4. Sparsely granulated Prolactin cell adenoma: diffusely arranged cells with focal immunoreactions of Prolactin ("Golgi pattern"). Prolactin-immunostaining-hematoxylin, Magnification: X250.

a. Densely granulated Prolactin cell adenomas are very rare. They are composed of large acidophilic elongated cells with large nuclei showing moderate chromatin and small nucleoli. The immunostaining for Prolactin is strong and diffuse in cytoplasm. They are more aggressive than the sparsely granulated ones [18].

b. Sparsely granulated Prolactin cell adenomas show a diffuse, trabecular or pseudo-papillar pattern of large chromophobe or slightly basophilic, often elongated cells. The nuclei are large, oval and moderate in chromatin. Mitoses are very rare or lacking. Calcifications, often of psammoma bodies-type can be present. Amyloid of endocrine type is demonstrable in up to 75% of these adenomas [19].

5.3. GH and Prolactin Secreting Adenomas

There are three adenoma types secreting GH and Prolactin (Table 1). They have a proportion of 7.2%. The production of both hormones can be concentrated on different adenoma cells or on nearly all adenoma cells. Bicellular GH and Prolactin adenomas are more aggressive than the monohormonal adenomas [20].

a. The *bicellular GH and Prolactin cell adenomas* are composed of densely or sparsely granulated GH cells and sparsely granulated Prolactin cells. Mostly, the GH positive adenoma cells are more frequent than the Prolactin-positive adenoma cells. The microscopic and ultrastructural features of these adenoma cell types do not differ from those of the monocellular adenoma types.

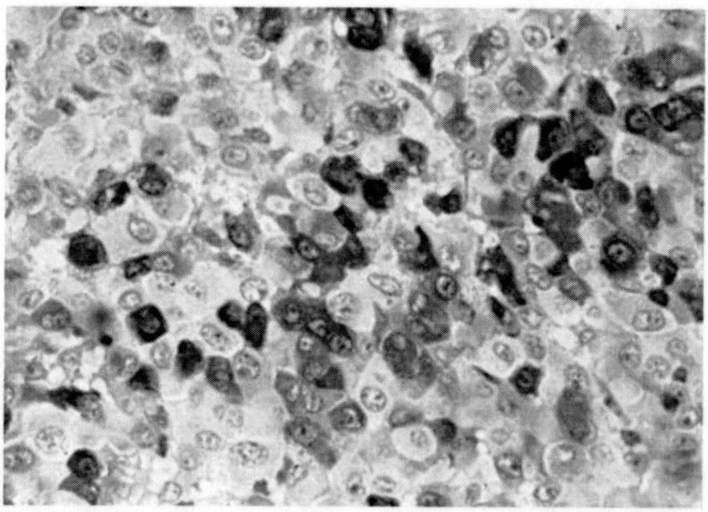

Figure 5. Mixed GH-Prolactin cell adenoma: diffusely arranged medium-sized cells with GH immunostaining in about 40% of cells. GH-immunostaining-hematoxylin, Magnification: X480.

b. The *mammosomatotroph adenoma* is in the light and electron microscope structurally identical with the densely granulated GH cell adenoma but shows a strong common immunostaining for GH and Prolactin in fast most adenoma cells.

c. The very rare *acidophilic stem cell adenoma* has a diffuse pattern of mostly monomorphic, rarely pleomorphic cells with moderately acidophilic cytoplasm. Next to many nuclei, vacuoles of same size as nuclei are found, which are negative in immunostaining for hormones and keratin and correspond to giant mitochondria in the electron microscope. Other cells contain fibrous bodies with keratin-positive globules, looking like those in sparsely granulated GH cell adenomas [11]. Immunostaining for GH is mostly weak, whereas it is distinctly stronger for Prolactin.

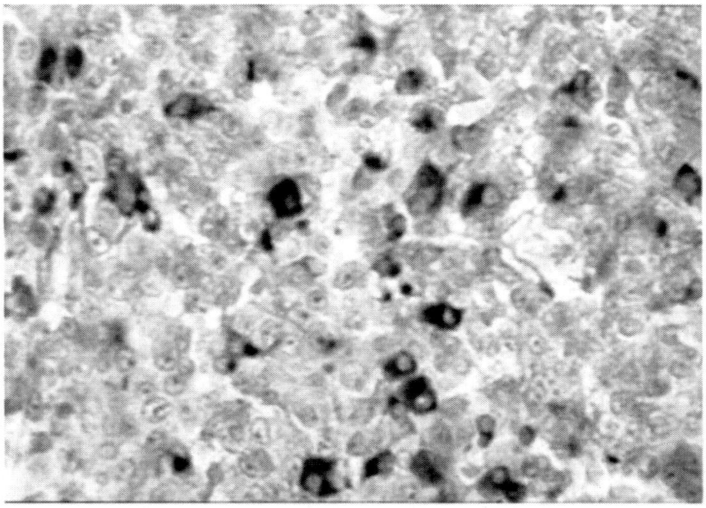

Figure 6. Mixed GH-Prolactin cell adenoma: diffusely arranged medium-sized often spindle-like cells with Prolactin immunostaining in about 30% of cells. Prolactin-immunostaining-hematoxylin, Magnification: X480.

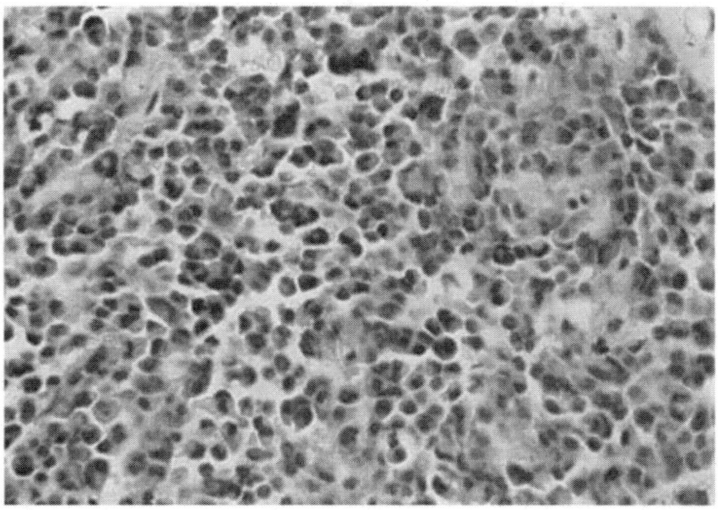

Figure 7. Acidophil stem cell adenoma: diffusely arranged pleomorphic cells with often doubled nuclei and large vacuoles in the cytoplasm by giant mitochondria. Hematoxylin-eosin stain, Magnification: X250.

5.4. ACTH Secreting Adenomas

ACTH-positive adenomas having a proportion of 15.8% are subclassified into densely and sparsely granulated types (Table 1), whereas the very rare third type is composed of Crooke's cells that are strongly suppressed ACTH cells. In the tumor-free pituitary, these Crooke's cells are typical for a hypercortisolism and therefore can be found in all cases with Cushing's syndrome or Morbus Cushing. They may be rarely found also as single cells in densely or sparsely granulated ACTH cell adenomas.

a. Densely granulated ACTH cell adenomas present a diffuse or sinusoidal growth pattern. The cells are monomorphic and medium-sized. The cytoplasm is basophilic. ThePAS-positivity is concentrated at the cellular membrane, where most secretory granules are localized. The nuclei are monomorphic oval and moderate in chromatin. The nucleoli are small. Immunostaining for ACTH is mostly strong. Other hormones of the POMC complex may also be demonstrable [21].

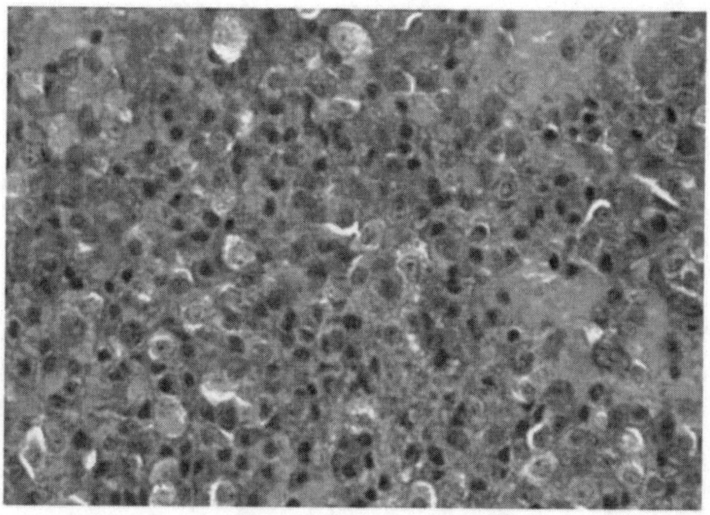

Figure 8. Densely granulated ACTH cell adenoma: diffusely arranged medium-sized monomorphic cells with PAS-positive cytoplasm. PAS-reaction-hematoxylin stain, Magnification: X440.

b. Sparsely granulated ACTH cell adenomas looking similar to the densely granulated ones but pleomorphism of nuclei and cytoplasm may be higher and some mitoses may be found. The cytoplasm is chromophobe or only slightly basophilic. The PAS-reaction is weak or negative.

c. The very rare *Crooke cell adenomas* are composed of Crooke's cells in a diffuse or sinusoidal pattern. The adenoma cells are characterized by a broad cytoplasm with a hyaline ring around the nuclei, being positive for keratins. Next to the nuclei, "enigmatic bodies" [11] with vacuoles and some PAS-positive secretory granules are demonstrable and represent large lysosomes. Other secretory granules are found along the cellular membrane. All these features are also characteristic for the Crooke cells in the tumor-free pituitary. Crooke cell adenomas must be composed of more than 50% Crooke's cells, otherwise they should better be classified as ACTH cell adenomas with Crooke cell parts.

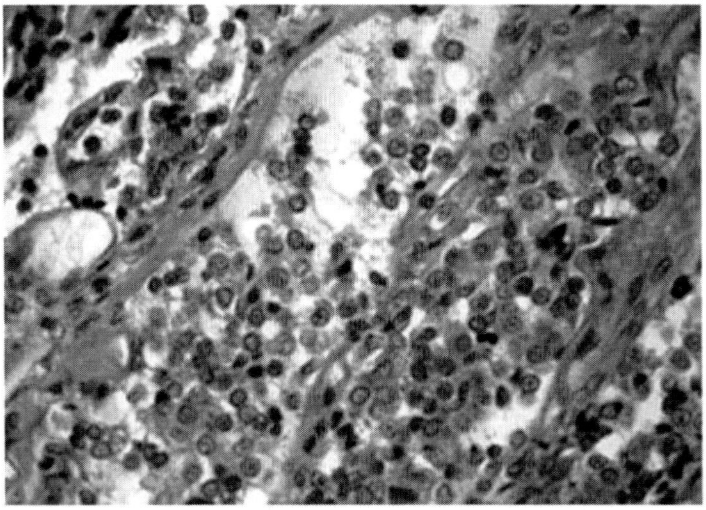

Figure 9. Sparsely granulated ACTH cell adenoma: solid complexes of slightly pleomorphic cells with weakly PAS-positive cytoplasm. PAS-reaction-hematoxylin stain, Magnification: X440.

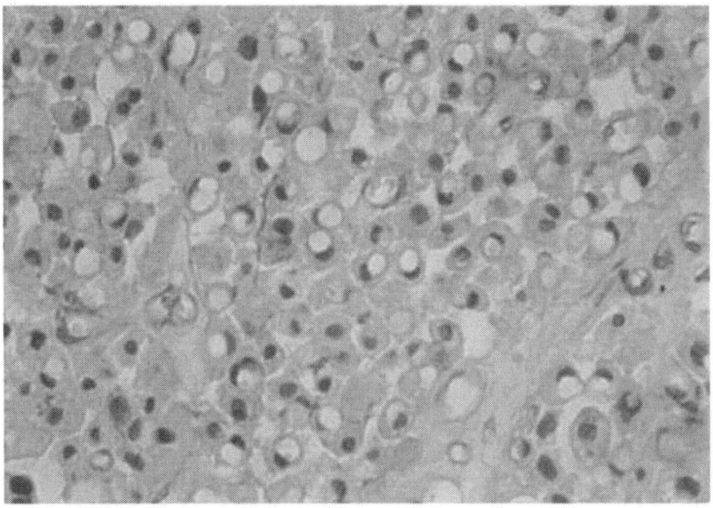

Figure 10. Crooke's cell adenoma: large cells with large vacuoles and sparse PAS-positive granulation pattern. PAS-reaction-hematoxylin stain, Magnification: X480.

5.5. TSH Cell Adenomas

TSH cell adenomas comprehending a proportion of 1.4% are not subclassified (Table 1). The growth pattern is mostly sinusoidal. The cells are medium-sized and chromophobe. Pleomorphism is not rare. Single adenoma cells may harbour PAS-positive globules of lysosomal type. Immunostaining for TSH is differently strong and may be negative [22]. In those rare cases more than one TSH antibody should be used.

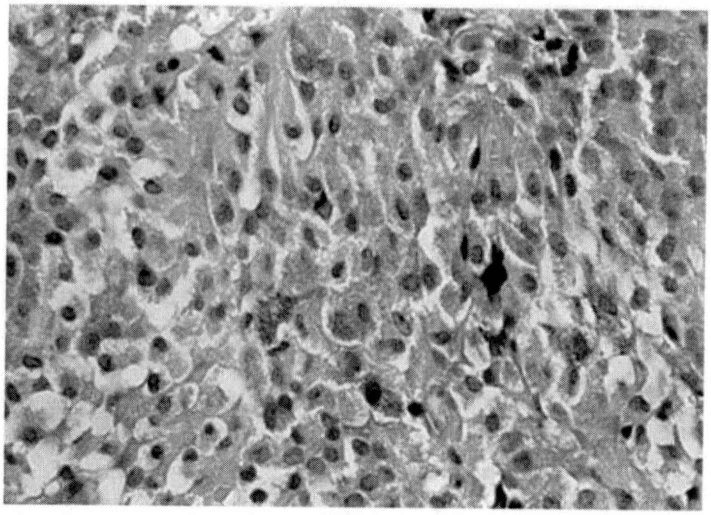

Figure 11. TSH adenoma: diffusely arranged partly spindle-like cells with partly weak TSH-immunostaining in about 20% of cells. TSH-immunostaining-hematoxylin, Magnification: X440.

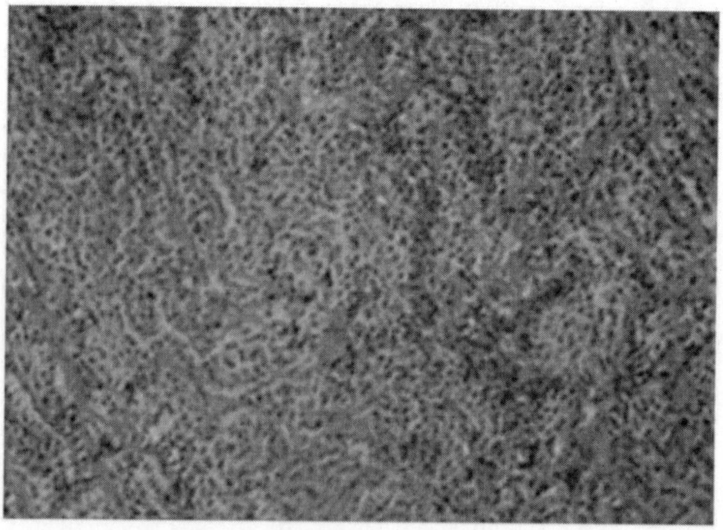

Figure 12. FSH/LH cell adenoma: sinusoidally arranged medium-sizedmonomorphic chromophobic cells. Hematoxylin-eosin stain, Magnification: X180.

5.6. FSH/LH Cell Adenomas

FSH/LH cell adenomas (gonadotroph adenomas) (Table 1) with a proportion of 30% present a sinusoidal growth pattern and pseudorosettes around capillaries. The cells are often large and cylindrical and always chromophobe. The nuclei are mostly oval and monomorphic and poor in chromatin. Many of these adenomas have oncocytic areas with larger more diffusely eosinophilc cells, but this is not accepted as a special adenoma subtype.

Immunostaining for FSH and LH is different. Some adenomas express only one of these both hormones. In some tumors the rate of positive cells is very low (less than 5% of cells). Nevertheless, these adenomas should not be classified as null cell adenomas, since the latter are definitively hormone-negative. In cases with difficult differential diagnosis to null cell adenomas, immunostaining for the transcription factor SF-1 should be used. SF-1 is positive only in the nuclei of FSH/LH cell adenomas.

5.7. Null Cell Adenomas

Null cell adenomas comprehending a proportion of 19.5% (Table 1) are clinically inactive pituitary adenomas without expression of pituitary hormones. They show a diffuse or sinusoidal growth pattern of chromophobe cells. These are small to medium-sized and monomorphic. The nuclei are oval and moderate in chromatin. Mitoses may be rarely found. Immunostaining for neuroendocrine markers is positive, but for pituitary hormones definitively negative, although the alpha-subunit of gonadotropins may be denonstrable. These adenomas had been classified as "alpha-subunit only adenomas." That was not accepted as a special adenoma type in the WHO classification. This applies also for the hormone-negative oncocytic adenomas.

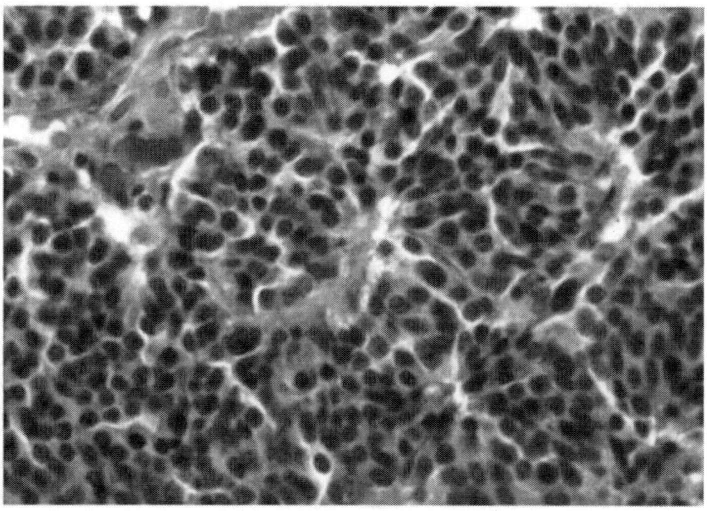

Figure 13. Null cell adenoma: rosettes of small cells with monomorphic chromatin-rich nuclei. Hematoxylin-eosin stain, Magnification: X250.

5.8. Plurihormonal Adenomas

Plurihormonal adenomas are defined as monomorph (frequently) or plurimorph (rarely) adenomas with two or more cell types and immunostaining for more than two pituitary hormones. They have a proportion of 1.0% (Table 1). The improvement of immunostaining with more specific antibodies led to a decrease of positive immunostaining for more than one or two hormones. Furthermore, it is known that one secretory granule can contain more than one pituitary hormones. The bihormonal production of GH and Prolactin in one adenoma is not a sign of plurihormonality, since GH- and Prolactin cells can transform into each other, whereas the not very rare combined production of GH, Prolactin, TSH and alpha-subunit is found in a plurihormonal adenoma.

Another plurihormal adenoma is a polymorph adenoma with expression of FSH, LH, alpha-subunit and TSH or GH and/or Prolactin. A rare third plurihormonal adenoma is the so-called *silent subtype 3 adenoma,* which is always clinically inactive. It is definetively endocrine inactive, but may show a slight hyperprolactinemia. The light microscopic structure [23] shows large chromophobic cells in diffuse arrangement. Some blotchy acidophilia and PAS positive granulation can be seen. Immunostainings [23] reveal mostly hormone-negative parts but also areas with GH-, Prolactin- or TSH-positive cells. ACTH-, FSH- or LH-positive cells are rarely found. The amount of Prolactin-positive cells does not correlate to the level of hyperprolactinemia. For an unequivocal evidence of this adenoma type, electron microscopy is necessary.

5.9. Unclassified Adenomas

The following condtions makes it impossible to subclassify a pituitary: (a) the specimens are mechanically damaged, (b) the specimens are necrotic, (c) the specimens are to small, (d) the specimens show structural and/or immuohistological features, which allow the identification of adenoma but not its subclassification. Unclassified adenomas (Table 1) comprehend 1.7% of all adenomas.

Table 2. Atypical Pituitary Adenomas in surgical specimens 2005 - 2014 (German Pituitary Tumor Registry)

Atypical Adenoma type	**N**	**%**
Atypical densely granulated GH cell adenoma	5	3.2%
Atypical sparsely granulated GH cell adenoma	14	9.0%
Atypical mixed GH-Prolactin cell adenoma	9	5.8%
Atypical mammosomatotropic adenoma	0	0.0%
Atypical acidophil stem cell adenoma	1	0.6%
Atypical densely granulated Prolactin cell adenoma	1	0.6%
Atypical sparsely granulated Prolactin cell adenoma	48	30.8%
Atypical densely granulated ACTH cell adenoma	13	8.3%
Atypical sparsely granulated ACTH cell adenoma	33	21.2%
Atypical Crooke's cell adenoma	0	0.0%
Atypical TSH cell adenoma	2	1.3%
Atypical FSH/LH cell adenoma	8	5.1%
Atypical null cell adenoma	21	13.4%
Atypical plurihormonal adenoma	1	0.6%
Adenomas, not classified	0	0,0%
All atypical adenomas	**156**	**100.0%**

5.10. Atypical Adenomas

Atypical adenomas are defined in the WHO classification of 2004 by an invasive growth, a Ki-67 index of more than 3%, demonstration of mitoses, and a significant nuclear expression of p53. Disregarding these parameters of proliferation, atypical adenomas are classified by the same parameters as the usual adenomas (Table 2). A proportion of atypical adenomas, within the series of adenomas, between 3% and 15% is reported. These great differences can be explained by different interpretations of p53 expression. Whereas in some collections a demonstration of clearly p53-positive nuclei is accepted for the diagnosis [24], in others 4% or more p53-positive nuclei are demanded. A cellular pleomorphism is not a criterion for atypical adenomas, and can be found only in rare atypical adenomas.

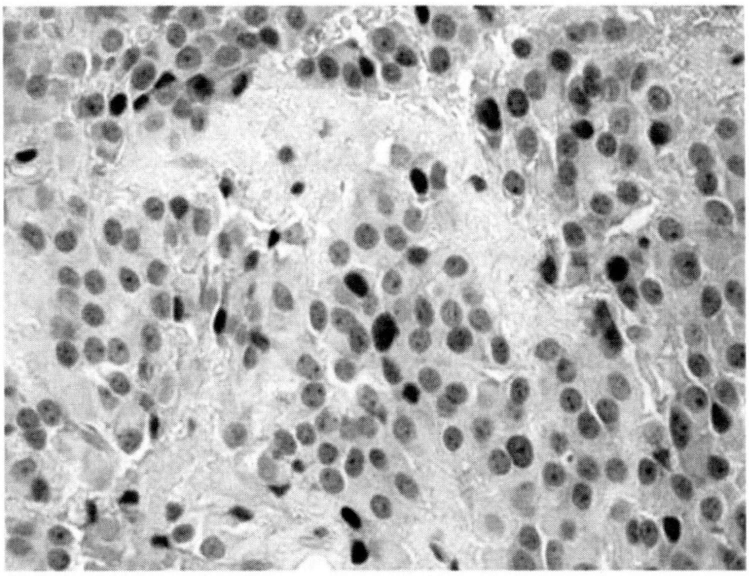

Figure 14. Atypical sparsely granulated ACTH cell adenoma: significant number of p53-positive nuclei. P53-immunostaining-hematoxylin, Magnification: X440.

6. Pituitary Carcinomas

Pituitary carcinomas are defined by demonstration of metastases that must be structurally identical with the intrasellar tumor. The subclassification (Table 3) is identical to that of atypical and ordinary adenomas. Most cases show a high rate of Ki-67 and increased mitoses, but carcinomas with not elevated proliferation parameters are described [25]. The rate of pituitary carcinomas is very low. Their incidence in our material is less than 0.1%.

Table 3. Pituitary Carcinomas (incl. their Metastases) Surgical specimens 1970-2014 (German Pituitary Tumor Registry) (Adenomas N=10,323, Carcinomas N=21, Relation Carcinoma: Adenoma 1: 491)

Case	Type	Clinic	Metastasis
1	ACTH cell carcinoma	Nelson's syndrome	Cerebral
2	ACTH cell carcinoma	Cushing's disease	Spinal
3	Prolactin cell carcinoma	Hyperprolactinemia	Spinal
4	Prolactin cell carcinoma	Hyperprolactinemia	Liver
5	ACTH cell carcinoma	Cushing's disease	Liver
6	ACTH cell carcinoma	Cushing's disease	Liver
7	ACTH cell carcinoma	Cushing's disease	Spinal
8	ACTH cell carcinoma	Cushing's disease	Liver
9	Densely granulated GH-cell carcinoma	Acromegaly	Infiltration of brain
10	ACTH cell carcinoma	Cushing's disease	Cerebral
11	Sparsely granulated GH-cell carcinoma	Acromegaly	Infiltration of brain
12	Metastasis of Prolactin cell carcinoma	Hyperprolactinemia	Spinal
12	Prolactin cell carcinoma	Hyperprolactinemia	Spinal
12	Metastasis of ACTH cell carcinoma	Inactive	Cerebral
13	Metastasis of ACTH cell carcinoma	Cushing's disease	Spinal
14	Metastasis of ACTH cell carcinoma	Inactive	Cerebral
15	Metastasis of ACTH cell carcinoma	Hyperprolactinemia	Spinal
16	Metastasis of Prolactin cell carcinoma	Hyperprolactinemia	Spinal
17	Metastasis of Prolactin cell carcinoma	Hyperprolactinemia	Spinal
18	ACTH cell carcinoma	Cushing's disease	Cerebral
19	Prolactin cell carcinoma	Hyperprolactinemia	Brain ventricle

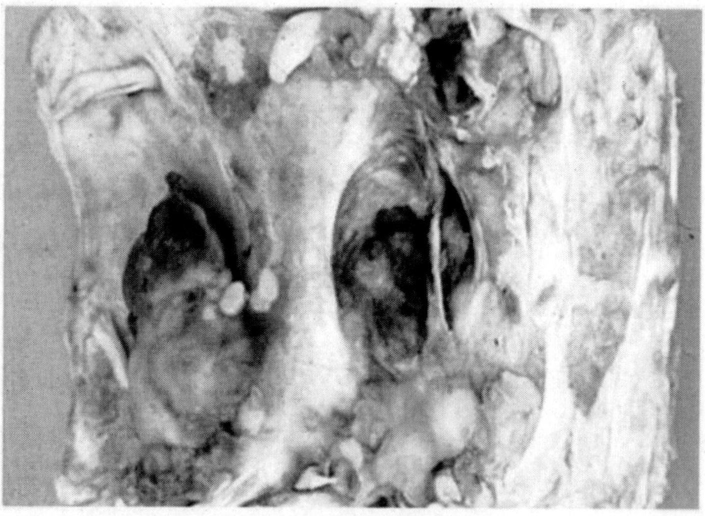

Figure 15. ACTH cell carcinoma: recurrent tumor in the sella, metastases around the sella and the clivus. Macroscopy of autopsy specimen.

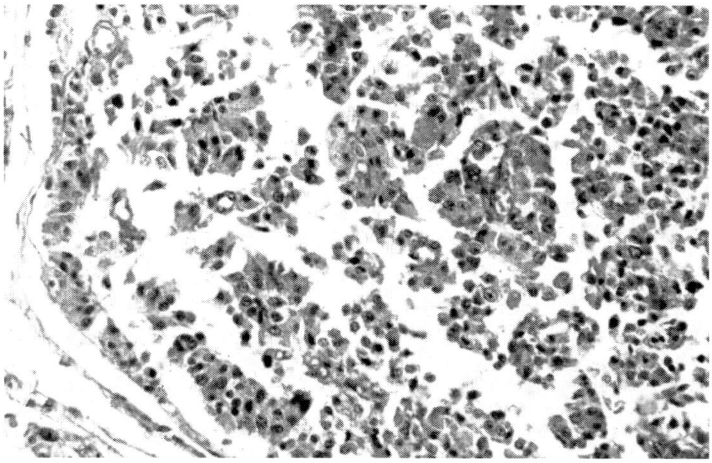

Figure 16. ACTH cell carcinoma: solid formations of slightly pleomorphic cells in the subarachnoid space. Hematoxylin-eosin stain, Magnification: X250.

7. Endocrine Functions of Pituitary Adenomas

The four main types of pituitary hyperfunctions base on a relatively specific spectrum of pituitary adenoma types.

In *acromegaly* (Table 4), we find monohormonal densely and sparsely granulated GH cell adenomas (together 62%), bihormonal (GH and Prolactin) adenomas (together 30.1%), plurihormonal adenomas (4.7%), atypical adenomas of different subtypes (1.2%), and very rarely GH cell carcinomas (0.1%). Due to different biological significance this subclassification is important. Generally, densely granulated GH cell are the only type with enough SST Receptors 2a for successful therapy with somatostatin analogues.

Table 4. Pituitary Tumors in Acromegaly
Surgical specimens 1991-2014 (German Pituitary Tumor Registry)

Adenoma type	N	%
Densely granulated GH cell adenomas	792	38.1%
Atypical densely granulated GH cell adenomas	6	0.3%
Sparsely granulated GH cell adenomas	496	23.9%
Atypical sparsely granulated GH cell adenomas	11	0.5%
Mixed GH-Prolactin cell adenomas	534	25.7%
Atypical mixed GH-Prolactin cell adenomas	7	0.4%
Mammosomatotropic adenomas	88	4.2%
Acidophil stem cell adenomas	4	0.2%
Plurihormonal adenomas	98	4.7%
Adenomas, unclassified	40	1.9%
GH cell carcinomas	2	0.1%
All pituitary tumors in acromegaly	**2,078**	**100.0%**
Additional GHRH Gangliocytoma	15	0.7%

In *isolated hyperprolactinemia,* with exclusion of concomittant hyperprolactinemia, mostly monohormonal Prolactin cell adenomas are found (85%) (Table 5). Bihormonal GH- and Prolactin-secreting adenomas and plurihomonal adenomas (2.1% resp. 3.1%) are rare. Atypical adenomas comprehend 7.1%, Prolactin cell carcinomas 2%. Most sparsely granulated Prolactin cell adenomas are sensible for dopamin agonists, whereas the others are not.

Table 5. Pituitary Tumors in Hyperprolactinemia (without concomitant hyperprolactinemia) Surgical specimens 1991-2014 (German Pituitary Tumor Registry)

Adenoma type	N	%
Densely granulated Prolactin cell adenomas	10	1.7%
Sparsely granulated Prolactin cell adenomas	480	83.3%
Atypical sparsely granulated Prolactin cell adenomas	40	6.9%
Sparsely granulated Prolactin cell adenoma/Prolactin gangliocytoma	1	0.2%
Sparsely granulated GH cell adenoma	1	0.2%
Acidophil stem cell adenoma	6	1.0%
Mixed GH-Prolactin cell adenoma	11	1.9%
Atypical mixed GH-Prolactin cell adenoma	1	0.2%
Mammosomatotropic adenoma	1	0.2%
Plurihormonal adenoma	18	3.1%
Adenoma, not classified	1	0.2%
Prolactin cell carcinoma	6	1.0%
All pituitary tumors in hyperprolactinemia	**576**	**100.0%**

In *Cushing's disease* (Table 6), 54.9% are densely granulated ACTH cell adenomas and 35.2% sparsely granulated ACTH cell adenomas. Atypical ACTH cell adenomas comprehend 1.3%, ACTH cell carcinomas 0.6%. As sign of hypercortisolism the adjacent tumor-free pituitary contains Crooke's cells [26].

Table 6. Pituitary Tumors in Cushing's disease Surgical specimens 1991-2014 (German Pituitary Tumor Registry)

Adenoma type	N	%
Densely granulated ACTH cell adenomas	677	54.9%
Atypical densely granulated ACTH cell adenomas	7	0.6%
Sparsely granulated GH cell adenomas	434	35.2%
Atypical sparsely granulated GH cell adenomas	9	0.7%
Crooke's cell adenomas	3	0.2%
Plurihormonal adenomas	4	0.3%
Adenomas, not classified	91	7.4%
ACTH cell carcinomas	7	0.6%
All pituitary tumors in Cushing's disease	**1,232**	**100.0%**

In *Nelson's syndrome* (Table 7), more sparsely (57.9%) than densely (26.3%) granulated ACTH cell adenomas are found, and due to a not any longer existing hypercortisolism, Crooke's cells are lacking.

In *TSH hyperfunction*, TSH cell adenomas and some plurihormonal adenomas are the result of the oversecretion.

Table 7. Pituitary Tumors in Nelson's syndrome Surgical specimens 1991-2014 (German Pituitary Tumor Registry)

Adenoma type	N	%
Densely granulated ACTH cell adenomas	15	26.3%
Atypical densely granulated ACTH cell adenomas	1	1.8%
Sparsely granulated ACTH cell adenomas	33	57.9%
Atypical sparsely granulated ACTH cell adenomas	7	12.3%
Adenomas, not classified	1	1.8%
ACTH cell carcinomas	0	0.0%
All pituitary tumors in Nelson's syndrome	**57**	**100.0%**

The following adenomas are considered **inactive adenomas** (Table 8): FSH/LH cell adenomas and null cell adenomas, although some FSH/LH cell adenomas induce increased hormone levels. 0.2% resp. 0.7% of them are atypical adenomas.

Table 8. Inactive Pituitary Tumors Surgical specimens 1991-2014 (German Pituitary Tumor Registry)

Adenoma type	N	%
FSH/LH adenomas	2,301	59.7%
Atypical FSH/LH adenomas	8	0.2%
Null cell adenomas	1,524	39.5%
Atypical null cell adenomas	18	0.5%
All inactive pituitary tumors	**3,851**	**100.0%**

Silent adenomas are by immunostaining hormone-positive adenomas that do not lead to an endocrine hyperfunction. The reason for that may be the result of the production of a biologically inactive hormone, which is found by immunostaining. Most of them (Table 9) correspond to sparsely granulated ACTH cell adenomas (37.1%), followed by densely granulated ACTH cell adenomas (12.9%) and sparsely granulated Prolactin cell adenomas (11.2%), TSH cell adenomas (6.8%) and sparsely granulated GH cell adenomas (6.4%). Atypical adenomas account for 6.7%. Generally, the prognosis of silent adenomas is worse than inactive adenomas and the correponding active adenomas. Sparsely granulated ACTH cell adenomas are prone in increased manner to necroses and bleedings.

Table 9. Clinically silent Pituitary Tumors
Surgical specimens 1991-2014 (German Pituitary Tumor Registry)

Adenoma type	**N**	%
Densely granulated GH cell adenomas	6	1.1%
Atypical densely granulated GH cell adenoma	1	0.2%
Sparsely granulated GH cell adenomas	35	6.4%
Atypical sparsely granulated GH cell adenomas	3	0.6%
Mixed GH-Prolactin cell adenomas	10	1.8%
Atypical mixed GH-Prolactin cell adenomas	2	0.4%
Acidophil stem cell adenoma	1	0.2%
Densely granulated Prolactin cell adenomas	4	0.7%
Sparsely granulated Prolactin cell adenomas	61	11.2%
Atypical sparsely granulated Prolactin cell adenomas	12	2.2%
Densely granulated ACTH cell adenomas	70	12.9%
Atypical densely granulated ACTH cell adenomas	4	0.7%
Sparsely granulated ACTH cell adenomas	202	37.1%
Atypical sparsely granulated ACTH cell adenomas	14	2.6%
TSH cell adenomas	37	6.8%
Plurihormonal adenomas	40	7.3%
Adenomas, not classified	40	7.3%
Metastases of ACTH cell carcinoma	2	0.4%
All clinically silent pituitary tumors	**544**	**100.0%**

8. Transcription Factors

The main transcription factors for pituitary adenomas are the same that were identified for the normal pituitary cells. In adenoma pathology, pit-1 is expressed in GH-, Prolactin-, and/or TSH-positive adenomas [27]. NeuroD1 and T-pit are found in ACTH adenomas [28] and SF-1(steroidogenic factor) and GATA-2 in FSH/LH adenomas [29]. These nuclear factors can be used for classification of adenomas when the usual immunostainings for hormones fail.

9. Regressive Changes and Reactions of Drug Therapy

Nearly every adenoma shows regressive changes (fibroses, scars, necroses, necrobioses), some contain fresh or old bleedings in combination with necroses. The cause for these changes is often not demonstrable. In some of these cases a surgery preceded. Radiotherapy does not lead to acute lesions but acute bleedings (so-called “pituitary apoplexia”) are followed by extensive necroses of adenomas. Silent ACTH cell adenomas develope much more frequently such bleedings than all other adenoma types [30].

Dopamine agonists induce a shrinkage of Prolactin adenoma cells and fibroses in the intercellular spaces [31]. After therapy of dopamine responders, the adenoma cells are much smaller and are sometimes similar to lymphocytes. The immunoreactivity for Prolactin is not changed by the therapy. In non-responders for domine agonists, the adenoma cells are unchanged or only some areas of smaller cells are demonstrable. Somatostatin analogues induce only low-grade changes mostly in densely granulated GH cell adenomas: slight perivascular and interstitial fibroses, a stronger acidophilia of the cytoplasm, a stronger GH immunoreactivity and a lower Ki-67 index [32]. Sparsely granulated adenomas and bihormonal GH-Prolactin positive adenomas mostly do not show such changes after therapy. As expected, GH receptor antagonists are without effect on the structure of GH adenomas.

10. Invasive Adenomas

Between 40 and 60% of adenomas are enclosed and non-invasive, about 50% invade surrounding tissues (capsule, dura, bone and/or sphenoid sinus). Macroadenomas (diameter more than 10 mm) are far more frequently invasive than microadenomas (diameter less than 10 mm) [33]. All adenoma types can be invasive, but some show more often an inasive growth: sparsely granulated GH cell macroadenomas (86%), sparsely granulated Prolactin cell macroadenomas (67%), silent ACTH cell macroadenomas (82%), ACTH cell macroadenomas in Nelson's syndrome (70%)[44], and silent subtype 3 adenomas (92%) [34]. All non-functional adenoma types (FSH/LH cell adenomas and null cell adenomas) together are invasive in 28%, all silent adenoma types, that means adenoma types being usually endocrine active, together are invasive in 70% [34].

An invasive growth is biologically insignificant if the tumor can be resected in the first surgery [35]. In those cases, the recurrence rate is not increased in comparison with non-invasive types, after complete resection.

11. Aggressive Adenomas

Some adenoma types, the sparsely granulated GH cell adenoma, the acidophilic stem cell adenoma, the densely granulated Prolactin cell adenoma, the TSH cell adenoma, the sparsely granulated ACTH adenoma, the Crooke's cell adenoma, and the silent subtype 3-adenoma are distinctly more often aggressive than the other types [18, 25]. Also, null cell adenomas may belong to this group [18]. They grow faster and recur more often.

The biological significance of the atypical adenomas is not yet clarified, although signs of increased proliferation are evident. Whether or not they are precursors of pituitary carcinomas is doubtful, although some authors believe that [34]. The fact that in series of atypical adenomas and in series of pituitary carcinomas the Prolactin secreting and the ACTH secreting tumors are over-represented speaks in favour for a sequence from atypical adenoma to carcinoma, but this has to be proved.

Adenomas with increased parameters of proliferation, especially with increased Ki-67 index, mitoses and invasion cannot be designated as atypical adenomas, if nuclear p53 expression is lacking. Some authors reported that adenomas with increased Ki-67 index show an increased rate of recurrences [18, 36], others doubt this [37]. In our opinion, it appears to be important to pay attention to this group. Therefore, in our reports we designate these tumors as adenomas with signs of increased proliferation but unclear significance.

Trouillas et al. [38] created a new clinicopathological classification with grades based on invasion and proliferation. This retrospective multicentric case-control study comprised 410 patients who had surgery for a pituitary tumour with long-term follow-up. Using pituitary magnetic resonance imaging, for diagnosis of cavernous or sphenoid sinus invasion, immunocytochemistry, markers of the cell cycle (Ki-67, mitoses) and p53, tumors were classified according to size (micro, macro and giant), type (PRL, GH, FSH/LH, ACTH and TSH) and grade (grade 1a: non-invasive, 1b: non-invasive and proliferative, 2a: invasive, 2b: invasive and proliferative, and 3: metastatic). The association between patient status at 8-year follow-up and age, sex, and classification was evaluated by two multivariate analyses, assessing disease- or recurrence/progression-free status. At 8 years after surgery, 195 patients were disease-free (controls) and 215 patients were not (cases). In 125 of the cases the tumors had recurred or progressed. Analyses of disease-free and recurrence/progression-free status revealed the significant prognostic value ($p < 0.001$, $p < 0.05$) of age, tumor type, and grade across all tumor types and for each tumor type independently. Invasive and proliferative tumors (grade 2b) had a poor prognosis, with an increased probability of tumor persistence or progression of 25- and 12-fold, respectively, as compared to non-invasive tumors (grade 1a). This new, easy to use clinicopathological classification of pituitary endocrine tumors has demonstrated its prognostic worth by strongly predicting the probability of post-operative complete remission or tumor progression, and so could help clinicians choose the best post-operative therapy [38].

12. PANCH (Pituitary Adenoma Neuronal Choristoma)

A common intrasellar presence of gangliocytoma and pituitary adenoma is called PANCH. Far most cases show gangliocytomas with GHRH expression, in combination with sparsely granulated GH and Prolactin secreting adenomas in acromegaly [39, 40]. Combinations of CRH positive gangliocytomas and ACTH [40] and of gangliocytomas and Prolactin positive adenomas [41] are also reported. The gangliocytomas and the adjacent adenomas are not sharply bordered to each other and transitions from one to the other appear to be present [32, 42]. The biological significance is similar to common adenomas. Their prognosis is not worse.

13. Other Pituitary Tumors

13.1. TTF-1 positive Spindle Cell Tumors

TTF-1 positive Spindle Cell Tumors is a new term for a group of tumors in the sellar region with the common features positivity for TTF-1, S100 protein and spindle cell shape. Three subtypes are defined: the spindle cell oncocytoma subtype, the oncocytic pituicytoma subtype, and the granular cell subtype [43]. All tumors have nuclear positivity for TTF-1 and are negative for CAM5.2, chromogranin-A, and NF. GFAP, vimentin, S100, galectin-3, EMA, and CD68 are variably positive in the majority of the three tumor subtypes [43]. Whereas granular cell tumors were negative for bcl-2 and CD56, pituicytomas and spindle cell oncocytomas showed variable positivity. All tumors were negative with the IDH1-R132H mutation-specific antibody, and none had evidence of BRAF alterations [BRAF(V600E)] mutation and BRAF-KIAA fusion] [43].

a. The *spindle cell oncocytoma subtype* (former spindle cell oncocytoma) is considered to arise from folliculostellate cells, which are sustentacular cells of the adenohypophysis, but recent data suggest that, although pituicytes and all three tumor types are positive for TTF-1, folliculostellate cells are negative for this marker [43]. The spindle cell oncocytoma subtype is composed mainly of fascicles of spindle cells with eosinophilic, granular cytoplasm [44]. Pseudopapillary features and multiple rudimentary to well-formed, follicle-like cavities are possible. The nuclei have spindle shape, the nucleoli are small.

Mitoses are rare and necrosis is absent.

b. The *pituicytoma subtype* (former pituicytoma) arises from pituicytes, which are specialized glia of the posterior pituitary [43]. Pituicytes have five ultrastructural variants: light, dark, granular, ependymal, and oncocytic [27]. The oncocytic pituicytoma subtype shows bundles of cells with delicate eosinophilic extensions around blood vessels.

c. The *granular cell subtype* (former granular cell tumor) of the pituitary gland is thought to arise from granular pituicytes and ultrastructural features are needed to refine their classification [43]. The granular cell subtype [45, 46] shows a mostly medullary pattern or whirl-like shapes. In the broad cytoplasm, granular acidophilic features and fine-grained PAS reactions are demonstrable.

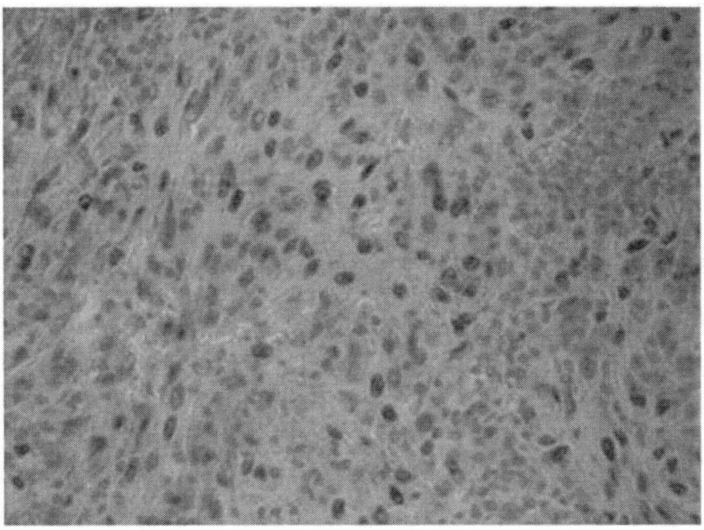

Figure 17. Spindle cell oncocytoma: moderate amount of spindle cells TTF-1-positive nuclei. TTF-1-immunostaining-hematoxylin, Magnification: X440.

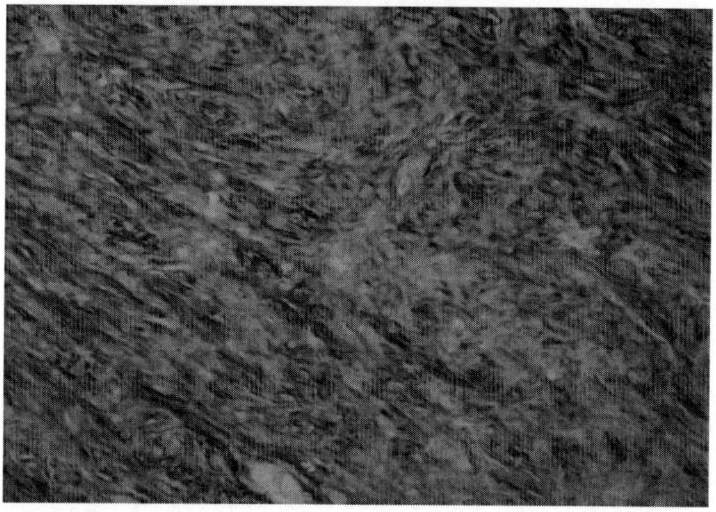

Figure 18. Pituicytoma: fascicles of strongly S100 protein-positive cells. S100-immunostaining-hematoxylin, Magnification: X440.

13.2. Craniopharyngiomas

Craniopharyngiomas are benign squamous epithelial cystic or solid tumors of the sellar region [47]. It is supposed that they develop from Erdheim's epithelia at the pituitary stalk resp. from remnants of the Rathke's pouch, but it may also be possible that they originate from squamous metaplasias of adenohypophysial cells especially of FSH/LH- and ACTH-type [48, 49]. Their proportion of tumors, in the chiasma region, is 22-30%. 45% develop before the age of 20. After the age of 55 they are rare. The prognosis is worse than that of common pituitary adenomas.

Craniopharyngiomas are localized in the suprasellar region (54%), intrasellar (15%) or combind intra- and suprasellar (31%) [50].

Two types have to be considered in the diagnosis: the more frequent adamantinomatous craniopharyngioma and the papillary craniopharyngioma.

13.2.1. Adamantinomatous Craniopharyngiomas

About one half of adamantinomatous craniopharyngiomas are mainly cystic and only 15% are solely solid. The cysts develop from tumor regressions. Their wall shows scars, calcifications and crystals of cholesterol. The vital intact tumor is composed of solid nests of layered squamous epithelia. The basal layer shows palisading, the intermediate layer is acanthoid and the surface layer shows irregular keratosis and parakeratosis. Regressive changes lead to scars, calcifications, siderosis, crystals of cholesterol, and giant cells of foreign body type. Lymphocytes, macrophages, and granulocytes are found in different amounts and distributions. In some craniopharyngiomas the regressions are so extensive that tumor cell remnants are not found by microscopy. In those cases, immunostainings for keratins are helpful to find remnants of squamous epithelia. Beta-Catenin is a good marker for differentiaton of adamantinomatous craniopharyngiomas from other squamous lesions and papillary craniopharyngiomas, since only in adamantinomatous craniopharyngiomas β-

Catenin is not only demonstrated at the cellular membranes, but also in a proportion of nuclei [51].

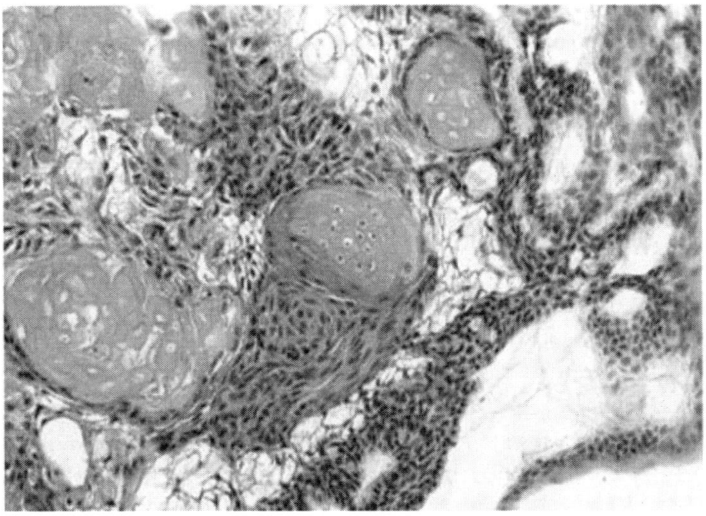

Figure 19. Adamantinomatous craniopharyngioma: solid, stripe-like and pseudoglandular pattern of squamous epithelia with abnormal keratinization. Hematoxylin-eosin stain, Magnification: X250.

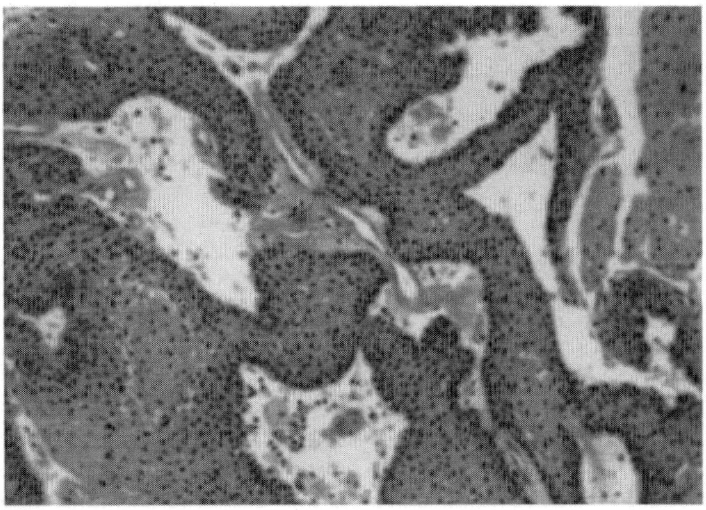

Figure 20. Papillary craniopharyngioma: papillary formations of monomorphic cells, loose connective tissue. Hematoxylin-eosin stain, Magnification: X250.

13.2.2. Papillary Craniopharyngiomas

Papillary craniopharyngiomas are localized in the suprasellar region. They are composed of typical papillary complexes of spinocellular squamous epithelia. A cylindrical basal cell layer is not developed. Keratinization, regressive changes and secondary inflammations are lacking. The adjacent brain tissue develops gliosis. The marker spectrum of keratins is similar to adamantinomatous craniopharyngiomas, but cytokeratin is in contrast to adenomantinomatous craniopharyngiomas expressed only in the surface layer. Beta-catenin is demonstrated only at the cellular membranes but not in nuclei.

14. Metastases in the Pituitary Gland

In unselected postmortem series, metastases in the pituitary are found in 0.2 to 0.3% of all cases. In collections of cases with malignant tumors, postmortem pituitaries showed metastases in 2.6%. They are always combined with bone metastases and are presumably secondary metastases, thus they are not related to the primary metastases of the bone.

In surgical collections (Table 10), metastases of breast cancers are most frequent (25%), followed by cancers of the kidneys (13%), of the prostate (12%), and of the lung (9%). Within the pituitary, metastases are found more frequent in the capsule (85%), than in the neurohypophysis (62%) and in the adenohypophysis (31%).

Table 10. Origin of resected pituitary metastases 1970-2014 (German Pituitary Tumor Registry: All specimens N=12,227, Adenomas N=10,640, Carcinomas N=21)

Primary tumor	N	%
Breast cancer	21	24.7%
Renal cancer	11	12.9%
Prostate cancer	10	11.8%
Cancer of bronchus	8	9.4%
Plasmacytoma	4	4.7%
Gastrointestinal adenocarcinoma	2	2.4%
Salivary gland carcinoma	1	1.2%
Nasal sinus carcinoma	2	2.4%
Urinary bladder cancer	1	1.2%
Malignant melanoma	2	2.4%
Large cell diffuse Non-Hodgkin-Lymphoma	2	2.4%
Unknown primary	21	24.7%
All pituitary metastases	**85**	**100.0%**

Acknowledgments

The studies within this work were mainly financed by Novartis Pharma GmbH (Nuremberg), Novo Nordisk Pharma GmbH (Mainz), Phizer Pharma GmbH (Karlsruhe), and Ipsen Pharma GmbH (Ettlingen).

REFERENCES

[1] Buurman H, Saeger W. Subclinical adenomas in postmortem pituitaries: classification and correlations to clinical data. *Exper Clin Endocr Metab* 2006;114 (Abstract P04-044):S 29.

[2] Saeger W, Schmidt W. Classification and immunohistology of clinically silent adenomas in postmortem pituitaries. In Levy E (editor): Advances in Pathology (anatomic and clinical). Pergamonn Press, Oxford-New York-Toronro-Sydney-Paris-Frankfurt 1994, Vol. 2, pp 343-347.

[3] Tomita,T., Gates, E. Pituitary adenomas and granular cell tumors - Incidence, cell type, and location of tumor in 100 pituitary glands at autopsy. *Am J Clin Pathol* 1999;111:817-825.

[4] Gold EB. Epidemiology of pituitary adenomas. *Epidemiol Rev* 1981;3:163-183.

[5] Shimon I, Melmed S. Pathogenesis and molecular biology of pituitary tumors. In Thapar K, Kovacs K, Scheithauer BW, Lloyd RV (editors): Diagnosis and management of pituitary tumors, Humana Press, Totowa, NJ 2001, Ed. 1, pp 71-80.

[6] Asa SL, Kovacs K, Stefanean L, Horvath E, Billestrup N, Gonzalez-Manchon C, et al. Pituitary adenomas in mice transgenic for growth hormone-releasing hormone. *Endocrinology* 1992;131:2083-2089.

[7] McCabe CJ, Boelaert K, Tannahill LA, Heaney AP, Strattford AL, Khaira JS et al. Vascular endothelial growth factor, its receptor KDR/Flk-1, and pituitary tumor transforming gene in pituitary tumors. *J Clin Endocrinol Metab* 2002;87:4238-4244.

[8] Levy A, Lightman S. Molecular defects in the pathogenesis of pituitary tumours. *Front Neuroendocrinol* 2003;24:94-127.

[9] Ma W, Ikeda H, Yoshimoto T. Clinicopathologic study of 123 cases of prolactin-secreting pituitary adenomas with special reference to multihormone production and clonality of the adenomas. *Cancer* 2002;95:258-266.

[10] Saeger W. Latent hyperplasias and adenomas in post-mortem pituitaries. *Endocr Pathol* 1995;6:379-380.

[11] Asa SL. "Tumors of the pituitary gland." Armed Forces Institute of Pathology, Washington DC 1998, pp 1-210.

[12] George DH, Scheithauer BW, Kovacs K, Horvath E, Young WF Jr, Lloyd RV, et al. Crooke's cell adenoma of the pituitary: an aggressive variant of corticotroph adenoma. *Am J Surg Pathol* 2003;2:1330-1336.

[13] Kovacs K, Horvath E. "Tumors of the pituitary gland." Armed Forces Institute of Pathology, Washington DC, pp 1-269.

[14] Saeger W. "Hypophysenadenome im Operations material." Daten aus dem Hypophysentumorregister 1996-2003. Unveröffentlicht (2004). ["Pituitary adenomas in the operating material." Data from the pituitary Register 1996-2003. Unpublished].

[15] Scheithauer BW. "The pituitary and sellar region." In Sternberg SS (editor): Diagnostic surgical pathology. Raven Press, New York 1989, pp 371-393.

[16] Saeger W. "Die Hypophysentumoren. Cytologische und ultrastrukturelle Klassifikation, Pathogenese, endokrine Funktionen und Tierexperiment" G. Fischer, Stuttgart - New York 1977, pp 1-240.

[17] DeLellis RA, Lloyd RV, Heitz PU. Pathology and genetics: Tumours of endocrine organs (World Health Organization classification of tumours). *International Agency for Research and Cancer (IARC),* Lyon 2004, Ed. 1, pp 1-311.

[18] Mete O, Asa SL. Therapeutic implications of accurate classification of pituitary adenomas. *Semin Diagn Pathol* 2013;30:158-164.

[19] Saeger W, Gerigk C, Missmahl PH, Lüdecke DK. Amyloidablagerungen in Hypophysenadenomen. Polarisationsoptische, immunhistologische und elektronen mikroskopische Untersuchungen. *Pathologe* 1983;4:183-189.

[20] Kreutzer J, Vance ML, Lopes MB, Laws ER Jr. Surgical management of GH-secreting pituitary adenomas: an outcome study using modern remission criteria. *J Clin Endocrinol Metab* 2001;86:4072-4077.

[21] Lloyd RV. Surgical pathology of the pituitary gland. WB Saunders Comp, Philadelphia-London-Toronto-Montreal-Sydney-Tokyo 1993, pp 1-256.

[22] Horvath E, Kovacs K. The adenohypophysis. In Kovacs K, Asa SL (editors): Functional endocrine pathology. Blackwell Scientific Publ, Oxford, London, Edinburgh, Melbourne, Paris, Berlin, Vienna 1991, pp 245-282.

[23] Horvath E, Kovacs K, Smyth HS, Cusimano M, Singer W. Silent adenoma subtype 3 of the pituitary - Immunohistochemical and ultrastructural classification: a review of 29 cases. Ultrastruct Pathol 2005;29:511-524.

[24] Miermeister CP, Petersenn S, Buchfelder M, Fahlbusch R, Lüdecke DK, Hölsken A, et al. Histological criteria for atypical adenomas - data from the German pituitary adenoma registry suggests modifications. Acta Neuropathol Commun 2015;3:50.doi: 10.1186/s40478-015-0229-8.

[25] Di Ieva A, Rotondo F, Syro LV, Cusimano MD, Kovacs K. Aggressive pituitary adenomas-diagnosis and emerging treatments. Nat Rev Endocrinol 2014;10:423-435.

[26] Crooke AC. A change in the basophil cells of the pituitary gland common to conditions which exhibit the syndrome attributed to basophil adenoma. J Pathol Bacteriol 1935;41:339-349.

[27] Asa SL, Puy LA, Lew AM, Sundmark VC, Elsholtz HP. Cell type-specific expression of the pituitary transcription activator pit-1 in the human pituitary and pituitary adenomas. J Clin Endocrinol Metab 1993;77:1275-1280.

[28] Suzuki M, Egashira N, Kajiya H, Minematsu T, Takekoshi S, Tahara S, et al. ACTH and alpha-subunit are co-expressed in rare human pituitary corticotroph cell adenomas proposed to originate from ACTH-committed early pituitary progenitor cells. Endocr Pathol 2008;19:17-26.

[29] Asa SL. Practical pituitary pathology: what does the pathologist need to know? Arch Pathol Lab Med 2008;132:1231-1240.

[30] Lopez JA, Kleinschmidt-Demasters Bk, Sze CI, Woodmansee WW, Lillehei KO. Silent corticotroph adenomas: further clinical and pathological observations. Hum Pathol 2004;35:1137-1147.

[31] Scheithauer BW, Horvath E, Lloyd RV, Kovacs K. Pathology of pituitary adenomas and pituitary hyperplasia. In Thapar K, Kovacs K, Scheithauer BW, Lloyd RV (editors): Diagnosis and management of pituitary tumors, Humana Press, Totowa NJ 2001, Ed. 1, pp 91-154.

[32] Stefaneanu L, Kovacs K, Horvath E, Scheithauer BW. The adenohypophysis. In Stefaneanu L, Sasano H, Kovacs K (editors): Molecular and cellular endocrine pathology. Arnold, London 2000, Ed. 1, pp 75-118.
[33] Scheithauer BW, Kovacs KT, Laws ER Jr, Randall RV. Pathology of invasive pituitary tumors with special reference to functional classification. J Neurosurg 1986;65:733-744.
[34] Scheithauer BW, Gaffey TA, Lloyd RV, Kovacs KT, Horvath E, Yapicier O, et al. Pathobiology of pituitary adenomas and carcinomas. Neurosurgery 2006;59:341-353.
[35] Roelfsema F, Biermasz NR, Pereira AM. Clinical factors involved in the recurrence of pituitary adenomas after surgical remission: a structured review and meta-analysis. Pituitary 2012;15:71-83.
[36] Chiloiro S, Doglietto F, Trapasso B, Lacovazzo D, Giampietro A, Di Nardo F, et al. Typical and atypical pituitary adenomas: a single-center analysis of outcome and prognosis. Neuroendocrinology 2015;101:143-150.
[37] de Aguiar PH, Aires R, Laws ER, Isolan GR, Logullo A, Patil C, Katznelson L. Labeling index in pituitary adenomas evaluated by means of MIB-1: is there a prognostic role? A critical review. Neurol Res 2010;32:1060-1071.
[38] Trouillas J, Roy P, Sturm N, Dantony E, Cortet-Rudelli C, Viennet G, et al. A new prognostic clinicopathological classification of pituitary adenomas: a multicentric case-control study of 410 patients with 8 years post-operative follow-up. Acta Neuropathol 2013;126:123-135.
[39] Kurosaki M, Saeger W, Lüdecke DK. Intrasellar gangliocytomas associated with acromegaly. Brain Tumor Pathol 2002;19:63-67.
[40] Scheithauer BW, Kovacs K, Randall RV, Horvath E, Laws ER Jr. Pathology of excessive production of growth hormone. Clin Endocrinol Metab 1986;15: 655-681.
[41] Puchner MJ, Lüdecke DK, Valdueza JM, Saeger W, Willig RP, Stalla GK, et al. Cushing's disease in a child caused by a corticotropin-releasing hormone-secreting intrasellar gangliocytoma associated with an adrenocorticotropic hormone-secreting pituitary adenoma. Neurosurgery 1993;33:920-925.
[42] Mikami S, Kameyama K, Takahashi S, Yoshida K, Kawase T, Sano T, et al. Combined gangliocytoma and prolactinoma of the pituitary gland. Endocr Pathol 2008;19:117-121.
[43] Mete O, Lopes MB, Asa SL. Spindle cell oncocytomas and granular cell tumors of the pituitary are variants of pituicytoma. Am J Surg Pathol 2013;37:1694-1699.
[44] Roncaroli F, Scheithauer BW, Cenacchi G, Horvath E, Kovacs K, Lloyd RV, et al. 'Spindle cell oncocytoma' of the adenohypophysis: a tumor of folliculostellate cells? Am J Surg Pathol 2002;26:1048-1055.
[45] McKeever PE, Blaivas M, Sima AAF. Neoplasms of the sellar region. In Lloyd RV (editor): Surgical pathology of the pituitary gland. WB Saunders Company, Philadelphia 1993, pp 141-210.
[46] Saeger W. Hypophyse. In Doerr W, Seifert G (editors): Pathologie der endokrinen Organe. Springer, Berlin-Heidelberg-New York 1981, Teil 2, pp 1-226.
[47] Janzer RC, Burger PC, Giangaspero F, Paulus W, Warzok RW, Vogelgesang S, Feiden W, Shuangshoti S. Tumours of the sellar region. In Kleihues P, Cavenee WK (editors): Pathology and genetics: Tumours of the nervous system. International Agency for Research and Cancer (IARC), Lyon 2000, Ed. 1, pp 243-248.

[48] Asa SL, Kovacs K, Bilbao JM. The pars tuberalis of the human pituitary. A histologic, immunohistochemical, ultrastructural and immunoelectron microscopic analysis. Virchows Arch A Pathol Anat Histopathol 1983;399:49-59.

[49] Thapar K, Kovacs K. Neoplasms of the sellar region. In Bigner DD, McLendon RE, Bruner JM, Tamariz AS (editors): Russell and Rubinstein's pathology of tumors of the nervous system. Arnold, London-Sydney-Auckland 1998, Vol. 2, Part II Pathologic Anatomy, Ed. 6, pp 561-680.

[50] Tönnis W. Kraniopharyngiome. In Olivecrona H, Tönnis W (editors): Klinik und Behandlung der raumbeengenden intrakraniellen Prozesse. Springer, Berlin-Göttingen-Heidelberg 1962, pp 186-196.

[51] Buslei R, Nolde M, Hofmann B, Meissner S, Eyupoglu IY, Siebzehnrubl F, et al. Common mutations of beta-catenin in adamantinomatous craniopharyngiomas but not in other tumours originating from the sellar region. Acta Neuropathol 2005;109:589-597.

In: Pituitary Adenoma
Editor: Dimitrios N. Kanakis
ISBN: 978-1-63484-985-2

Chapter 8

IMAGING OF PITUITARY ADENOMAS

Antonios Drevelegas, MD, PhD,
Elissabet Papadopoulou**, *MD, PhD,
and Danai Chourmouzi, MD, PhD
Interbalcan European Medical Center, Thessaloniki, Greece

ABSTRACT

Pituitary Adenomas (PAs) can be classified as functioning and non-functioning adenomas depending of their hormone-secreting activity. In diagnostic imaging adenomas are mainly classified according to their size as microadenomas and macroadenomas, each category displaying specific imaging characteristics.

Imaging of PAs plays a crucial role in diagnosis (especially of non-functioning adenomas), in accurate delineation of tumor extend and determination of its relationship to the adjacent structures. Imaging is also used in the assessment of pharmaceutical therapy and it is most valuable in preoperative surgical planning, evaluation of postoperative status and assessment of tumor recurrence.

MultiDetector Computed Tomography (MDCT) allows aquisition of multiple images during a single rotation of the x-ray tube, which improoves image quality and provides highly diagnostic multiplanar reformations. MDCT can accurately detect bony sellar erosion and tumor calcification, findings most useful in differentiating PAs from other sellar/paraseller masses.

Imaging modality of choice for the evaluation of sellar region is Magnetic Resonance (MR) imaging because of its superior soft tissue contrast differentiation, that enables optimum delineation of sellar and parasellar strustures.

In this chapter the CT/MR anatomy of sellar/parasellar region and the characteristic changes in size and shape of the pituitary gland according to the age and sex are described. Imaging findings of microadenomas and macroadenomas in MR/MDCT are discussed in detail, as well as the more recent applications of advanced MR techniques. Furthermore, emphasis is given on imaging findings differentiating PAs from other sellar/parasellar masses. Postsurgical imaging findings and residual/recurrent tumor features are also discussed.

* Corresponding author: Elissabet Papadopoulou, MD, PhD, Papanikolaou Str. 6, 55238 Panorama, Thessaloniki, Greece, E-mail: antwnis.kol@hotmail.com.

Keywords: pituitary adenoma, CT, MR

1. Changes in Size and Shape of the Pituitary Gland Related to Age and Gender

The pituitary gland undergoes dynamic changes in size and shape during life, reflecting hormonal fluctuations related to age and gender. The radiologist must be familiar with these changes before assessing pituitary pathology.

In neonates, both the anterior and posterior pituitary gland show high signal intensity on T1-weighted images and more globular shape. The high signal intensity of the anterior lobe, which is believed to reflect increased hormonal activity, decreases gradually by about 6 weeks of age. The high signal intensity of the posterior lobe is attributed to the presence of neurosecretory granules, neurophysin, or phospholipids and does not change. As the child grows the pituitary gland decreases in height and increases in width and anteroposterior diameter, obtaining the more flat figure seen in childhood [1].

In childhood the height of the gland in sagittal MR plane is up to 6mm, with no significant differences according to sex.

In adolescence, the gland undergoes physiologic hypertrophy reaching a height up to 10mm in girls and up to 7mm in boys. In pubertal girls the pituitary gland frequently obtains a more spherical shape or a convex upper margin [2] (Figure 1).

Physiologic hypertrophy of the gland is also seen during pregnancy and the immediate postpartum period, when the gland volume is reported to increase by 20-136% [3].

After the age of 20 years the pituitary height decreases [4]. Hormonal factors (e.g., oral contraceptives uptake), female cycle phase, number of given births and menopause, do not significantly influence pituitary volumes (when corrected for age) [5].

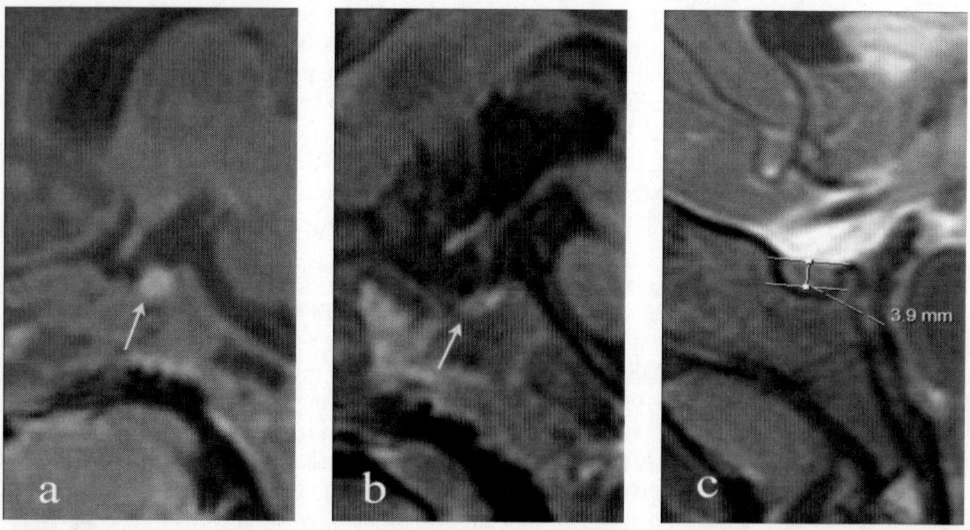

Figure 1. (Continued).

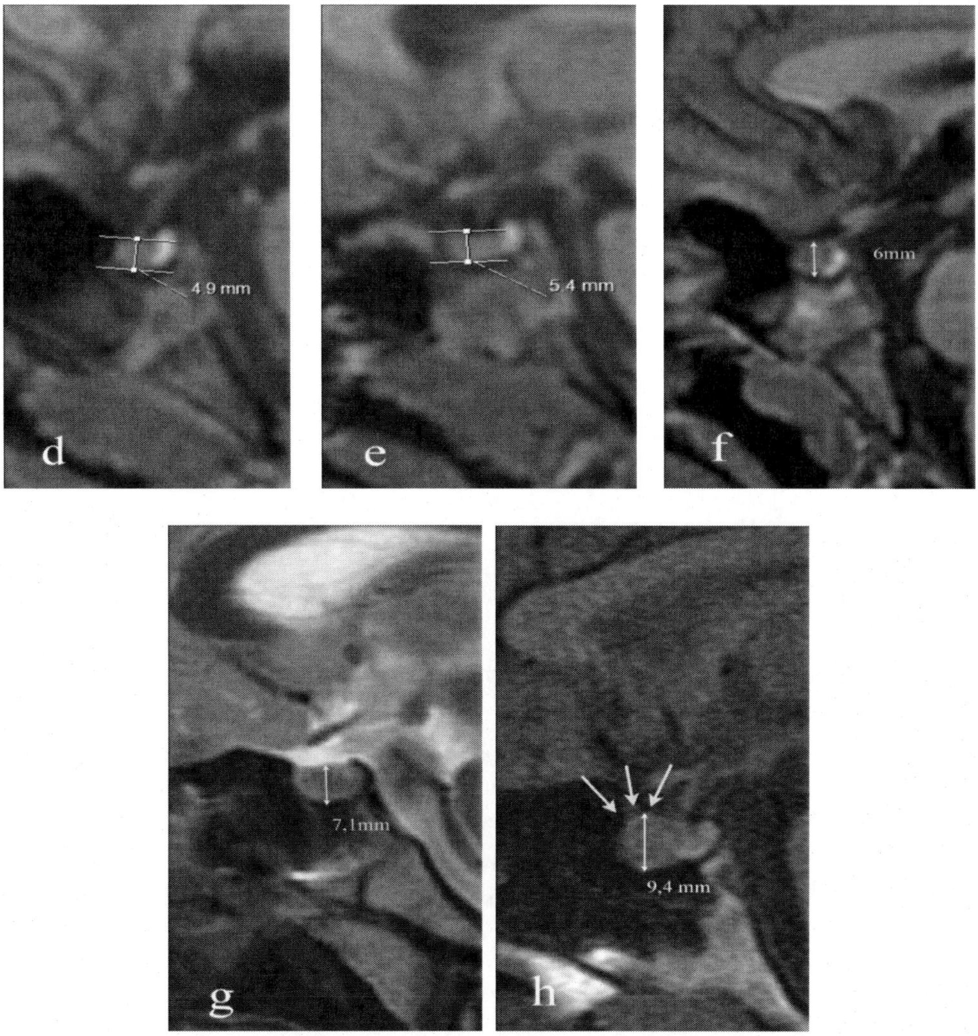

Figure 1. Normal changes in size and shape of the pituitary gland during life: High-signal intensity can be seen in adenohypophysis (arrow) of the neonates (a), while gradually the signal decreases in infants (b). Note the increases signal intensity of the posterior pituitary lobe (arrowhead). Progressive enlargement of the pituitary gland as seen in 2- (c), 4- (d), 6- (e), 10- (f) and 14 year-old child (g). In teenage girls the height of the pituitary gland can normally reach 10mm, sometimes with convex upper border (arrows) (h).

Occasionally, marked flattening of the pituitary gland can be seen, associated with cerebrospinal fluid herniation from the suprasellar cistern, an anatomic variant (and post-operative finding) called "empty sella."

2. Imaging Protocol of the Pituitary Gland

Computed Tomography (CT) scan is not routinely used for the evaluation of sellar-parasellar region. CT images can sometimes add valuable information about presence of calcifications or bone destruction or remodeling, but expose patients to ionizing radiation and lack soft tissue characterization compared to Magnetic Resonance (MR) imaging. CT scan is mainly performed as the initial modality in brain evaluation and sellar/parasellar evaluation when MR is contraindicated (patients with pacemakers, metallic implants, etc). In these cases, high resolution images, with 1mm thickness are obtained in both axial and coronal planes, before and after intravenous administration of contrast medium [6]. Multidetector CT (MDCT) scanners provide highly diagnostic multiplanar reconstruction from axial images only.

MR imaging is the modality of choice for the evaluation of sellar/parasellar region, mainly due to its multiplanar capability and superior soft-tissue characterization. High resolution images are acquired using thin slices (≤3mm), with minimal (1mm) or no gap, small field of view (FOV 20x25cm) and high resolution matrix (256x256 or 256x512). Precontrast and postcontrast MR images are acquired in both sagittal and coronal plane. Dynamic contrast MR imaging is usually applied for the detection of intrasellar pathology, with sometimes acquisition of delayed images, even after 30 minutes. T2-weighted spin echo or double-echo images with the same parameters are also acquired to increase diagnostic accuracy [6].

3. Normal MR Anatomy of the Pituitary Gland

The pituitary gland is composed of two lobes: a) the anterior lobe, which is larger (75% of pituitary volume) and appears homogeneous and isointense on non-contrast T1-weighted (T1W) and T2-weighted (T2W) images. In neonates and occasionally during pregnancy, the anterior pituitary appears hyperintense on T1W images, b) the posterior lobe, which is crescentic and hyperintense on T1W images ("bright spot"). Absence of the posterior pituitary hyperintensity may be caused by ectopic neurohypophysis, central diabetes insipidus, compressive lesions of the pituitary gland, or non-pathological factors [7].

The pituitary gland lies in the sella turcica, a deep depression of the superior surface of the body of the sphenoid bone. The sella turcica in the anteroposterior axis (best seen in sagittal images) is bounded by two elevations, anteriorly the tuberculum sellae and posteriorly the dorsum sellae [8]. Behind the dorsum sellae the clivus is seen, which forms the roof of the nasopharynx.

In the upper surface of the pituitary gland inserts the pituitary stalk (infundibulum), which originates from the hypothalamus, is vertically orientated and has a width of 3mm at its origin and 2mm near its insertion [9]. The infundibulum enhances homogeneously along with the anterior pituitary lobe on post-contrast T1W images, as both lack a blood-brain barrier. The diaphragma sellae, a thin dural membrane, forms the roof of the sella turcica and is not constantly identified on MR images.

In the suprasellar space the optic chiasm is clearly visualized on MR images, as a non-enhancing horizontal structure lying just in front of the pituitary stalk at the site of its origin.

Inferior to the sella turcica, two large irregular cavities with a variable degree of pneumatization, the sphenoid sinuses, are identified, normally demonstrating very low signal intensity on T1W and T2W images, separated by a bony septum.

On either side of the sella turcica lies the carotid groove, which lodges the internal carotid artery (ICA). The ICAs are clearly identified on coronal images next to the pituitary gland, as the rapid blood flow results in a signal void. The ICAs run through the cavernous sinuses, which are hypointense relative to the pituitary gland on non-enhanced images (and thus easier to recognize) and enhance along with the pituitary gland on post-contrast images. The medial dural margin of the cavernous sinuses is not well defined and can better be demarcated on non-enhanced images. The intracavernous neural structures are more hypointense and can sometimes be identified: the 3rd, 4th, V1 and V2 cranial nerves run near the lateral wall (from superior to inferior, respectively), while the 6th cranial nerve runs more proximally and caudally to the carotid artery (Figures 2-3).

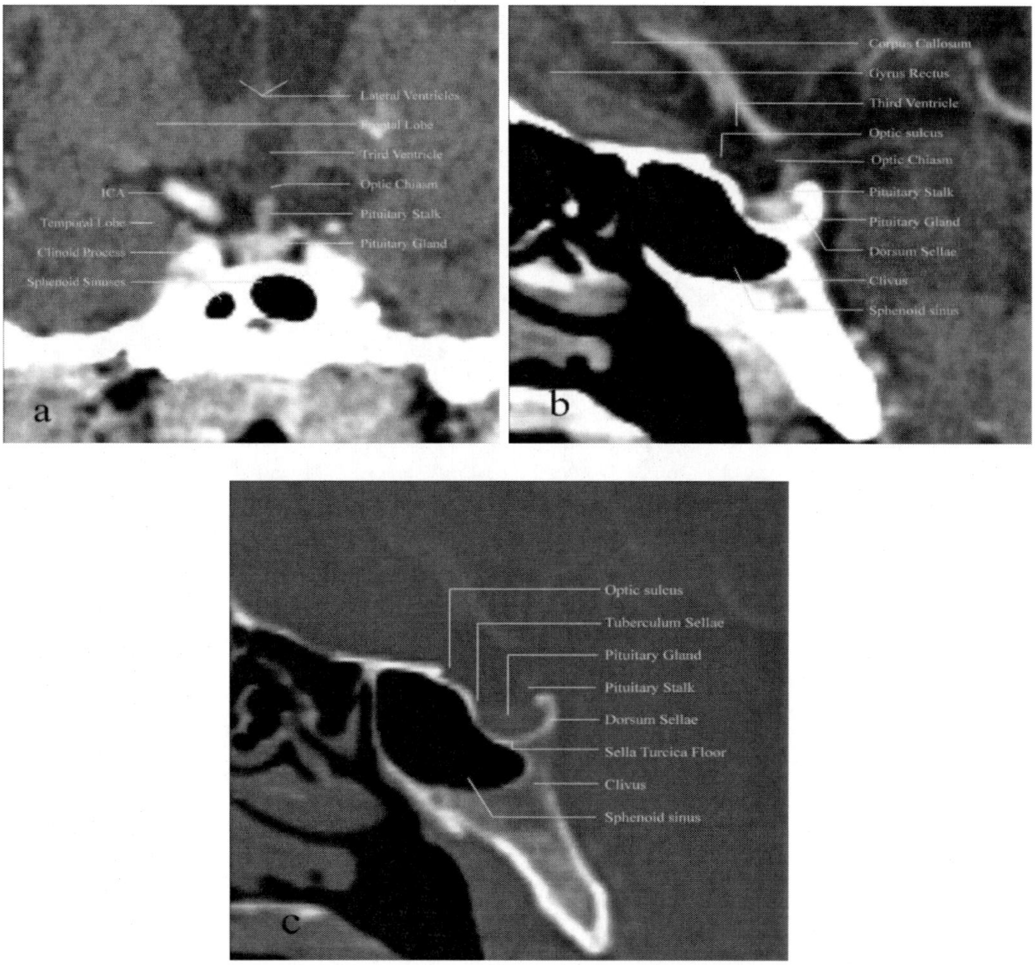

Figure 2. 3D reconstructions in coronal (a) and sagittal (b,c) plane of the sellar region in 128-slice CT scanner, in parenchymal (a,b) and bone (c) window.

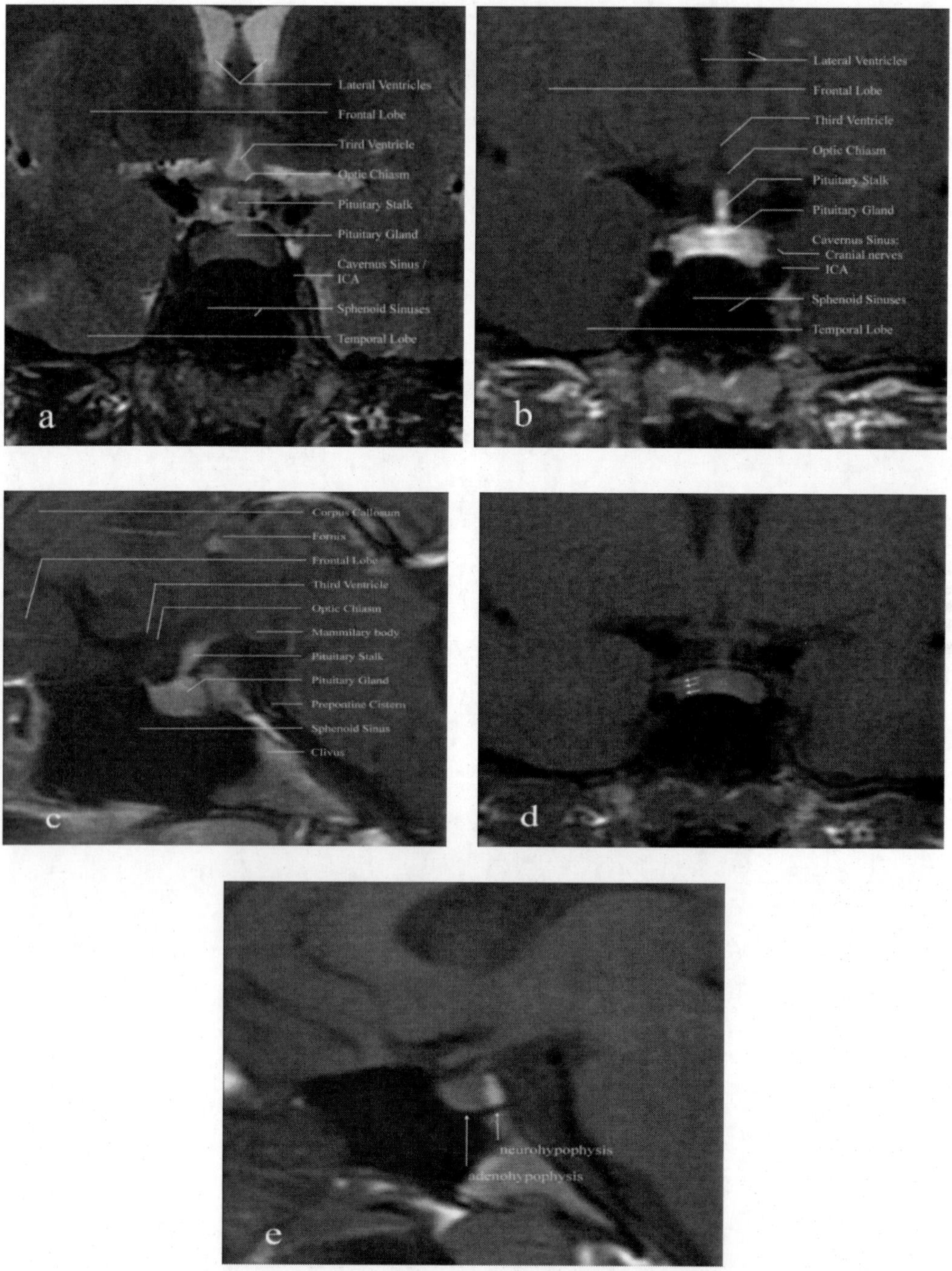

Figure 3. MR anatomy of the sellar region on coronal T2W (a) and post-contrast coronal (b) and sagittal (c) T1W images. On non-contrast T1W images the medial dural margin of the cavernous sinus (arrows) is better delineated as lower signal intensity linear structure (d). On sagittal non-contrast T1W images (e) neurohypophysis shows high signal intensity (short arrow) and can easily be differentiated from adenohypophysis (long arrow).

4. Imaging of Pituitary Adenoma

Pituitary adenomas (PAs) are classified as microadenomas, which are smaller than 10mm in height and macroadenomas, which are greater than 10mm in height.

Microadenomas are typically hypointense or isointense relative to the normal pituitary gland on unenhanced T1W images and show variable signal intensity on T2W images. After contrast administration they typically enhance less than the richly vascularized pituitary gland (Figure 4).

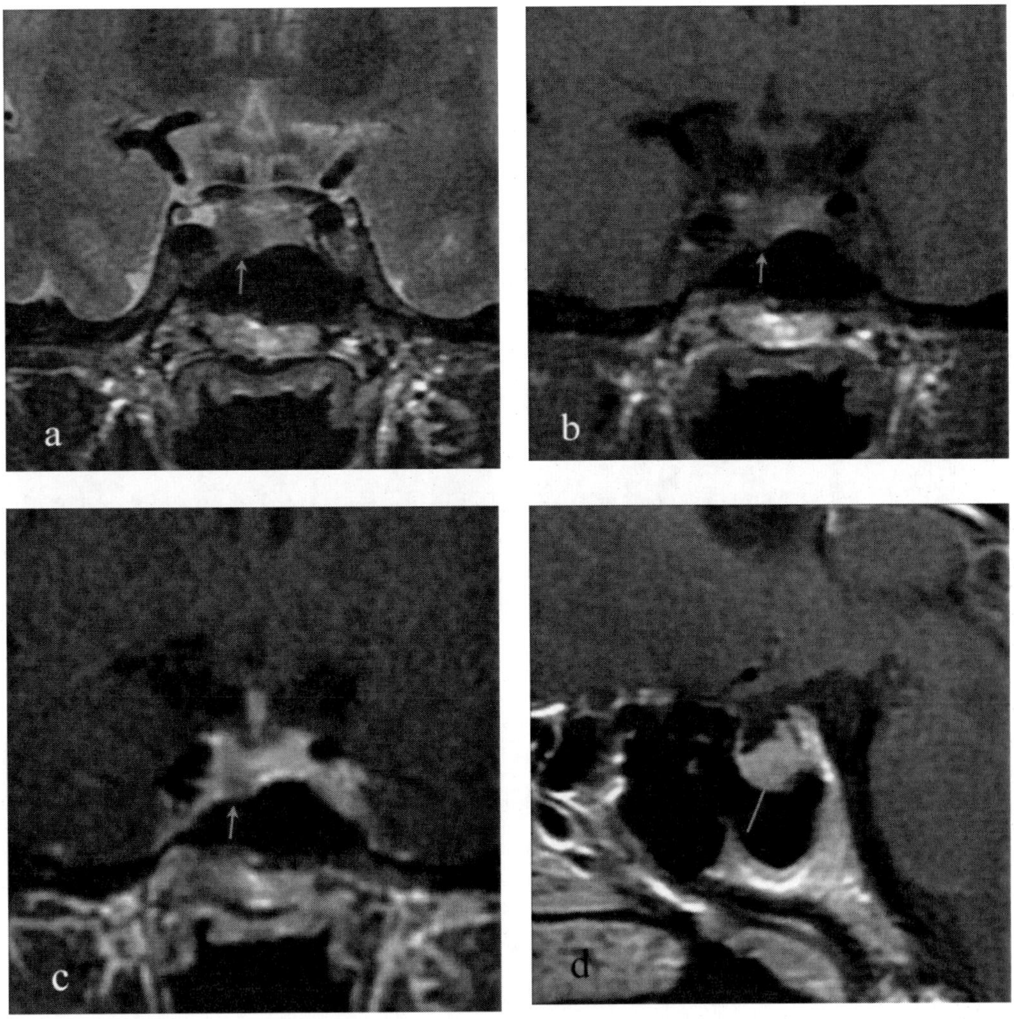

Figure 4. Pituitary microadenoma (arrows) with low signal intensity on coronal T2W (a) and T1W (b) images. On post-contrast T1W coronal (c) and sagittal (d) images, the microadenoma (arrow) shows less enhancement than the pituitary gland.

Due to the different blood supply of the pituitary gland and microadenomas, dynamic MR imaging after contrast administration improves visibility and increases sensitivity of MR in diagnosing pituitary microadenomas. Serial images are obtained every 20 to 30 seconds after gadolinium injection on coronal and sagittal planes. The earliest contrast enhancement is seen in the pars nervosa (supplied by the inferior hypophyseal artery) and the infundibulum (supplied by the superior hypophyseal artery), with the pars distalis enhancing latter (supplied by the portal system). The peak enhancement of the pituitary gland appears within the first two minutes [10-12]. Microadenomas are usually hypovascular, resulting in later peak enhancement, occurring between the second and forth minute. The pituitary gland "wash-out" phase is seen earlier, resulting in delineation of an enhanced microadenoma in an non-enhancing pituitary gland on delayed scan (30-60 minutes) after gadolinium administration (Figure 5). Time for optimal delineation of microadenomas from the pituitary gland is reported to be 1-2 minutes after contrast injection. Early enhancement of microadenomas has also been reported [13, 14] implying a direct arterial blood supply.

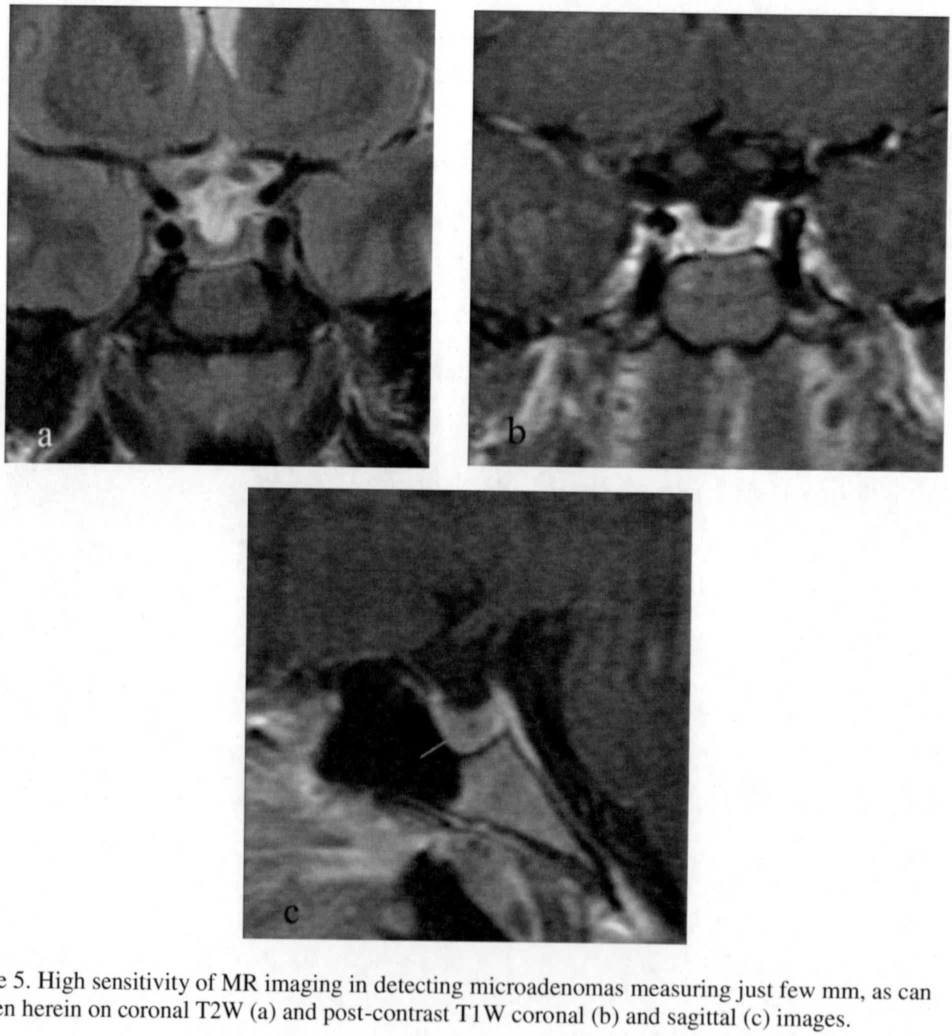

Figure 5. High sensitivity of MR imaging in detecting microadenomas measuring just few mm, as can be seen herein on coronal T2W (a) and post-contrast T1W coronal (b) and sagittal (c) images.

In all cases, dynamic serial MR imaging has proven to be the best imaging technique in diagnosing pituitary microadenomas, increasing the detection rate by an additional 5-20% (compared to conventional non-dynamic contrast-enhanced images) and raising the sensitivity of MR imaging up to 90% [15] (Figure 6).

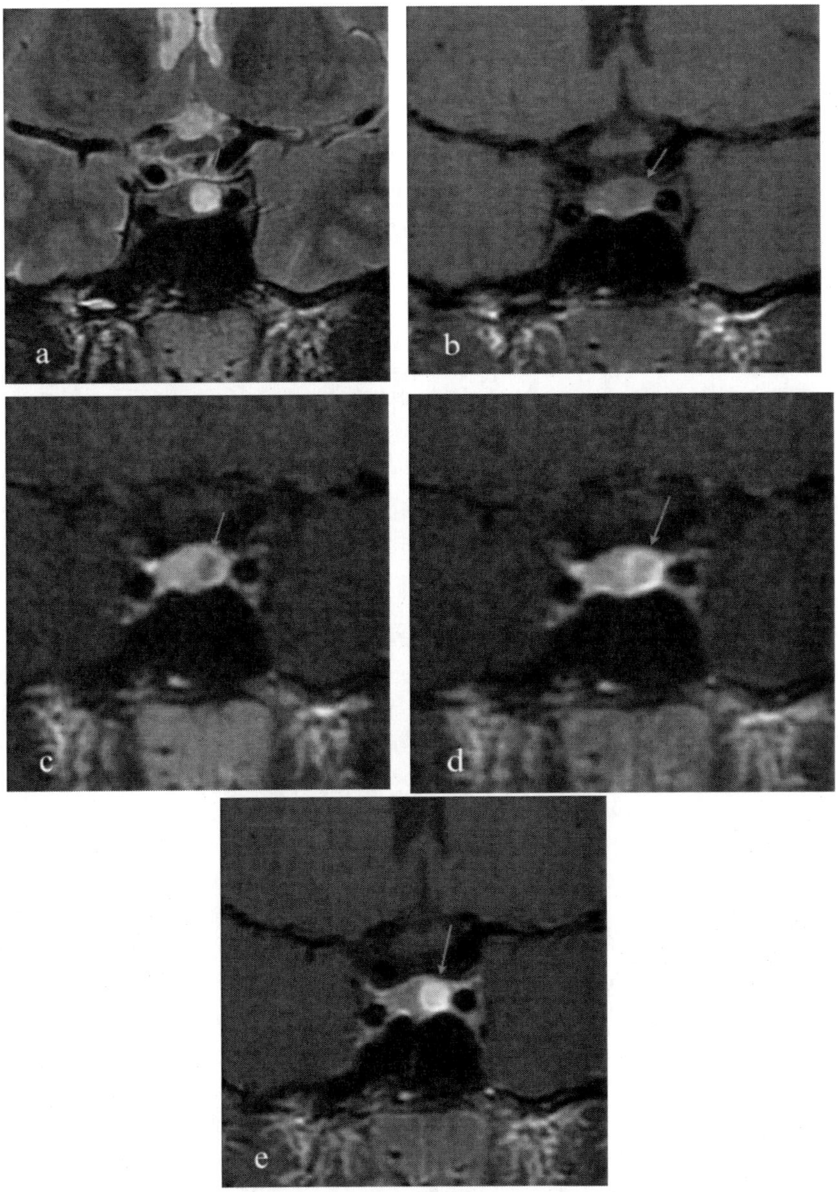

Figure 6. Dynamic MR imaging of a pituitary microadenoma (arrows) with high signal intensity on coronal T2W image (a) and low on coronal T1W image (b). After the intravenous administration of gadolinium the microadenoma in early phase appears hypointense compared to the pituitary gland (c). As the microadenoma begins to enhance (d), its margins are less clearly seen, while on delayed scan (e) the microadenoma becomes hyperintense within the washed-out pituitary gland.

Secondary signs of microadenoma include asymmetrical upward convexity of the gland, lateral displacement of the infundibulum and focal protrusion of the sellar floor.

Secondary signs can also be assessed with CT imaging, which has a less optimal soft-tissue contrast and consequently a lower detection rate of microadenomas. These signs are not diagnostic, since upward convexity can also be seen in adolescent girls and pregnant women and an infundibular deviation can be due to eccentric position of the pituitary gland or ectopic infundibular insertion into the pituitary gland [16, 17]. Thus, CT scan is only used when MR scan is contraindicated and its main role is the detection of calcifications or bony erosions, findings that can orientate differential diagnosis.

Recently, with the introduction of MDCT, multiplanar images of the sellar region are acquired with satisfactory spatial and temporal resolution, which improves the detection of microadenomas [18, 19] and add useful preoperative information about anatomy and integrity of osseous structures [20].

Double or multiple synchronous pituitary adenomas are rare, with an incidence reported to be 0,2-1,8% in surgical reports and 0,9-5,4% in autopsy reports [21]. They are typically microadenomas, the majority secreting growth hormone and either prolactin/ adenocorticotropin/non-secreting adenomas, while the co-existence of ACTH-secreting adenomas and prolactinomas is also reported to be common [21, 22].

Macroadenomas on CT/MR imaging appear as enhancing soft-tissue masses originating in the sella, which cause expansion, remodeling or erosion of the sella floor. On T1W images they are usually isointense relative to the gray matter, while on T2W images they show variable signal intensity. After contrast administration enhancement is typically seen, rendering macroadenomas indistinguishable from the normal pituitary gland (Figure 7). Hemorrhage is not infrequent, with a prevalence reported to be 14-17%. It can be clinically occult or may cause the clinical syndrome of pituitary apoplexy [16, 23]. Subacute hemorrhage is seen with high signal intensity on T1W images (Figure 8), while acute and chronic hemorrhage are best seen on T2*W images as marked low signal intensity [23]. Cystic changes can be seen in up to 18% of macroadenomas, while calcifications are rare [6].

The most common route of extension of pituitary macroadenomas is towards the suprasellar region, where constriction by the diaphragma sellae produces o "figure-of-eight" configuration. Further superior extension can cause optic nerve/chiasm compression. Contrast-enhanced FIESTA MR sequence is reported to provide optimum delineation of the optic nerve and chiasm, when compressed by large suprasellar tumors [24]. Optic nerve hyperintensity on T2W images and edema-like changes along the optic pathway have also been reported in patients with suprasellar extension of pituitary macroadenomas [25, 26]. The infundibulum can be laterally displaced or compressed upwardly against the inferior hypothalamus.

Infrasellar extension causes remodeling or erosion of the sellar floor and protrusion of the adenoma into the sublying sphenoid sinus/bone, imaging findings better assessed with CT.

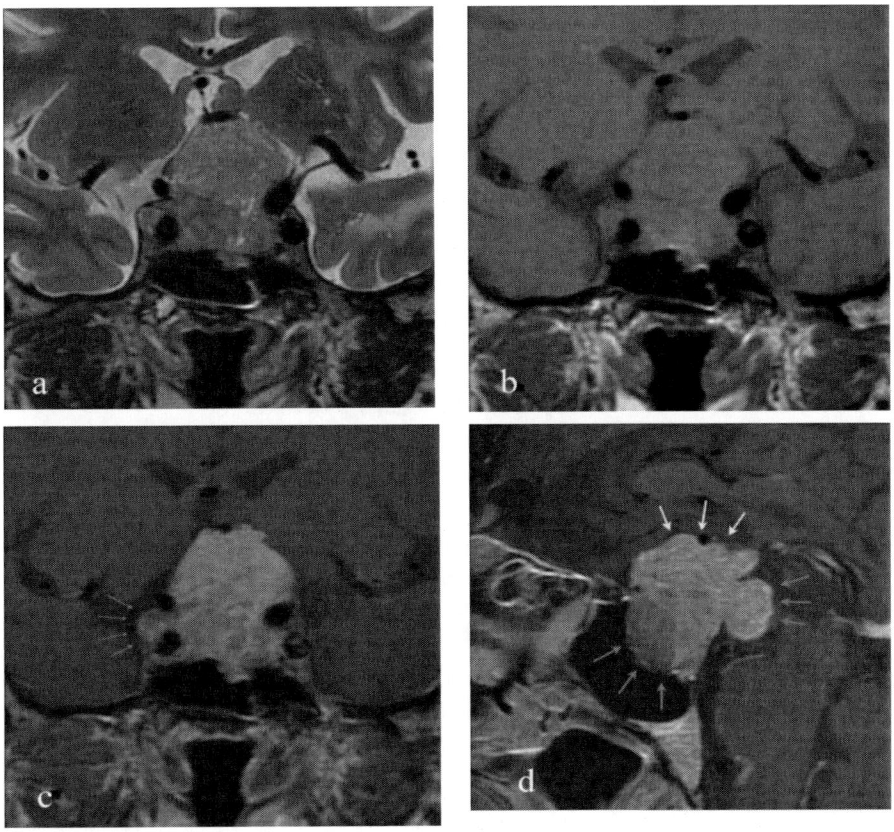

Figure 7. Pituitary macroadenoma isointense on coronal T2W (a) and T1W (b) images, with intense enhancement on post-contrast T1W coronal (c) and sagittal (d) images. Typical "figure-of-eight" configuration, with a constriction at the level of the diaphragm sellae. Encasement of the right cavernous sinus is clearly seen on coronal post-contrast T1W image (red arrows). The macroadenoma extends upwards in the suprasellar region, compressing the hypothalamus (yellow arrows), as well as posteriorly in the interpenduncular cistern (red arrows). Down slopping of the adenoma to the sphenoid sinus is also seen (blue arrows).

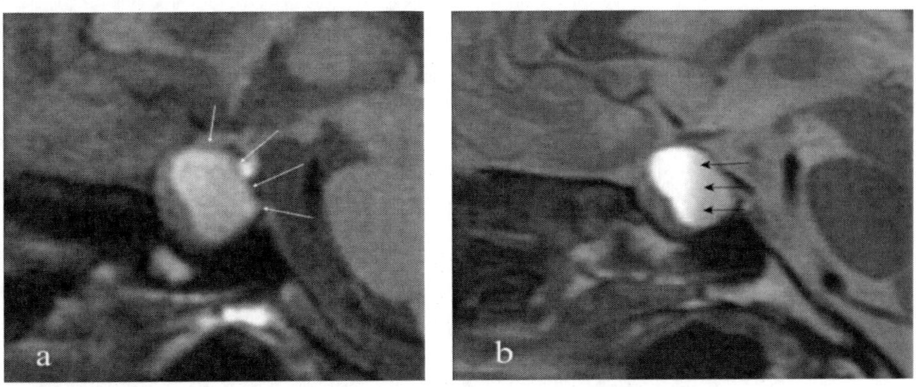

Figure 8. Subacute hemorrhage in a pituitary macroadenoma on sagittal T1W (a) and T2W (b) images. On T1W image the hemorrhage shows high signal intensity (white arrows) and on T2W image fluid-fluid level (black arrows).

Lateral extension of a pituitary macroadenoma can cause compression or invasion of the cavernous sinus. Invasion of a cavernous sinus by a pituitary macroadenoma is reported to occur in 6-10% of cases and is often associated with a more difficult and less efficient surgery, as well as with more increased frequency of postoperative complications [27]. Since the medial wall of the cavernous sinuses is not clearly delineated neither by CT, nor by MR imaging, the differential diagnosis of compression or invasion can be difficult. Encasement of the intracavernous ICA by more than two thirds of its diameter is reported to be a specific sign of cavernous sinus invasion, while invasion is highly probable when the adenoma obscures the carotid sulcus venous compartment or extends beyond the line joining the lateral wall of the intracavernous and supracavernous ICA [27].

Posterior extension is the less common route of extension of pituitary macroadenomas, with clival invasion reported to occur in 8% of patients [28].

There are no characteristic imaging findings correlating with hormonal activity of adenomas, though infrasellar extension, hypointensity on T2W images and smaller tumor size are reported to be more common in somatotropin macroadenomas, while suprasellar extension is reported to be more common in non-functioning adenomas [29-32]. Additionally, somatotropin microadenomas are reported to be more commonly associated with empty sella [33]. Giant adenomas compressing the brain parenchyma and causing seizures are reported to be typically prolactinomas [34].

Aggressive pituitary adenomas are rare and can cause dissemination within the neuroaxis via subarachnoid and hematogenous spread. They are typically histologically benign, with multiple relapses. Dissemination can occur without residual or recurrent intrasellar tumor [35] and prognosis is usually, but not always [36], poor.

5. Imaging at 3 Tesla

High field MR imaging is reported to have a significantly improved spatial resolution compared to 1,5 Tesla imaging. Higher resolution offers better delineation of sellar and parasellar anatomy.

Detailed anatomy of the pituitary stalk [37], better visualization of normal or invaded cavernous sinuses, as well as increased sensitivity and specificity, with ability to depict very small adenomas (even 2mm in diameter) have been reported with the application of 3 Tesla MR imaging [38-40].

Three Tesla MR imaging has also been applied intraoperatively. It is reported to provide accurate information about the extent of resection and it can often lead to additional tumor resection [41, 42].

6. Advanced MR Imaging

Advanced MR imaging has evolved the last years to a widespread diagnostic tool, that provides morphologic, as well as biologic information. Cellularity (Diffusion Weighted Imaging), hemodynamics (Perfusion Weighted Imaging), metabolism (MR-Spectroscopy), function (Functional MR Imaging) and cytoarchitecture (Diffusion Tensor Imaging) are parameters evaluated by advanced MR techniques, increasing diagnostic accuracy [43].

- **Diffusion Weighted Imaging** (DWI) evaluates water diffusivity within the extracellular space. Reduction of water diffusivity within the extracellular space implies increased cellularity. Quantitative assessment of diffusivity is expressed by Apparent Diffusion Coefficient (ADC): The lower the ADC, the higher the cellularity.

The ADC of pituitary macroadenomas is reported to be lower than that of craniopharyngiomas, with an ADC value of 0.6 x 10^{-3} mm^2 /sec reported to be highly suggestive of macroadenoma [44, 45].

DWI is also reported to assist in the early detection of acute pituitary apoplexy-infarction, characterized by restricted water diffusion [46].

The ability of DWI to evaluate the consistency of a pituitary macroadenoma has become the "apple of Eris" between many researchers, since soft macroadenomas are successfully treated by transsphenoidal surgery, while hard tumors may demand a transcranial approach. While some researchers support the absence of correlation of ADC with tumor consistency [47], most of the reported studies describe ADC values of 0.6 - 0.8 x 10^{-3} mm^2 /sec indicative of soft or intermediate macroadenomas, while ADC values of 1.3 x 10^{-3} mm^2 /sec suggestive of hard macroadenomas [48-51]. Lu et al. [52] reports the correlation of ADC values to the collagen content of macroadenomas in an aligned relationship: the more the collagen content in a macroadenoma, the lower the ADC ratio.

Finally, ADC values of the pituitary gland are reported to predict pituitary function in patients with traumatic brain injury [53].

- **Diffusion Tensor Imaging** (DTI) is an application of DWI characterized by its sensitivity to directionally depended diffusion (anisotropy) and provides information about the integrity of white matter tracts. Nichols et al. [54] describe the study of optic pathway with DTI in patients with pituitary tumors.
- **MR Spectroscopy** (MRS) is a technique that enables identification and quantification of metabolites. The most common brain metabolites are: N-acetylaspartate (NAA), which is a marker of neuronal density and integrity, Choline (Cho), which is a marker of cellular proliferation, Lactate (Lac), which is the end-product of anaerobic glycolysis, Lipids (Lip), which are components of cell membranes and are increased in cellular membrane destruction and necrosis, and Creatine (Cr), which is a marker of intracellular energy-metabolism and is relatively constant [43].

Faten et al. report that on MRS macroadenoma is usually characterized by a significant reduction of NAA, moderate elevation of Cho, frequent small Lip/Lac peaks and reduced Cr [48]. Stadlbeuer et al. report the absence of Cho in hemorrhagic macroadenomas [55]. Furthermore, Chaudhory et al. report the increased Cho in gliomas, dominant lipid peak in craniopharyngiomas and germinomas and increased myoinositol in hypothalamic hamartomas

[56]. Thus, MRS data can contribute to differential diagnosis of sellar/parasellar masses and provide information about hemorrhage in pituitary adenomas.

- **Perfusion Weighted Imaging** (PWI) is a method used to estimate capillary permeability and vasculature by measuring the contrast agent concentration over time. PWI is reported to assess the vascular density of non-functioning macroadenomas, related to the risk of intra- and post-operative tumor hemorrhage [57]. Pituitary gland perfusion delay is reported in idiopathic growth hormone deficiency [58] and secondary to dural arteriovenous fistulas in the cavernous sinus [59].
- **Functional MR Imaging** (fMRI) is a technique that studies cortical activity in response to stimuli or actions. Song et al. [60] report the decrease in visual cortex activation after eye stimulation in patients with pituitary macroadenomas, with a correlation between the decrease in visual cortex activation and the visual field defect [60]. Furthermore, fMRI in association with DTI can be used for the correlation of anterior optic pathway compression with functional vision and thus prediction of postoperative visual recovery [61].
- **Magnetization Transfer** (MT) is a technique used to evaluate tissues containing macromolecules, since they can transfer magnetization more efficiently. The quantitative marker is the MT Ratio (MTR), which is related to the difference in signal intensity between a sequence with and one without application of MT. The MTR of prolactinomas is reported to be higher than the normal pituitary gland and the normal pituitary gland has higher MTR than non-secreting adenomas. Furthermore, MTR is reported to be able to detect postoperative residual tumor when conventional MR imaging is negative [62].

7. Differential Diagnosis of Pituitary Adenoma

Differential diagnosis of pituitary adenoma should include:

- **Meningiomas**: differential diagnostic problems are usually encountered from meningiomas arising from the diaphragma sellae, since meningiomas from other origin with intra- or suprasellar extension are usually characterized by broad dural base, dural tail sign and/or hyperostosis. The main finding suggestive of a meningioma of the diaphragma sellae with intrasellar extension versus pituitary adenoma is that the epicenter of the lesion is not seen in the sella and the detection of the compressed and/or deviated pituitary gland (Figure 9). Meningiomas are usually hyperdense on CT scan, isointense on T1W and T2W images and enhance strongly after the intravenous administration of contrast medium. Calcifications are not rare. On MRS meningiomas show a characteristic alanine peak [43].

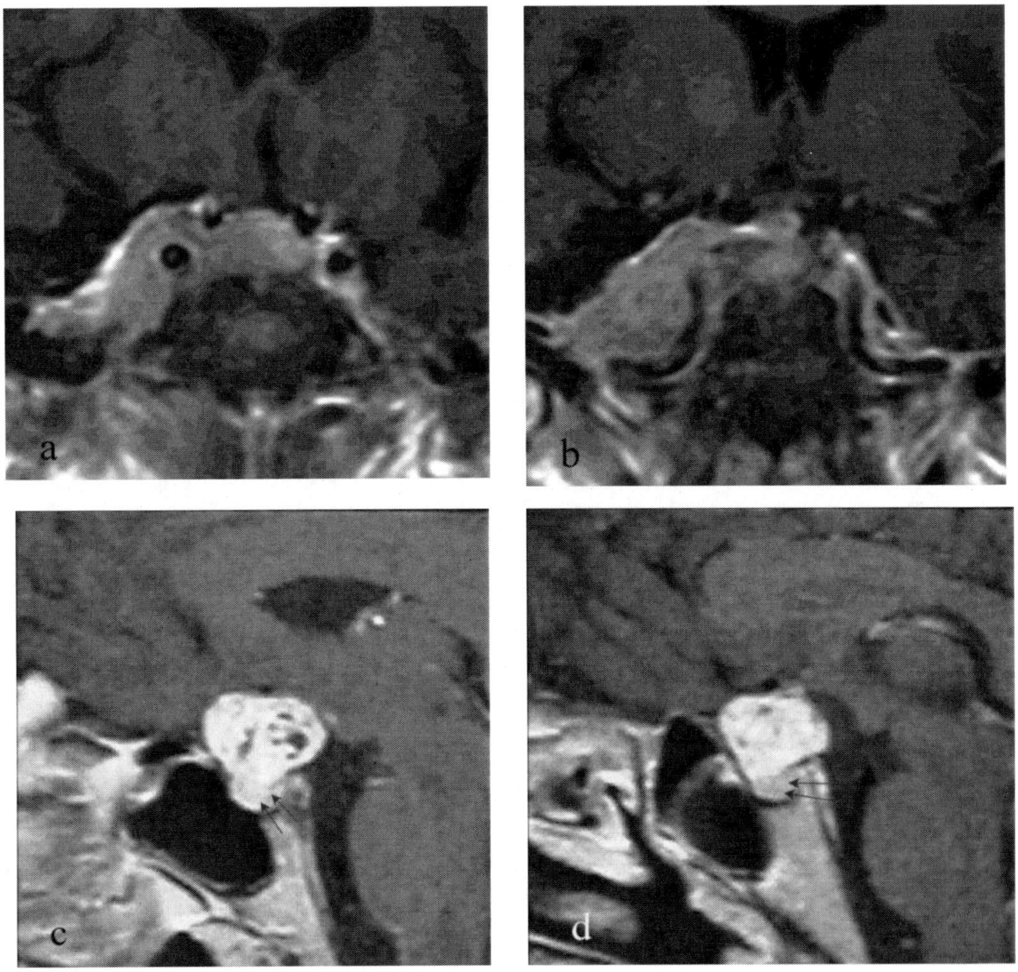

Figure 9. Pituitary macroadenomas can sometimes be difficult to differentiate from meningiomas (a,b) or craniopharyngiomas (c,d), as seen herein in coronal (a,b) and sagittal (c,d) contrast-enhanced T1W images. The best diagnostic clue is the recognition of the compressed/deviated pituitary gland in the pituitary fossa (arrows).

- **Craniopharyngiomas**: Intrasellar and/or suprasellar in location, craniopharyngiomas are divided in two histologic types: (i) the adamantinomatus, more common in children and young adults, typically with cystic (serous or mucoid) and solid enhancing components and calcifications, and (ii) the squamous papillary, usually in older adults, predominately solid (Figure 9). On DWI the ADC of craniopharyngiomas is typically higher than the ADC of pituitary adenomas [44, 45].
- **Hypophysitis**: Granulomatous, inflammatory and infectious hypophysitis (e.g., from sarcoidosis, tuberculosis, Wegener granulomatosis, lymphocytic hypophysitis, Langerhans cell histiocytosis, cysticercosis) cause symmetric enlargement of the pituitary gland with homogenous appearance and enhancement, thickened pituitary stalk, loss of posterior pituitary bright spot, while autoimmune hypophysitis is

usually associated with late pregnancy and early postpartum. Clinical signs of systematic disease can also be present. Leptomeningeal enhancement can sometimes be seen [63].

- **Chiasmatic gliomas**: They usually arise from the optic nerve/chiasm, may contain cystic areas and are locally invasive. Association with neurofibromatosis type 1 is common.
- **Metastatic disease**: An enhancing pituitary or infundibular mass, in a patient with a history of carcinoma is typical.
- **Cystic lesions**: a cystic/necrotic pituitary adenoma should be differentiated from other cystic pituitary lesions: **Rathke cleft cysts** are usually intrasellar or both intrasellar and suprasellar, with serous (hypointense on T1W images) or mucoid (hyperintense on T1W images) content, while 50% of them show rim enhancement. **Arachnoid cysts** have signal intensity similar to cerebrospinal fluid in all sequences and may compress adjacent structures. **Epidermoid cysts** have signal intensity slightly higher than cerebrospinal fluid on T1W images and lower on T2W images. On DWI they display high signal intensity, which differentiates them from other non-inflammatory cystic lesions. Engulfment of neurovascular cisternal structures can be seen, while 10-25% show calcifications. **Dermoid cysts** have signal intensity similar to fat in all sequences. Calcifications are common [16].

8. Postoperative MR Imaging of the Sella

Interpretation of postoperative (p.o) MR images can be difficult, because of anatomic changes, surgical interventions and implanted material. In order to assess possible residual tumor and remnant pituitary tissue and detect possible complications, familiarity with early and late p.o imaging findings is imperative.

Nowadays, the most commonly applied surgical approach for pituitary adenomas is the transsphenoidal approach. In the immediate p.o period after transsphenoid tumor resection, the sellar appearance is characterized by a combination of edema, hemorrhage, fluid collections, implanted fat or hemostatic material, with or without residual tumor. Thus, absent or minimal decrease, or even increase of pituitary mass height can be seen [64, 65]. A marked decrease in height of the pituitary mass is typically observed on late p.o studies.

Deoxyhemoglobin (with low signal intensity on T2W images) and methemoglobin (with high signal intensity on T1W and T2W images), sometimes with a fluid-fluid level are suggestive of hemorrhage in the immediate p.o period [66].

Packing material can be implanted in the sella and the sphenoid sinuses in order to prevent hemorrhage and leakage of cerebrospinal fluid (Figure 10).

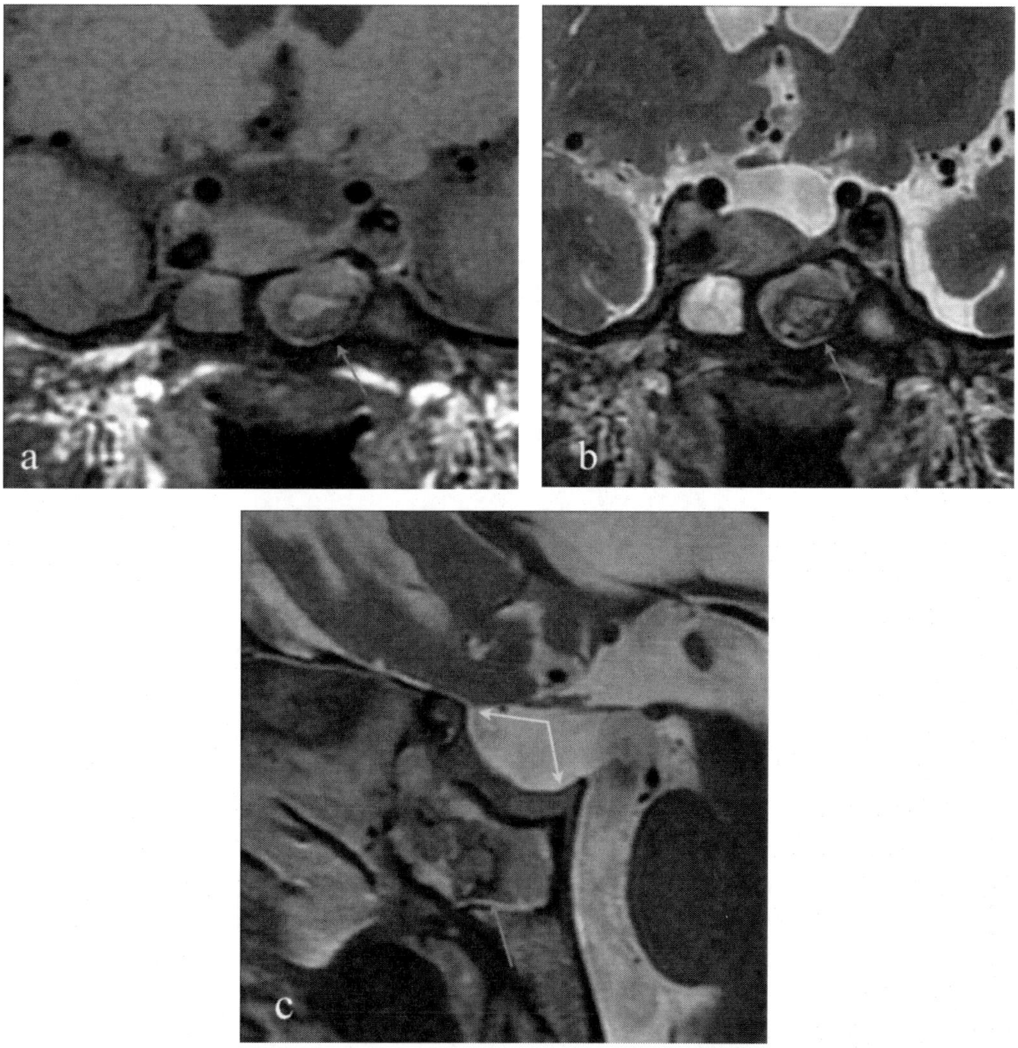

Figure 10. MR scan after transsphenoid resection of a pituitary macroadenoma. Coronal T1W (a) and T2W (b) images show surgical material filling the left sphenoid sinus (red arrows). Note the distension of the pituitary fossa on sagittal T2W (c) images (yellow arrows).

Fatty material is easily recognized by its high signal intensity in T1W images. Time of total absorption depends on the volume of the implanted fat and fat is reported to have been seen in MR scan even 29 years after surgery [67]. Except from fat packing, T1 signal hyperintensity can also be caused by reduction of venous flow from direct pressure to the cavernous sinus by excess embolic material, from an hypersecreting remnant of pituitary gland,[68] and, as already mentioned, from methemoglobin.

Hemostatic material (Oxycel or Surgicel) and spongostan (Gelfoam) display respectively low and iso signal intensity on T1W images. In the first p.o days air bubbles can be seen within the hemostatic material, while on early follow-up scan granulation tissue surrounding the material can be observed, as an enhancing peripheral rim. Differential diagnosis of an hypointense mass lesion with rim enhancement should also include necrotic residual tumor, fluid collection and scar tissue surrounded by granulation tissue [67]. Total absorption of hemostatic material is reported to require 3-6 months [69].

Implanted muscle with fascia is isointense on T1W images and has a peripheral enhancing border, which gradually decreases and vanishes after approximately 2 years [70]. On T2W images muscle with fascia has a characteristic appearance: the hyperintense degenerating muscle is surrounded by the linear, of very low signal intensity fascia [67].

In the early p.o period the sphenoid sinus usually shows opacification with fluid, fat and thickened mucosa, which resolves almost completely (sometimes except from fat packing) on later MR studies. After the intravenous administration of gadolinium, the sphenoid sinus filling material can show marginal enhancement, caused by the hypervascularized and edematous mucosa [70].

Nodular enhancement in the early p.o MR imaging of the sella is reported to be highly suggestive of residual tumor [66]. The most common sites of residual tumor are in the cavernous sinus, suprasellar area and clivus [66, 69], where surgical approach is most difficult.

Follow-up studies typically reveal a decrease in size of the pituitary mass, re-expansion of the pituitary gland, better visualization of a previously compressed pituitary stalk, reposition or even lowering of the optic chiasm and partial absorption of packing material [64, 69]. Reconstitution of the normal residual pituitary gland on p.o MR imaging is reported to correlate with preservation of the pituitary hormonal function [71].

Controversy exists about the optimum timing (early or late) for the reliable evaluation of the p.o sella, with supporters of early p.o MR imaging stating the accurate and easy detection of residual tumor, in order to decide about supplemental radiation therapy [66, 72, 73], while supporters of late p.o MR imaging claiming the improved assessment of the sella after regression of the p.o changes [65, 74].

Nevertheless, a reduction in size of an abnormal structure in the operative bed indicates to a p.o change, while the stability or even growth of such a lesion should alert for possible residual tumor.

REFERENCES

[1] Dietrich RB, Lis LE, Greensite FS, Pitt D. Normal MR appearance of the pituitary gland in the first 2 years of life. *AJNR* 1995;16:1413-1419.

[2] Elster AD, Chen MY, Williams DW 3rd, Key LL. Pituitary gland: MR imaging of physiologic hypertrophy in adolescence. *Radiology* 1990;174:681-685.

[3] Elster AD, Sanders TG, Vines FS, Chen MY. Size and shape of the pituitary gland during pregnancy and post partum: measurement with MR imaging. *Radiology* 1991;181:531-535.

[4] Suzuki M, Takashima T, Kadoya M, Konishi H, Kameyama T, Yoshikawa J, et al. Height of normal pituitary gland on MR imaging: age and sex differentiation. *J Comput Assist Tomogr*. 1990;14:36-39.

[5] Grams AE, Gempt J, Stahl A, Forschler A. Female pituitary size in relation to age and hormonal factors. *Neuroendocrinology* 2010;92:128-132.

[6] Bourekas EC, Miller JW, Christoforidis GA. Masses of the sellar and juxtasellar region. In Drevelegas A (editor): Imaging of brain tumors with histological correlations. *Springer* 2002, pp. 227-252.
[7] Evanson J. Imaging the pituitary gland. *Imaging* 2002;14:93-102.
[8] Soames RW. Skeletal system. In Gray's Anatomy. Thirty-eighth edition. Churchill Livingstone 1995, pp. 585-589.
[9] Saleem SN, Said AH, Lee DH. Lesions of the hypothalamus. MR imaging diagnostic features. *Radiographics* 2007;27:1087-1108.
[10] Tien RD. Sequence of enhancement of various portions of pituitary gland on gadolinium-enhanced MR images. *AJR* 1992;158:651-654.
[11] Bartynski WS, Lin L. Dynamic and conventional spin-echo MR of pituitary microlesions. *AJNR* 1997;18:965-972.
[12] Indrajit IK, Chidambaranathan N, Sundar K, Ahmed I. Value of dynamic MR imaging in pituitary adenomas. *Neuroradiology* 2001;11:185-190.
[13] Yuh WT, Fisher DJ, Nguyen HD, Tali ET, Gao F, Simonson TM, et al. Sequential MR enhancement pattern in normal pituitary gland and in pituitary adenoma. *AJNR* 1994;15:101-108.
[14] Bonneville JF, Cattin F, Gorczyca W, Hardy J. Pituitary microadenomas: early enhancement with dynamic CT-implications of arterial blood supply and potential importance. *Radiology* 1993;187:857-861.
[15] Elster AD. High-resolution, dynamic pituitary MR imaging: standard of care or academic pastime? *AJR* 1994;163:680-682.
[16] Johnsen DE, Woodruff WW, Allen IS, Cera PJ, Funkhouser GR, Coleman LL. MR imaging of the sellar and juxtasellar regions. *Radiographics* 1991;11:727-758.
[17] Steiner E, Imhof H, Knosp E. Gd-DTPA enhanced high resolution MR imaging of pituitary adenomas. *Radiographics* 1989;9:587-598.
[18] Kinoshita M, Tanaka H, Arita H, Goto Y, Oshino S, Watanabe Y. Pituitary-targeted dynamic contrast-enhanced multisection CT for detecting MR imaging-occult functional pituitary microadenoma. *AJNR* 2015;36:904-908.
[19] Abe T, Izumiyama H, Fujisawa I. Evaluation of pituitary adenomas by multidirectional multislice dynamic CT. *Acta Radiol* 2002;43:556-559.
[20] Miki Y, Kanagaki M, Takahashi JA, Ishizu K, Nakagawa M, Yamamoto A, et al. Evaluation of pituitary macroadenomas with multidetector-row CT (MDCT): comparison with MR imaging. *Neuroradiology* 2007;49:327-333.
[21] Zielinski G, Maksymowicz M, Podgorski J, Olszewski WT. Double, synchronous pituitary adenomas causing acromegaly and Cushing's disease. A case report and review of literature. *Endocr Pathol* 2013;24:92-99.
[22] Iacovazzo D, Bianchi A, Lugli F, Milardi D, Giampietro A, Lucci-Cordisco E, et al. Double pituitary adenomas. *Endocrine* 2013;43:452-457.
[23] Tosaka M, Sato N, Hirato J, Fujimaki H, Yamaguchi R, Kohga H, et al. Assessment of hemorrhage in pituitary macroadenoma by T2*-weighted gradient-echo MR imaging. *AJNR* 2007;28:2023-2029.
[24] Watanabe K, Kakeda S, Yamamoto J, Watanabe R, Nishimura J, Ohnari N, et al. Delineation of optic nerves and chiasm in close proximity to large suprasellar tumors with contrast-enhanced FIESTA MR imaging. *Radiology* 2012;264:852-858.

[25] Tokumaru AM, Sakata I, Terada H. Optic nerve hyperintensity on T2-weighted images among patients with pituitary macroadenoma: correlation with visual impairment. *AJNR* 2006,27:250-254.

[26] Saeki N, Uchino Y, Murai H, Kubota M, Isobe K, Uno T, et al. MR imaging study of edema-like change along the optic tract in patients with pituitary region tumors. *AJNR* 2003,24:336-342.

[27] Cottier JP, Destrieux C, Brunereau L, Bertrand P, Moreau L, Jan M, et al. Cavernous sinus invasion by pituitary adenoma: MR imaging. *Radiology* 2000;215:463-469.

[28] Chen X, Dai J, Ai L, Ru X, Wang J, Li S, et al. Clival invasion on multi-detector CT in 390 pituitary macroadenomas: correlation with sex, subtype and rates of operative complication and recurrence. *AJNR* 2011;32:785-789.

[29] Hagiwara A, Inoue Y, Wakasa K, Haba T, Tashiro T, Miyamoto T. Comparison of growth hormone-producing and non-growth hormone-producing pituitary adenomas: imaging characteristics and pathologic correlation. *Radiology* 2003;228:533-538.

[30] Bakhtiar Y, Hanaya R, Tokimura H, Hirano H, Oyoshi T, Fujio S, et al. Geometric survey on magnetic resonance imaging of growth hormone producing pituitary adenoma. *Pituitary* 2014;17:142-149.

[31] Zada G, Lin N, Laws ER Jr. Patterns of extrasellar extension in growth hormone-secreting and nonfunctional pituitary macroadenomas. *Neurosurg Focus* 2010;29(4):E4.

[32] Potorac I, Petrossians P, Daly AF, Schillo F, Ben Slama C, Naqi S, et al. Pituitary MRI characteristics in 297 acromegaly patients based on T2-weighted sequences. *Endocr Relat Cancer* 2015;22:169-177.

[33] Liu W, Zhou H, Neidert MC, Schmid C, Bernays RL, Ni M, et al. Growth hormone secreting pituitary microadenomas and empty sella - An under-recognized association? *Clin Neurol Neurosurg* 2014;126:18-23.

[34] Chenti F, Akkache L, Daffeur K, Azzouq S. General seizures revealing macroadenomas secreting prolactin or prolactin and growth hormone in men. *Indian J Endocrinol Metab* 2014;18:361-363.

[35] O'Brien DP, Phillips JP, Rawluk DR, Farrell MA. Intracranial metastases from pituitary adenoma. *Br J Neurosurg* 1995;9:211-218.

[36] Lehman NL, Horoupian DS, Harsh GR 4th. Synchronous subarachnoid drop metastases from a pituitary adenoma with multiple recurrences. Case report. *J Neurosurg* 2003;98:1120-1123.

[37] Satogami N, Miki Y, Koyama T, Kataoka M, Togashi K. Normal pituitary stalk: high-resolution MR imaging at 3T. *AJNR* 2010;31:355-359.

[38] Pinker K, Ba-Ssalamah A, Wolfsberger S, Mlynarik V, Knosp E, Trattnig S. The value of high field MRI (3T) in the assessment of sellar lesions. *Eur J Radiol* 2005;54:327-334.

[39] WolfsbergerS, Ba-Ssalamah A, Pinker K, Mlynarik V, Czech T, Knosp E, et al. Application of three-tesla magnetic resonance imaging for diagnosis and surgery of sellar lesions. *J Neurosurg* 2004;100:278-286.

[40] Erickson D, Erickson B, Watson R, Patton A, Atkinson J, Meyer F, et al. 3 Tesla magnetic resonance imaging with and without corticotropin releasing hormone stimulation for the detection of microadenomas in Cushing's syndrome. *Clin Endocrinol* (Oxf) 2010;72:793-799.

[41] Netuka D, Masopust V, Belsan T, Kramar F, Benes V. One year experience with 3.0 T intraoperative MRI in pituitary surgery. *Acta Neurochir Suppl* 2011;109:157-159.

[42] Berkmann S, Schlaffer S, Nimsky C, Fahlbusch R, Buchfelder M. Intraoperative high-field MRI for transsphenoidal reoperations of nonfunctioning pituitary adenoma. *J Neurosurg* 2014;121:1166-1175.

[43] Chourmouzi D, Papadopoulou E, Marias K, Drevelegas A. Imaging of brain tumors. *Surg Oncol Clin N Am* 2014;23:629-684.

[44] Yamasaki F, Kurisu K, Satoh K, Arita K, Sugiyama K, Ohtaki M, et al. Apparent diffusion coefficient of human brain tumors at MR Imaging. *Radiology* 2005;235:985-991.

[45] Faten FM, Doaa IH, Mohamed GA. MR spectroscopy and diffusion MR imaging in characterization of common sellar and supra-sellar neoplastic lesions. *The Egyptian Journal of Radiology and Nuclear Medicine* 2014;45:859-867.

[46] Rogg JM, Tung GA, Anderson G, Cortez S. Pituitary apoplexy: early detection with diffusion-weighted MR imaging. *AJNR* 2002;23:1240-1245.

[47] Mahmoud OM, Tominaga A, Amatya VJ, Ohtaki M, Sugiyama K, Sakoguchi T, et al. Role of PROPELLER diffusion-weighted imaging and apparent diffusion coefficient in the evaluation of pituitary adenomas. *Eur J Radiol* 2011;80:412-417.

[48] Faten FM, Abouhashem S. Diagnostic value of apparent diffusion coefficient (ADC) in assessment of pituitary macroadenoma consistency. *The Egyptian Journal of Radiology and Nuclear Medicine* 2013;44:617-624.

[49] Pierallini A, Caramia F, Falcone C, Tinelli E, Paonessa A, Ciddio AB, et al. Pituitary macroadenomas: preoperative evaluation of consistency with diffusion-weighted MR imaging-initial experience. *Radiology* 2006;239:223-231.

[50] Suzuki C, Maeda M, Hori K, Kozuka Y, Sakuma H, Taki W, et al. Apparent diffusion coefficient of pituitary macroadenoma evaluated with line-scan diffusion-weighted imaging. *J Neuroradiol* 2007;34:228-235.

[51] Boxerman JL, Rogg JM, Donahue JE, Machan JT, Goldman MA, Doberstein CE. Preoperative MRI evaluation of pituitary macroadenoma: imaging features predictive of successful transsphenoidal surgery. *AJR* 2010;195:720-728.

[52] Lu Y, Yin B, Geng D. Prediction of consistency of pituitary adenoma: a comperative study on diffusion-weighted imaging and pathological results. *ECR* 2015/C-0807.

[53] Zheng P, He B, Guo Y, Zeng J, Tong W. Decreased apparent diffusion coefficient in the pituitary and correlation with hypopituitarism in patients with traumatic brain injury. *J Neurosurg* 2015;123:75-80.

[54] Nichols AD, Moffat B, Danesh-Meyer H, Kaye AH. fMRI and diffusion tensor imaging biomarkers for assessing optic pathway structure and function in patients with pituitary tumours. *Proc Intl Soc Mag Reson Med.* 2011;19:2339.

[55] Stadlbauer A, Buchfelder M, Nimsky C, Saeger W, Salomonowitz E, Pinker K, et al. Proton magnetic resonance spectroscopy in pituitary macroadenomas: preliminary results. *J Neurosurg* 2008;109:306-312.

[56] Chaudhary V, Bano S. Imaging of the pituitary: Recent advances. Indian *J Endocrinol Metab* 2011;15(Suppl 3):S216-S223.

[57] Sakai N, Koizumi S, Yamashita S, Takehara Y, Sakahara H, Baba S, et al. Arterial spin-labeled perfusion imaging reflects vascular density in nonfunctioning pituitary macroadenomas. *AJNR* 2013;34:2139-2143.

[58] Wang CY, Chung HW, Cho NY, Liu HS, Chou MC, Kao HW, et al. Idiopathic growth hormone deficiency in the morphologically normal pituitary gland is associated with perfusion delay. *Radiology* 2011;258:213-221.

[59] Shigematsu Y, Korogi Y, Kitajima M, Ishii A, Liang L, Yamura M, et al. Abnormal perfusion of the pituitary gland secondary to dural arteriovenous fistulas in the cavernous sinus: dynamic MR findings. *AJNR* 2003;24:930-936.

[60] Song X, Wang G, Zhang T, Feng L, An P, Zhu Y. Functional magnetic resonance imaging evaluation of visual cortex activation in patients with anterior visual pathway lesions. *Neural Regen Res* 2012;7:692-696.

[61] Rosiene J, Liu X, Imielinska C, Ferrera J, Bruce J, Hirsch J, D'Ambrosio A. Structure-function relationships in the human visual system using DTI, fMRI and visual field testing: pre- and post-operative assessments in patients with anterior visual pathway compression. *Stud Health Technol Inform* 2006;119:464-466.

[62] Argyropoulou MI, Kiortsis DN. Magnetization transfer imaging of the pituitary gland. *Hormones* 2003;2:98-102.

[63] Gutenberg A, Larsen J, Lupi I, Rohde V, Caturegli P. A radiologic score to distinguish autoimmune hypophysitis from nonsecreting pituitary adenoma preoperatively. *AJNR* 2009;30:1766-1772.

[64] Dina TS, Feastler SH, Laws ER Jr, Davis D. MR of the pituitary gland postsurgery: serial MR studies following transsphenoidal resection. *AJNR* 1993;14:763-769.

[65] Rajaraman V, Schulder M. Postoperative MRI appearance after transsphenoidal pituitary tumor resection. *Surg Neurol* 1999;52:592-598.

[66] Yoon PH, Kim DI, Jeon P, Lee SI, Lee SK, Kim SH. Pituitary adenomas: early postoperative MR imaging after transsphenoidal resection. *AJNR* 2001;22:1097-1104.

[67] Bladowska J, Bednarek-Tupikowska G, Sokolska V, Badowski R, Moron K, Bonicki W, et al. MRI image characteristics of materials implanted at sellar region after transsphenoidal resection of pituitary tumors. *Pol J Radiol* 2010;75:46-54.

[68] Bonneville F, Cattin F, Marsot-Dupuch K, Dormont D, Benneville JF, Chiras J. T1 signal hyperintensity in the sellar region: spectrum of findings. *Radiographics* 2006;26:93-113.

[69] Steiner E, Knosp E, Herold CJ, Kramer J, Stiglbauer R, Staniszewski K, et al. Pituitary adenomas: findings of postoperative MR imaging. *Radiology* 1992;185:521-527.

[70] Rodriguez O, Mateos B, de la Pedraja R, Villoria R, Hernando JI, Pastor A, et al. Postoperative follow-up of pituitary adenomas after trans-sphenoidal resection: MRI and clinical correlation. *Neuroradiology* 1996;38:747-754.

[71] Di Maio S, Biswas A, Vezina JL, Hardy J, Mohr G. Pre- and postoperative magnetic resonance imaging appearance of the normal residual pituitary gland following macroadenoma resection: Clinical implications. *Surg Neurol Int* 2012;3:67.

[72] Kilic T, Ekinci G, Seker A, Elmaci I, Erzen C, Pamir MN. Determining optimal MRI follow-up after transsphenoidal surgery for pituitary adenoma: scan at 24 hours postsurgery provides reliable information. *Acta Neurochir* (Wien) 2001;143:1103-1126.

[73] Patel KS, Kazam J, Tsiouris AJ, Anand VK, Schwartz TH. Utility of early postoperative high-resolution volumetric magnetic resonance imaging after transsphenoidal pituitary tumor surgery. *World Neurosurg* 2014;82:777-780.

[74] Kremer P, Forstling M, Ranaei G, Wuster C, Hamer J, Sartor K, et al. Magnetic resonance imaging after transsphenoidal surgery of clinically non-functional pituitary macroadenomas and its impact on detecting residual adenoma. *Acta Neurochir* (Wien) 2002;144:433-443.

In: Pituitary Adenoma
Editor: Dimitrios N. Kanakis

ISBN: 978-1-63484-985-2

Chapter 9

RADIONUCLIDE IMAGING AND THERAPY OF PITUITARY ADENOMAS

Efstratios Moralidis**, MD, PhD
Associate Professor of Nuclear Medicine,
School of Health Sciences, Medical Faculty,
Aristotle University of Thessaloniki, Thessaloniki, Greece

ABSTRACT

Pituitary adenomas can be imaged with somatostatin analogues or dopamine D2 receptor agonists labeled with radionuclides and also positron emission tomography agents. Although radionuclide pituitary scintigraphy does not outperform radiological imaging, it may provide supplementary diagnostic information. Radionuclide pituitary imaging does not provide reliable predictive information with respect to the response to medical treatment of pituitary adenomas, but it may be particularly useful in the localization of ectopic sources of hormone secretion and in cases of disease recurrence after surgery. Somatostatin receptor radionuclide therapy of pituitary tumors may offer a benefit when other treatment modalities have failed.

Keywords: pituitary adenoma, pituitary tumor, somatostatin receptor scintigraphy, dopamine D2 receptor scintigraphy, positron emission tomography, peptide receptor radionuclide therapy

1. INTRODUCTION

The pituitary gland (hypophysis cerebri) lies within the sella turcica of the sphenoid bone and lacks the blood-brain barrier. It consists of an anterior lobe (adenohypophysis) and a posterior lobe (neurohypophysis), separated by an intermediate lobe (pars intermedia) [1]. The normal pituitary gland weighs approximately 0.6 gr, it is usually less than 10 mm in

* Corresponding author: Efstratios Moralidis, MD, PhD, Nuclear Medicine Department, AHEPA University Hospital, S. Kyriakidi Str. 1, 54636, Thessaloniki, Greece, E-mail: emoral@med.auth.gr.

height and is generally larger in females than in males [2, 3]. The adenohypophysis secretes adrenocorticotropic hormone (ACTH), growth hormone (GH), thyroid-stimulating hormone (TSH), follicle-stimulating hormone (FSH), luteinizing hormone (LH), prolactin and from the pars intermedia, melanocyte-stimulating hormone. The neurohypophysis is effectively a projection of the hypothalamus with which is connected via the infundibulum and stores and releases antidiuretic hormone and oxytocin [1]. Most hypothalamic hormones stimulate anterior pituitary cell secretion, as for example the corticotropin-releasing hormone (CRH) and the growth hormone-releasing hormone (GHRH). However, dopamine confers inhibitory effect on prolactin secretion and somatostatin exerts a similar inhibitory action on the secretion of GH and TSH.

Pituitary adenomas arise from the anterior lobe and they are the most common neoplasms near the sella turcica, accounting for 10- 15% of all intracranial tumors in neurosurgical series [1, 2, 4]. They are benign, slow growing tumors and according to size they can be divided into microadenomas (<1cm in diameter) and macroadenomas (≥1cm in diameter) [1]. Pituitary adenomas also can be divided into functioning (57%) and non-functioning (43%) [5]. Functioning adenomas can be further characterized by the hormone they secrete: prolactin (30% of all pituitary adenomas), GH (14%), ACTH (12%) and others such as TSH-producing and gonadotropin-producing (<1%-2%) [4, 5, 6]. Microadenomas typically manifest with endocrine disturbances, whereas macroadenomas usually extend beyond the sella turcica and result in manifestations related to the local mass effect on structures surrounding the hypophyseal fossa. Malignant adenomas and pituitary carcinomas are very rare [1, 7].

Prolactinomas are the most common functioning microadenomas in women whereas in men prolactinomas are nearly always diagnosed at the macroadenoma stage [1]. ACTH-secreting adenomas are very small microadenomas in 90% of cases and they are the most difficult pituitary tumors to visualize in imaging [1, 8]. Conversely, 70-90% of GH-secreting tumors are macroadenomas with invasiveness in approximately 30% of cases [1].

The diagnosis of a pituitary adenoma is based on blood hormones and pituitary imaging. The radiological appearance of pituitary adenomas is nonspecific regarding its histological inferences. However, anatomic imaging can define the extent of the lesion, contribute in differential diagnosis and reveal any structural variations, thus providing information that is essential prior to surgery. Venous sampling of the inferior petrosal or cavernous sinus can be used for the detection of a suspected adenoma and in particular in the differentiation of Cushing's disease due to a pituitary microadenoma from ectopic ACTH syndrome, in patients with negative imaging [9].

Treatment options include surgery (commonly performed through a transsphenoidal route), radiotherapy, and medical treatment. Surgery is generally recommended for the treatment of macroadenomas and is also preferred for functioning, non-prolactin-secreting adenomas as in those tumors the response to medical management is inconsistent. Surgery can restore pituitary endocrinopathies and relieve compressive symptoms. However, incomplete resection of tumor may occur, particularly in cases of fibrous tumors or in situations where tumor invades the cavernous sinus [10]. Control rates of approximately 50–80% have been reported after transsphenoidal resection [1]. Adjuvant radiation can be considered for patients with macroscopic residual disease, whereas patients with minimal amounts of residual disease may be followed with serial imaging. For prolactinomas medical management is preferred as it can suppress prolactin levels and induce tumor shrinkage quite rapidly. Surgery and radiation therapy is usually reserved for refractory tumors or for patients intolerant to medical treatment [1]. Somatostatin receptor ligands have a pivotal role in the treatment of GH-secreting adenomas and they are also effective in TSH-omas [11, 12].

2. IMAGING

Imaging in pituitary pathologies aims to (1) localize, characterize and define the extent of a tumor and (2) provide functional information [13].

Magnetic resonance imaging (MRI) is the single most useful diagnostic imaging modality for the diagnosis of pituitary adenomas because it can delineate precisely the pituitary gland and small lesions in the pituitary sella and also surrounding soft tissue structures and the bone marrow. Computed tomography (CT) has a low sensitivity in detecting pituitary microadenomas, but it is superior for the evaluation of osseous structures and calcifications and is useful in preoperative planning [1, 5].

The use of MRI and CT enables the detection of macroadenomas and a substantial portion of microadenomas and the combination of high resolution imaging with a syndrome of hormone hypersecretion can readily reach a diagnosis. However, problems may be encountered in cases of pituitary tumors with no overt endocrinopathy, or in patients with pituitary hormone overproduction with no pituitary mass identified with conventional radiological techniques. In such cases, functional imaging with radionuclides may be useful.

3. SOMATOSTATIN RECEPTOR IMAGING

3.1. Technical Details

Endogenous somatostatin is secreted by neuroendocrine cells, activated immune cells and inflammatory cells and it is a key regulator of anterior pituitary hormone production [14, 15]. The predominant physiologically active forms of somatostatin are a 14-amino and a 28-amino polypeptide [16]. This hormone affects antisecretory and antiproliferative functions by binding to somatostatin receptors, which are constantly expressed in all subtypes of pituitary adenomas, both functioning and non-functioning [15]. Five different subtypes of somatostatin receptors have been cloned (SSTR1- SSTR5), which are integral membrane glycoproteins. SSTR2 is the most commonly expressed subtype, followed by SSTR1 and SSTR3, while inactive pituitary adenomas frequently express SSTR3 [16, 17].

Naturally occurring somatostatin is unsuitable for medical use mainly because of its very short half-life of <3 minutes after intravenous injection due to rapid enzymatic degradation [18]. Hence, somatostatin analogues have been synthesized that are more resistant to enzymatic degradation. Octreotide is a synthetic octapeptide with a high affinity to SSTR2, moderate affinity to SSTR5 and SSTR3 and a similar affinity profile of its ^{111}In labeled derivative [19, 20]. The presence of octreotide-binding sites on tumors allows their in vivo visualization after the injection of a radionuclide-labeled somatostatin analogue [21, 22].

^{123}I-Tyr-3-octreotide was used initially for somatostatin receptor-based imaging, but for practical and economical reasons it was replaced by ^{111}In-DTPA-D-Phe-1-octreotide (^{111}In-pentetreotide) [23]. This compound can provide whole-body planar (two-dimentional) images, but single photon emission computed tomography (SPECT) increases the target-to-background ratio and it is particularly advantageous in the assessment of deeply lying structures. Alternatively, the newer compound ^{99m}Tc-EDDA-hydrazinonicotinyl(HYNIC)-Tyr3-octreotide or ^{99m}Tc EDDA/HYNIC-octreotate can be used (Figure 1) [24, 25].

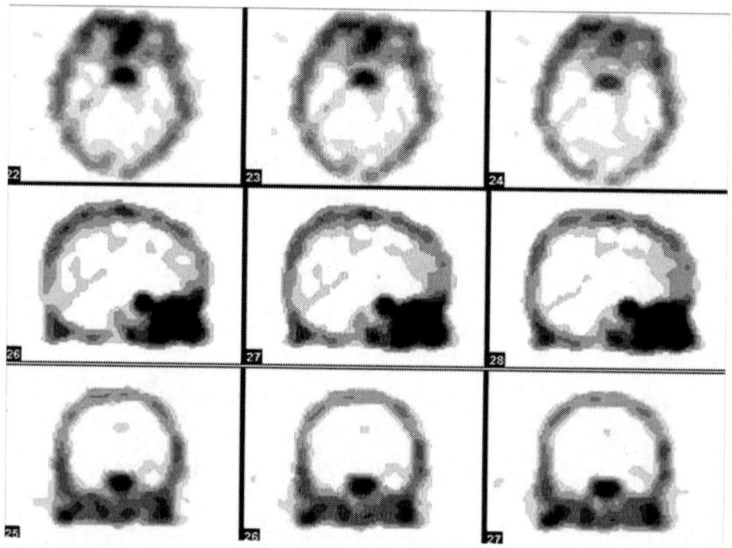

Figure 1. Normal appearance of the pituitary gland with ^{99m}Tc-EDDA-HYNIC-octreotide SPECT in a patient with ectopic ACTH secretion (upper row, transverse images, middle row, sagittal images, bottom row, coronal images).

Several studies have supported that this agent possesses improved imaging characteristics in comparison to ^{111}In-pentetreotide scintigraphy, although only few patients with pituitary lesions were included in those publications [26-28]. Nevertheless, almost all clinical data are based upon ^{111}In-octreotide imaging.

3.2. Clinical Applications

Early studies have correlated the uptake of ^{123}I-labeled Tyr-3-octreotide in the pituitary fossa with GH suppression after administration of a single dose of octreotide [29]. It is important to note that, unlike ^{123}I-labeled Tyr-3-octreotide, the normal anterior pituitary gland takes up ^{111}In-pentetreotide or the newer imaging agents (Figure 1) [29]. Many studies were based on visual assessment, but conflicting results, especially in clinically non-functioning pituitary adenomas, may be caused by differences in the subjective evaluation of these images. An uptake index calculated from the uptake of radioactivity in the pituitary region divided by the uptake in a background region in the brain can be used as a measure of the pituitary concentration of ^{111}In-pentetreotide and may contribute in the discrimination of somatostatin receptor positive tumors from the normal pituitary gland [30-32].

Virtually all GH-producing pituitary adenomas express SSTRs (particularly SSTR2 and also SSTR5) in vitro, and as expected in most cases (up to 89%) they were found positive in ^{111}In-pentetreotide scintigraphy [33-39] (Figure 2).

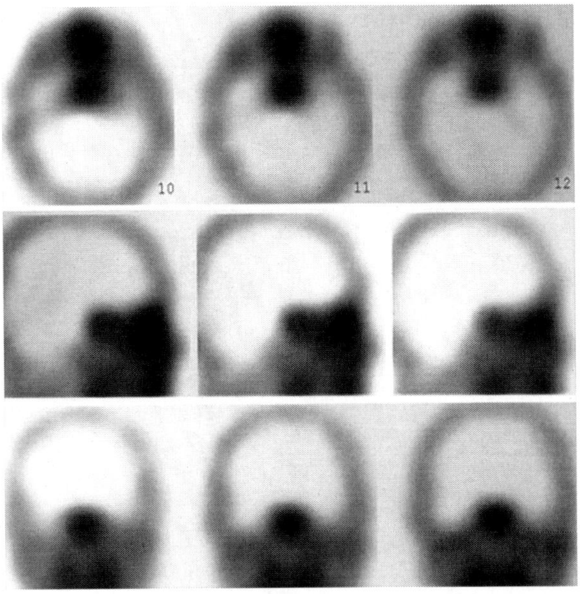

Figure 2. Somatostatin receptor scintigraphy with ^{99m}Tc-EDDA-HYNIC-octreotide SPECT in a patient with a growth hormone-secreting pituitary adenoma.

In a number of studies ^{111}In-pentetreotide pituitary uptake was associated with inhibition of the GH hypersecretion by somatostatin analogues [40-44], but other series could not confirm such a relationship [25, 29, 35, 37, 38, 44, 45]. Although a high tracer uptake in the pituitary fossa was associated with hormone suppression on octreotide treatment, half of patients with low or no pituitary tracer uptake also experienced a therapeutic benefit with this type of treatment [40]. A somoatostatin receptor density index, calculated from the previously described uptake index and the tumor volume obtained with MRI, was found to predict both tumor shrinkage and GH suppression on octreotide treatment [44].

In the postoperative setting the role of somatostatin receptor scintigraphy in the evaluation of patients with persistent hypersecretion of GH remains controversial. In a series of nine unoperated acromegalic patients, ^{111}In-pentetreotide predicted GH response to octreotide treatment. Post-operatively, however, six of those patients had evidence of residual tumor and acromegaly and they all responded to octreotide therapy, although ^{111}In-pentetreotide was positive in only one case [34]. Thus, the usefulness of somatostotatin receptor scintigraphy in predicting therapy was least in patients that gained from octreotide treatment [34, 46].

TSH-secreting pituitary tumors can be visualized with nearly 100% sensitivity [16, 46, 47]. However, existing data do not show an unequivocal relationship between ^{111}In-pentetreotide uptake in TSH-secreting pituitary adenomas and inhibition of TSH overproduction by acute or chronic administration of somatostatin analogues [25, 47, 48].

Patients with both positive and negative pituitary scintigraphy responded to octreotide treatment [48].

Non-functioning pituitary tumors express SSTRs and a substantial proportionof them (up to 75%) can be visualized by somatostatin receptor scintigraphy (Figure 3) [16, 21, 30, 37, 49-51]. On immunohistochemistry these adenomas frequently stain for gonadotropins (FSH, LH or glycoprotein hormone subunits) and they may secrete these substances, although this is not commonly reflected in serum concentrations [13, 46, 52]. Most investigators could not find a substantial effect of octreotide therapy on tumor shrinkage in such adenomas [37, 38, 46, 49], whereas, unlike GH secreting adenomas, MRI tumor volume was not related to uptake in ^{111}In-pentetreotide imaging [38]. Nevertheless, several studies with clinically non-functioning pituitary adenomas have reported a correlation between pituitary uptake of ^{111}In-pentetreotide and inhibition of tumor growth and gonadotropin secretion or improvement in visual field defects by somatostatin analogue therapy (without necessarily appreciable tumor volume reduction on CT scans) [30, 40, 44, 49]. Quantification of pituitary radioactivity has been suggested to be helpful in the diagnosis of pituitary adenomas and the determination of somatostatin receptor density in nonsecreting adenomas as a potential predictor of the response to cold octreotide treatment [30, 44, 50].

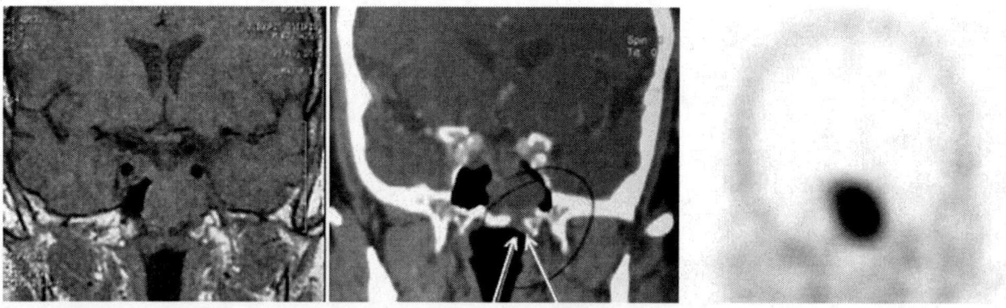

Figure 3. Coronal T1 weighted MRI (left), CT (middle) and ^{99m}Tc-EDDA-HYNIC-octreotide SPECT (right) images of a patient with a non-functioning lobulated pituitary macroadenoma, extending into the left cavernous sinus. CT clearly shows bone loss of the floor of the sella turcica (white arrows) and protrusion of the tumor into the sphenoid sinus.

^{111}In-pentetreotide scintigraphy was negative in cases of microprolactinomas and ACTH-secreting pituitary microadenomas, but it was positive in patients with infiltrating macroprolactinomas and invasive ACTH-secreting macroadenomas [29, 40, 53]. In cases of hyperprolactinemia with normal pituitary MRI scans, it is reasonable to treat with dopamine agonists, assuming the presence of a microadenoma, as resistance to these agents is extremely rare [46]. Concerning ACTH-secreting pituitary adenomas, surgery is the preferred therapy and medical treatment to restore hypercortisolism may also be used [54].

^{111}In-pentetreotide scintigraphy allows post-surgical differentiation between scar tissue or radionecrosis and residual pituitary tumor or tumor recurrence [46, 53, 55]. In this respect MRI does not display high sensitivity because material implanted to promote hemostasis and also adipose and muscle tissue, used to fill the cavity in the pituitary fossa, cannot be distinguished from tumor remnants, unless serial MRI is used [56].

Several lesions in and around the pituitary fossa express SSTR2,3 and 5 receptors and hence they can be visualized by radiolabeled somatostatin analogues. Parasellar meningiomas, grade III-IV gliomas, metastases from breast carcinomas and other adenocarcinomas, osteosarcomas, lymphomas, abscesses and granulomatous lesions, angioleiomyomas, chordomas, hemangiopericytomas and fibrous dysplasia may be positive [51, 57, 58]. Thus, the diagnostic specificity and the clinical value of somatostatin receptor scintigraphy in pituitary tumors is limited [13, 34, 40], although it has been suggested that differences in tracer uptake of the skull base tumors may aid in diagnosis [59].

3.3. Ectopic Sources of Hormone Secretion

Somatostatin receptor scintigraphy may be useful in the localization of ectopic tissue secreting ACTH, CRH, GH and GHRH [46]. Furthermore, it could help in identifying receptor positive patients for subsequent therapy with somatostatin analogues. Whole-body scintigraphy should be followed by conventional imaging focused on the regions with abnormal uptake of ^{111}In octreotide.

Ectopic ACTH production accounts for approximately 10% of cases of Cushing's syndrome. It is commonly associated with lung tumors (bronchial carcinoids in 30% of cases and small cell lung cancer in about 20% of cases), but it may also originate from other neuroendocrine tumors, including thymic carcinoids (approximately 20%), gastroenteropancreatic tumors, pheochromocytomas, and medullary thyroid carcinomas [60, 61, 62]. CT and MRI are used most frequently to localize the source of ectopic ACTH production. However, the tumor cannot be found in a considerable number of cases (12-19%), despite repeated imaging over a prolonged follow-up period, because of the small size [60, 62].

Several series have showed that ^{111}In-pentetreotide scintigraphy can localize successfully ectopic tumors secreting ACTH and CRH and their metastases, even very small ones, and this was particularly helpful in cases in which conventional radiological imaging had failed [63-73]. However, published results are not always concordant [71]. In a prospective study somatostatin receptor scintigraphy detected ectopic ACTH secreting tumors equally well as CT (53% sensitivity for both techniques) and better than MRI (37% sensitivity) and ^{18}F-fluorodeoxyglucose (^{18}F-FDG) PET (35% sensitivity) and seemed to have a complementary role, mainly when CT or MRI results were equivocal [74]. Additionally, when somatostatin receptor scintigraphy with standard injected activity (i.e., 222 MBq) was negative, repeat imaging with a higher dose could occasionally localize the tumor [74]. In a retrospective analysis of data from the National Institute of Health (US), ^{111}In-octreotide imaging identified ectopic sources of ACTH production in 49% of examined patients, whereas CT and MRI in 74%, and there was only one case with positve scintigraphy and negative CT and MRI [75]. However, in authors' experience a single positive imaging study may represent a falsely positive result and more than one positive studies are required to confirm a true ACTH-secreting lesion [75]. In a prospective multimodality assessment of patients with resected or occult ectopic ACTH-secreting tumor the per patient sensitivity of CT, MRI, high and low dose ^{111}In-ocreotide scanning, ^{18}F-FDG and ^{18}F-dihydroxyphenylalanine (^{18}F-DOPA) PET were 93%, 90%, 57%, 50%, 64% and 55%, respectively, but at the expense of many falsely positive lesions with the anatomic modalities (50% and 31% of patients with CT and MRI, respectively) [76]. On a per lesion basis, the positive predictive values of those modalities were 66%, 74%, 79%, 53% and 100%, respectively [76].

Concerning the prediction of response to treatment, a positive correlation was found between ^{111}In-octreotide scintigraphy in Cushing's syndrome, due to ectopic ACTH or CRH secretion, and the response to octreotide therapy [63]. However, in a different study including a small number of patients with ectopic ACTH syndrome, ^{111}In-pentetreotide results were not related with hyper- or eucortisolism and they were not clearly predictive of response of plasma cortisol after octreotide therapy [71]. Nevertheless, it should be mentioned that drug therapy rarely controls adrenocortical hyperfunction completely in these patients [63].

Overall, anatomic modalities appear more sensitive than somatostatin receptor scintigraphy, but the combination of both increases the probability of identification of an ectopic ACTH-secreting lesion. ^{18}F-FDG and ^{18}F-DOPA PET may add in the diagnosis in isolated cases [77]. In this setting, CT/MRI plus ^{111}In-ocreotide scans is proposed for initial imaging with lesion confirmation by two modalities, since a single positive imaging study may represent a falsely positive result [75, 76].

In no more than 1-2% of cases, acromegaly results from GHRH-secreting neuroendocrine tumors usually located in the lungs, thymus and endocrine pancreas which can be localized with somatostatin receptor scintigraphy [78, 79]. Less frequent are cases of ectopic GH secretion by adenomas arising in embryological pituitary remnants in the sphenoid sinus [80]. In a French national survey of patients with acromegaly from ectopic secretion of GHRH (mostly pancreatic and bronchial primary tumors), CT had a sensitivity of 86% on a per patient basis for the detection of the tumor and/or metastases, whereas somatostatin receptor scintigraphy could visualize abnormal lesions in 81% of patients [81]. Different reports have also demonstrated the value of ^{111}In-pentetreotide in detecting ectopic GHRH-associated acromegaly from bronchial and thymic carcinoids and also a metastasis from a GH-secreting pituitary carcinoma [73, 82-84].

Ectopic TSH-secreting tumors are extremely rare and only few cases have been reported in the literature with the tumor invariably located in the nasopharynx [85]. There is evidence that these tumors express somatostatin receptors and respond to this type of treatment. A non-functioning ectopic pituitary tumor has also been found in the pharynx with ^{111}In-pentetreotide scintigraphy [86].

3.4. SPECT/CT

Tomographic images of somatostatin receptor scintigraphy can be fused with CT to provide anatomic detail, better registrate somatostatin-receptor avid structures and improve diagnostic accuracy [87, 88]. Although it has not been demonstrated that this type of hybrid imaging improves diagnostic accuracy in pituitary lesions, SPECT/CT may be particularly helpful after surgery because the anatomy may be altered and it becomes more difficult to localize precisely viable tumor remnants in a relatively small anatomical space [89]. The advantage of anatomic imaging (CT or MRI) in conjuction or fused with somatostatin receptor scintigraphy in the interpretation of images has been highlighted in guidelines [90, 91].

4. Dopamine Receptor Imaging

4.1. Technical Details

Dopamine receptors are divided into D1-like receptors (D1, D5) and D2-like receptors (D2, D3 and D4), but the D2-like receptor system has drawn much clinical attention [92, 93]. Dopamine D2 receptors are expressed in PRL-, GH-, ACTH-, TSH-secreting and clinically non-functioning pituitary tumors and this is the basis for pharmacological treatment with dopamine receptor agonists [94-98]. Pituitary dopamine receptor imaging is feasible with SPECT using ^{123}I-S-(K)-N-[(1-ethyl-2-pyrrolidinyl)-methyl]-2-hydroxy-3-iodo-6-methoxybenzamide (^{123}I-IBZM) [99, 100] or with the newer substituted benzamide derivative ^{123}I-(S)-N-[(1-ethyl-2-pyrrolidinyl) methyl]-5-iodo-2,3-dimethoxybenzamide (^{123}I-epidepride) [101, 102]. Compared to ^{123}I-IBZM, ^{123}I-epidepride offers a higher target-to-background ratio, improved image quality and an increased sensitivity in the visualization of D2 receptor bearing pituitary adenomas [102-104]. Therefore, ^{123}I-epidepride has been proposed to be the radioligand of choice for D2 receptor scans of pituitary tumors [13, 94, 103].

4.2. Clinical Applications

In studies with small numbers of patients ^{123}I-IBZM SPECT was positive in most patients with prolactinomas and in 25-50% of cases with non-functioning pituitary adenomas, but it was negative in microprolactinomas and GH and TSH secreting adenomas [99, 100, 105]. The response to quinagolide (a dopamine agonist) treatment was variable and it could not be predicted by pituitary radiotracer uptake. Among patients with prolactinomas and intense ^{123}I-IBZM pituitary uptake tumor shrinkage and decreased plasma levels of PRL was observed in a considerable proportion, but there were also patients with negative scans who experienced a benefit with this therapy [99, 100]. The results of quinagolide treatment were similarly unpredictable in non-functioning adenomas [99, 100, 105]. In case reports of patients with mixed GH/PRL-secreting pituitary tumors there was no clear association between ^{123}I-IBZM pituitary uptake and cabergoline or bromocriptine treatment, regarding blood hormone levels and tumor shrinkage [106, 107].

^{123}I-epidepride pituitary uptake was recorded in almost all patients with prolactinoma, in all patients with non-functioning pituitary adenomas and in half of patients with a GH-secreting adenoma [102]. In investigating the ability of ^{123}I-epidepride SPECT to assess the response to long-term dopaminergic treatment with either carbegoline or quinagolide in patients with non-functioning pituitary adenomas, the results indicated a limited predictive efficacy in terms of tumor stabilization or shrinkage [108]. In a different work ^{123}I-epidepride revealed extensive extracranial metastases of a previously operated malignant prolactinoma and guided the therapeutic approach [109].

Overall, these observations show a no more than moderate sensitivity of pituitary scintigraphy with ^{123}I-IBZM, but better results with ^{123}I-epidepride scanning. Concerning the clinical value of dopamine D2 receptor scintigraphy with respect to prediction of response to treatment the results are not encouraging [94].

5. Positron Emission Tomography

Positron emission tomography (PET) images typically are fused with CT, providing anatomic detail and an enhanced spatial registration of metabolically active lesions, and they have a substantially higher resolution (3-6mm) than conventional scintigraphy (10-15mm) and hence increased sensitivity [32, 110].

5.1. Somatostatin Receptor PET

Novel somatostatin analogues with a high affinity for SSTRs were linked to a macrocyclic chelator (DOTA) and were labeled with the positron emitter ^{68}Ga (half life of 68min), resulting in the stable conjugated peptides (^{68}Ga-DOTA^{0}-Tyr3) octreotide (^{68}Ga-DOTATOC), (^{68}Ga-DOTA^{0}-1NaI^{3}) octreotide (^{68}Ga-DOTANOC) and (^{68}Ga-DOTA^{0}-Tyr^{3}) octreotate (^{68}Ga-DOTATATE). ^{68}Ga can be produced by a ^{68}Ge-^{68}Ga generator, which may be available in departments without a cyclotron. Studies have demonstrated that ^{68}Ga-DOTATOC and ^{68}Ga-DOTATATE PET are more efficient than ^{111}In-DTPA-octreotide SPECT and ^{99m}Tc-EDDA/HYNIC-octreotide in the detection of small NET lesions [27, 32, 111, 112].

Several studies have evaluated the physiological biodistribution of ^{68}Ga-DOTATATE and ^{68}Ga-DOTATOC on PET/CT and consistently reported a high uptake in the pituitary gland [113-115]. However, standardized uptake values may vary and hence a cut-off value to differentiate normal pituitary glands from adenomas cannot be set [116].

^{68}Ga-DOTATOC PET showed three focal areas in the pancreatic tail in a patient with ectopic GHRH secretion, MEN I syndrome and negative CT, MRI and ^{111}In-pentetreotide [117]. ^{68}Ga-DOTANOC PET/CT was able to detect a sphenoidal ectopic pituitary macroadenoma in the setting of MEN 1 syndrome and a paranasal ectopic ACTH-secreting pituitary adenoma [116, 118]. In a different report of a low grade pituitary carcinoma, PET/CT scan showed increased ^{68}Ga-DOTATATE activity in the pituitary gland and posterior fossa metastases and it was also useful in monitoring the response to ^{177}Lu DOTATATE treatment [119]. Moreover, in a patient with acromegaly, post-operative radiotherapy planning was performed with MRI and PET/CT scanning with ^{68}Ga DOTATATE, which showed tracer uptake in the residual mass [120].

5.2. ^{18}F-Fluorodeoxyglucose PET

^{18}F-fluorodeoxyglucose (^{18}F-FDG) PET imaging in oncology is based on the increased transport and intracellular concentration of glucose in tumors. ^{18}F is a cyclotron product and its half-life (110min) allows delivery and use of the compound in departments within a reasonable distance. ^{18}F-FDG does not show sufficient uptake in well-differentiated neuroendocrine tumors, but it may provide complementary information in poorly differentiated and rapidly growing neuroendocrine tumors in which conventional somatostatin scintigraphy may be negative [121, 122]. However, benign pituitary adenomas were reported to avidly accumulate ^{18}F-FDG [123]. Moreover, in series of patients with pituitary tumors (mostly GH-secreting and non-functioning), ^{18}F-FDG PET was positive in all macroadenomas and in 50% of microadenomas, but no tracer uptake was noted in most cystic lesions [124]. In a small series of patients with Cushing's disease due to ACTH-secreting pituitary adenomas ^{18}F-FDG PET was positive in 60% of them and could identify an adenoma which remained undetected by MRI [125]. In a different study of patients with pituitary microadenomas ^{18}F-FDG PET had a sensitivity of 60%, which was comparable to that of MRI, it provided complementary information when MRI was negative and, in contrast to MRI, it showed no false-positive cases [126]. In patients having undergone transsphenoidal adenomectomy for non-functioning GH and ACTH secreting adenomas ^{18}F-FDG PET was positive in almost all cases and radiotracer uptake was relatively more intense in recurrent/residual pituitary tumor than that of ^{68}Ga DOTATATE, but the opposite occurred in the remaining (surrounding) pituitary tissue [127].

5.3. ^{11}C-Methionine PET

^{11}C-methionine PET has also been shown to detect effectively residual tumor or recurrent pituitary adenomas [127]. All non-functional adenomas were detected by both MRI and ^{11}C-methionine PET, but the latter visualized all ACTH-secreting adenomas, whereas MRI identified only 13% of these lesions [128]. In treatment monitoring, a considerable decrease in ^{11}C-methionine uptake was observed in all tumors that responded to treatment with dopamine agonist and somatostatin analogues, thus predicting the long-term effectiveness of medical therapy [129]. The combination of ^{11}C-methionine PET and 3 T MRI had up to 100% accuracy rates for the localization of ACTH producing pituitary microadenomas, whereas the accuracy rates for ^{18}F-FDG-PET/3 T MRI and conventional MRI were 73% and 40%, respectively [130]. It should be added, however, that the short half-life of ^{11}C (20min) prevents its wider clinical use.

5.4. ^{11}C-Labeled Dopamine D2 Antagonists PET

PET studies with the ^{11}C-labeled dopamine D2 antagonists ^{11}C-N-raclopride and ^{11}C-N-methylspiperone were performed in patients with pituitary adenomas [94, 129, 131]. They have demonstrated intense dopamine D2 binding in prolactinomas and some GH-secreting adenomas and also a significant correlation between high density of D2 receptors and a positive effect of dopamine agonist therapy [129].

5.5. ^{11}C-5-Hydroxy-Tryptophan and ^{18}F-Dihydroxyphenylalanine PET

Positive results have been reported with ^{11}C-5-hydroxy-tryptophan PET in patients with ACTH-producing foregut carcinoids [132]. In another case report a mid-jejunum ACTH-secreting tumor, undetectable with CT, MRI and ^{18}FDG-PET, was finally unmasked with ^{18}F-dihydroxyphenylalanine PET [133].

6. Clinical Implications of Pituitary Scintigraphy

The majority of clinical studies with somatostatin receptor scintigraphy were based on ^{111}In-octreotide and it is not known if newer ^{99m}Tc or PET imaging agents could perform better in assessing pituitary disorders. Moreover, the strength of evidence from the literature is limited by the very small numbers of patients in many studies, including several case reports, the heterogeneity of clinical scenarios and disease states of patiens enrolled, dissimilar imaging and interpretation standards in various institutions, variations in the management of patients and different criteria and monitoring periods for assessing the response to treatment. In addition, the inherent variability of the effects of medical treatment poses significant difficulties in planning and evaluating studies on the association of functional imaging with the therapeutic result. Nevertheless, the clinical value of pituitary imaging with radionuclides can be supported in certain clinical situations.

Since MRI can reliably discriminate non-functioning pituitary adenomas from other sellar and parasellar disorders, routine functional imaging does not add. ^{123}I-epidepride scintigraphymay be useful in few specific situations, such as the differentiation of pituitary tumors from metastases or meningiomas. Regarding the prediction of response to treatment, because of the limited effectiveness of somatostatin analogues and dopamine agonists in patients with non-functioning pituitary tumors, these types of therapy have a minor role and in this setting the clinical value of somatostatin receptor imaging has not been convincingly demonstrated [13, 31, 38, 64, 99, 100, 105].

Concerning prolactinomas, the treatment of choice is dopamine agonists and the assessment of the response to treatment may be based on symptomatology and serum prolactin levels. Since all patients respond to this type of therapy, additional tests for patient selection are superfluous and cost-increasing. In exceptional cases that no treatment response is recorded, dopamine receptor imaging might offer insights for the unresponsiveness [13].

In GH-secreting adenomas surgical excision and/or radiotherapy is the preferred treatment. Medical therapy may be required in cases of incomplete tumor removal or contraindications to surgery. In this respect somatostatin analogue treatment is more effective than dopamine agonists in suppressing hormone levels and attaining tumor shrinkage [13]. However, it is not widely accepted that somatostatin receptor scintigraphy can have an essential role in the decision to treat patients with GH-secreting adenomas with somatostatin receptor ligands [11, 13]. Dopamine agonists may be preferred because of lower treatment costs, but again there is no strong evidence to substantiate the clinical use of dopamine D2 receptor scintigraphy for this purpose [11, 13, 106, 107, 129]. Regarding the rarely occurring TSH-secreting adenomas, there are no data to support the use of radionuclide pituitary scintigraphy as a reliable guide for medical therapy decisions [48, 49].

^{18}F-FDG PET can add in the diagnostic work-up of ACTH secreting pituitary adenomas in conjuction with MRI [125, 126, 128]. In these lesions surgery is performed and medical therapy aims to control hypercortisolism [54]. Apparently, in treatment decisions a clinical role for somatostatin receptor scintigraphy cannot be supported.

Somatostatin receptor scintigraphy (and conceivably ^{18}F-FDG PET) can localize ectopic ACTH and CRH secreting lesions and their metastases which may be particularly useful in cases of unsuccessful conventional imaging [40]. Similarly, in ectopic GHRH secreting tumors somatostatin receptor scintigraphy can also add effectively on conventional imaging

[73, 81-84]. Regarding the rare ectopic TSH secreting lesions, somatostatin receptor scintigraphy may also be helpful [86]. Finally, radionuclide pituitary imaging may have a significant clinical role postoperatively for the differentiation of scar tissue from disease recurrence or residual viable tissue [94, 120].

In conclusion, currently accumulated evidence suggests that radionuclide pituitary imaging has a limited and complementary role in the diagnostic evaluation of pituitary adenomas, mainly in cases of discrepancies between clinical, biochemical and radiological findings. The use of receptor scintigraphy as a guide for medical therapy decisions is problematic because it is expensive and more complex than biochemical tests and insufficiently reliable in the prediction of the response to treatment [46]. However, this type of imaging may be particularly helpful when ectopic hormone secretion is suspected and in the postoperative assessment of tissue remnants and recurrent disease.

7. Peptide Receptor Radionuclide Therapy of Pituitary Tumors

The principle for this type of radionuclide therapy involves a somatostatin analogue which serves as carrier for a radioisotope emitter. Once the conjugate binds to tumor cells that express somatostatin receptors in their surface, it is internalized and delivers radiation energy which is able to destroy the targeted cells. Radiation can cause direct disruption of the DNA strands, but most often it acts through an increased acrivity of free radicals, leading to cell death. However, the density of the somatostatin receptors and internalization of the radioactive compound are not homogeneous. This necessitates proper selection of the therapeutic radiopharmaceutical (emitting particles, physical half-life and residence time of the isotope in the tumor) to ensure local irradiation tailored to the size of the lesion.

High activities of the diagnostic compound ^{111}In DTPA-octreotide have been employed initially to treat neuroendocrine tumors. The therapeutic effect of this compound is based upon emitted Auger and internal conversion electrons by ^{111}In. Auger electrons are low energetic particles with a tissue range of no more than few μm and as such Auger emitters are most effective when internalized by a cell to create locally multiple damage sites in the DNA [16, 134]. In phase I trials of patients with neuroendocrine tumors, however, ^{111}In DTPA-octreotide did not attain appreciable response in terms of tumor shrinkage, although symptomatic improvement was reported [135, 136]. No patients with a pituitary tumor were included in those series. Nevertheless, there is a published report of a patient with a giant prolactinoma, relapsing after surgery and not responding to dopamine agonists and octreotide treatment, who underwent four cycles of ^{111}In-DTPA-octreotide therapy with remarkable tumour shrinkage and a significant improvement of the clinical condition [137].

In Europe, ^{111}In-pentetreotide was replaced by the more efficient β-emitters ^{90}Y and ^{177}Lu. ^{90}Y is a pure β-emitter with a physical half-life of 64 h and a mean β-particle penetration in soft tissues of 3.9mm. ^{177}Lu has a physical half-life of 162 h and emits beta-particles with a mean soft-tissue penetration depth of 0.23mm. This isotope can destroy almost 100% of tumors with a diameter smaller than 1cm, but only 40-50% of the tumors with a higher diameter [138]. Hence it was proposed that ^{90}Y is more effective in larger tumors, whereas ^{177}Lu would be preferred for smaller tumors. These isotopes are linked to somatostatin analogues to form conjugates, such as ^{90}Y-[DOTA0,Tyr3]-octreotide (^{90}Y-DOTATOC) and ^{177}Lu-[DOTA0,Tyr3]-octreotate (^{177}Lu -DOTATATE) [138].

Both ^{90}Y-DOTATOC and ^{177}Lu-DOTATATE have been used extensively in patients treated with targeted radionuclide therapy, mainly for gastroenteropancreatic and lung neuroendocrine tumors. In those studies an objective response rate (complete and/or partial remission) ranged from 9% to 33% [135, 136, 139-141]. Very few patients with pituitary tumors were included in those series. Two patients with relapsed pituitary adenomas were treated with ^{90}Y-DOTATOC and disease stabilization was achieved for 4-19 months [51, 142]. In the European Institute of Oncology Group four patients with pituitary adenomas were treated with ^{90}Y-DOTATOC [143]. Although the overall objective response rate was >20%, the results in patients with pituitary tumors were not specifically mentioned.

Few published case reports presented the effects of peptide receptor radionuclide therapy in pituitary tumors. In a patient with a non-functioning pituitary adenoma and previous ineffective transsphenoidal surgery and gamma knife, therapy with ^{177}Lu-DOTATOC successfully relieved the local compressive effects of the tumor and stabilized the disease for more than eight years [144]. Treatment of a pituitary metastasis from a neuroendocrine tumour with radiolabeled somatostatin analogs (^{90}Y-DOTATOC and ^{177}Lu-DOTATATE) lead to a significant symptomatic relief and a considerable improvement in quality of life, together with a remarkable shrinkage of the sellar mass [145] In a different case of a patient with pituitary carcinoma and posterior fossa metastases, ^{177}Lu DOTATATE administration resulted in stabilization of the tumor over four years [119]. Mixed were the results of three patients with pituitary pathologies which were treated with ^{177}Lu-DOTATATE [146]. One patient with a metastatic pituitary carcinoma of low mitotic activity was stabilized after ^{177}Lu-DOTATATE therapy. In the other two patients, one with a GH/PRL-secreting macroadenoma and the second with a non-functioning macroadenoma (both lesions displaying a high mitotic activity), that had been submitted to debulking surgery, chemotherapy and radiotherapy, ^{177}Lu-DOTATATE was ineffective and was terminated early due to disease progression [146].

Apart from the acute effects from radiopharmaceutical administration and renal and bone marrow toxicity, no significant alteration in endocrine hormone function has been reported with therapeutic β-emitting somatostatin analogues [136, 147]. It should be noted, however, that in normal pituitary glands the uptake of radiolabeled somatostatin analogues is relatively low and the observations in patients with gastroenteropancreatic or lung neuroendocrine tumors may not apply in cases of pituitary adenomas receiving high therapeutic doses of β-radiation.

REFERENCES

[1] Lysack JT, Schaefer PW. "Imaging of the Pituitary Gland, Sella, and Parasellar Region." In Swearingen B, Biller BMK (editors): Contemporary Endocrinology: Diagnosis and Management of Pituitary Disorders. Humana Press, Totowa, NJ 2008, pp 45-91.

[2] Zierhut D. Pituitary Adenoma. In Seegenschmiedt MH, Makoski HB, Trott KR, Brady LW (editors): "Radiotherapy for Non-Malignant Disorders." Springer-Verlag, Berlin Heidelberg 2008, pp 653-663.

[3] Elster AD. Modern imaging of the pituitary. *Radiology* 1993;187:1-14.

[4] Ezzat S, Asa SL, Couldwell WT, Barr CE, Dodge WE, Vance ML, et al. The prevalence of pituitary adenomas: a systematic review. *Cancer* 2004,101:613-619.

[5] McCutcheon IE. Pituitary tumors in oncology. In M. D. Anderson Cancer Care Series: Tumors of the Brain and Spine. Springer 2007, pp 191-223.

[6] Asa SL, Ezzat S. The pathogenesis of pituitary tumors. *Ann Rev Pathol* 2009,4:97-126.

[7] Pernicone PJ, Scheithauer BW, Sebo TJ. Pituitary carcinoma. *Cancer* 1997;79:804-812.

[8] Buchfelder M, Nistor R, Fahlbusch R, Huk WJ. The accuracy of CT and MR evaluation of the sella turcica for detection of adrenocorticotropic hormone-secreting adenomas in Cushing disease. *AJNR Am J Neuroradiol* 1993;14:1183-1190.

[9] Bourekas EC, Slone HW, Ray-Chaudhury A. Masses of the Sellar and Junxtasellar Region. In Drevelegas A. (editor): Imaging of Brain Tumors with Histological Correlations. *Springer-Verlag,* Berlin Heidelberg 2011, pp 325-371.

[10] Greenman Y, Ouaknine G, Veshchev I, Reider-Groswasser II, Segev Y, Stern N. Postoperative surveillance of clinically non-functional pituitary macroadenomas: markers of tumor quiescence and regrowth. *Clin Endocrinol* (Oxf) 2003;58:763-769.

[11] Melmed S, Colao A, Barkan A, Molitch M, Grossman AB, Kleinberg D, et al. Acromegaly Consensus Group. Guidelines for acromegaly management: an update. *J Clin Endocrinol Metab* 2009;94:1509-1517.

[12] Zemskova MS, Skarulis MC. Thyrotropin-secreting pituitary adenomas. In Swearingen B, Biller BMK (editors): Contemporary Endocrinology: Diagnosis and Management of Pituitary Disorders. *Humana Press,* Totowa, NJ 2008, pp 237-270.

[13] Kwekkeboom DJ, de Herder WW, Krenning EP. Receptor imaging in the diagnosis and treatment of pituitary tumors. *J Endocrinol Invest* 1999;22:80-88.

[14] Patel YC. Somatostatin and its receptor family. *Front Neuroendocrinol* 1999;20:157-198.

[15] Maclean J, Aldridge M, Bomanji J, Short S, Fersht N. Peptide receptor radionuclide therapy for aggressive atypical pituitary adenoma/carcinoma: variable clinical response in preliminary evaluation. *Pituitary* 2014;17:530-538.

[16] Champaneria, Modlin IM, Latich I, Bornschein J, Drozdov I, Kidd M. Somatostatin Analogue Therapy. In Kaufman HL, Wadler S, Antman K (editors): Cancer Drug Discovery and Development: Molecular Targeting in Oncology. *Humana Press,* Totowa, NJ 2008, pp 585-637.

[17] Breeman WAP, de Jong M, Kwekkeboom DJ, Valkema R, Bakker WH, Kooij PP, et al. Somatostatin receptor-mediated imaging and therapy:basic science, current knowledge, limitations and future perspectives. *Eur J Nucl Med* 2001;28:1421-1429.

[18] Krenning EP, de Jong M, Kooij PPM, Breeman WAP, Bakker WH, de Herder WW, et al. Radiolabelled somatostatin analogue(s) for peptide receptor scintigraphy and radionuclide therapy. *Annals of Oncology* 1999;10(Suppl 2):S23-S29.

[19] Reubi JC, Schar JC, Waser B, Wenger S, Heppeler A, Schmitt JS, et al. Affinity profiles for human somatostatin receptor subtypes SST1–SST5 of somatostatin radiotracers selected for scintigraphic and radiotherapeutic use. *Eur J Nucl Med* 2000;27:273-282.

[20] Grozinsky-Glasberg S, Shimon I, Korbonits M, Grossman AB. Somatostatin analogues in the control of neuroendocrine tumours: efficacy and mechanisms. *Endocrine-Related Cancer* 2008;15:701-720.

[21] Krenning EP, Kwekkeboom DJ, Bakker WH, Breeman WA, Kooij PP, Oei HY, et al. Somatostatin receptor scintigraphy with [^{111}In-DTPA-DPhe1]- and [^{123}I-Tyr3]-octreotide: the Rotterdam experience with more than 1000 patients. *Eur J Nucl Med* 1993;20:716-731.

[22] Krenning EP, Valkema R, Kwekkeboom DJ, de Herder WW, van Eijck CH, de Jong M, et al. Molecular imaging as in vivo molecular pathology for gastroenteropancreatic neuroendocrine tumors: implications for follow-up after therapy. *J Nucl Med* 2005;46(Suppl 1):76S-82S.

[23] Laznicek M, Laznickova A, Maecke HR. Receptor affinity and preclinical biodistribution of radiolabeled somatostatin analogs. *Anticancer Res* 2012;32:761-766.

[24] Hubalewska-Dydejczyk A, Szybinski P, Fross-Baron K, Mikolajczak R, Huszno B, Sowa-Staszczak A. (99m)Tc-EDDA/HYNIC-octreotate - a new radiotracer for detection and staging of NET: a case of metastatic duodenal carcinoid. *Nucl Med Rev Cent East Eur* 2005;8:155-156.

[25] GabrielM, Hausler F, Bale R, Moncayo R, Decristoforo C, Kovacs P, et al. Image fusion analysis of (99m)Tc-HYNICTyr(3)-octreotide SPECT and diagnostic CT using an immobilization device with external markers in patients with endocrine tumours. *Eur J Nucl Med Mol Imaging* 2005;32:1440-1451.

[26] Decristoforo C, Mather SJ, Cholewinski W, Donnemiller E, Riccabona G, Moncayo R. ^{99m}Tc-EDDA/HYNIC-TOC: a new ^{99m}Tc-labelled radiopharmaceutical for imaging somatostatin receptor-positive tumours: first clinical results and intra-patient comparison with ^{111}In-labelled octreotide derivates. *Eur J Nucl Med* 2000;27:1318-1325.

[27] Gabriel M, Decristoforo C, Donnemiller E, Ulmer H, Watfah Rychlinski C, Mather SJ, et al. An intrapatient comparison of ^{99m}Tc-EDDA/HYNIC-TOC with ^{111}In-DTPA-octreotide for diagnosis of somatostatin receptor expressing tumors. *J Nucl Med* 2003;44:708-716.

[28] Plachcińska A, Mikolajczak R, Maecke HR, Mlodkowska E, Kunert-Radek J, Michalski A, et al. Clinical usefulness of ^{99m}Tc-EDDA/HYNIC-TOC scintigraphyin oncological diagnostics: a preliminary communication. *Eur J Nucl Med Mol Imaging* 2003;30:1402-1406.

[29] de Herder WW, Lamberts SW. Somatostatin analogs as radiodiagnostic tools. *Rev Endocr Metab Disord* 2005;6:23-27.

[30] Duet M, Mundler O, Ajzenberg C, Berolatti B, Chedin P, Duranteau L, et al. Somatostatin receptor imaging in non-functioning adenomas: value of an uptake index. *Eur J Nucl Med* 1994;21:647-650.

[31] Oppizzi G, Cozzi R, Dallabonzana D, Orlandi P, Benini Z, Petroncini M, et al. Scintigraphic imaging of pituitary adenomas: an in vivo evaluation of somatostatin receptors. *J Endocrinol Invest* 1998;21:512-519.

[32] Hofmann M, Maecke H, Borner R, Weckesser E, Schoffski P, Oei L, et al. Biokinetics and imaging with the somatostatin receptor PET radioligand ^{68}Ga-DOTATOC: Preliminary data. *Eur J Nucl Med Mol Imaging* 2001;28:1751-1757.

[33] Ur E, Mather SJ, Bomanji J, Ellison D, Britton KE, Grossman AB, et al. Pituitary imaging using a labelled somatostatin analogue in acromegaly. *Clin Endocrinol* (Oxf) 1992;36:147-150.

[34] Legovini P, De Menis E, Billeci D, Conti B, Zoli P, Conte N. ^{111}Indium-pentetreotide pituitary scintigraphy and hormonal responses to octreotide in acromegalic patients. *J Endocrinol Invest* 1997;20:424-428.

[35] Rieger A, Rainov NG, Elfrich C, Klaua M, Meyer H, Lautenschlager C, et al. Somatostatin receptor scintigraphy in patients with pituitary adenoma. *Neurosurg Rev* 1997;20:7-12.

[36] Reubi JC, Landolt AM. The growth hormone responses to octreotide in acromegaly correlate with adenoma somatostatin receptor status. *J Clin Endocrinol Metab* 1989;68:844-850.

[37] Plöckinger U, Reichel M, Fett U, Saeger W, Quabbe HJ. Preoperative octreotide treatment of growth hormone-secreting and clinically nonfunctioning pituitary macroadenomas: effect on tumor volume and lack of correlation with immunohistochemistry and somatostatin receptor scintigraphy. *J Clin Endocrinol Metab* 1994;79:1416-1423.

[38] Plöckinger U, Bäder M, Hopfenmüller W, Saeger W, Quabbe HJ. Results of somatostatin receptor scintigraphy do not predict pituitary tumor volume- and hormone-response to ocreotide therapy and do not correlate with tumor histology. *Eur J Endocrinol* 1997;136:369-376.

[39] de Herder WW, Kwekkeboom DJ, Feelders RA, van Aken MO, Lamberts SWJ, van der Lely AJ, et al. Somatostatin receptor imaging for neuroendocrine tumors. *Pituitary* 2006;9:243-248.

[40] Broson-Chazot F, Houzard C, Ajzenberg C, Nocaudie M, Duet M, Mundler O, et al. Somatostatin receptor imaging in somatotroph and non-functioning pituitary adenomas: Correlation with hormonal and visual responses to octreotide. *Clin Endocrinol* (Oxf) 1997;47:589-598.

[41] Colao A, Ferone D, Lastoria S, Marzullo P, Cerbone G, Di Sarno A, et al. Prediction of efficacy of octreotide therapy in patients with acromegaly. *J Clin Endocrinol Metab* 1996;81:2356-2362.

[42] Ferone D, Pivonello R, Lastoria S, Faggiano A, Del Basso de Caro ML, et al. In vivo and in vitro effects of octreotide, quinagolide and cabergoline in four hyperprolactinaemic acromegalics: Correlation with somatostatin and dopamine D2 receptor scintigraphy. *Clin Endocrinol* (Oxf) 2001;54:469-477.

[43] Panza N, Rambaldi PF, Battista C, Ambrosio G, Cascini GL, Schilliro F, et al. Receptor imaging with ^{111}In-pentreotide and ^{123}I-methoxybenzamide, and inhibition tests with octreotide and bromocriptine of mixed growth hormone/prolactin secreting pituitary tumors. *Biomed Pharmacother* 1999;53:319-322.

[44] Duet M, Ajzenberg C, Benelhadj S, Lajeunie E, Lormeau B, Guillausseau PJ, et al. Somatostatin receptor scintigraphy in pituitary adenomas: A somatostatin receptor density index can predict hormonal and tumoral efficacy of octreotide in vivo. *J Nucl Med* 1999;40:1252-1256.

[45] de Herder WW, Lamberts SWJ. Somatostatin analogs as radiodiagnostic tools. *Reviews in Endocrine and Metabolic Disorders* 2005;6:23-27.

[46] Moulik PK, Varma TR, Vora JP, Vinjamuri S. The role of somatostatin receptor scintigraphy in the management of pituitary tumours. *Nucl Med Commun* 2002;23:117-120.

[47] Losa M, Magnani P, Mortini P, Persani L, Acerno S, Giugni E, et al. Indium-111 pentetreotide single-photon emission tomography in patients with TSH-secreting pituitary adenomas: correlation with the effect of a single administration of octreotide on serum TSH levels. *Eur J Nucl Med* 1997;24:728-731.

[48] Socin HV, Chanson P, Delemer B, Tabarin A, Rohmer V, Mockel J, et al. The changing spectrum of TSH-secreting pituitary adenomas: diagnosis and management in 43 patients. *Eur J Endocrinol* 2003;148:433-442.

[49] de Bruin TW, Kwekkeboom DJ, Van'tVerlaat JW, Reubi JC, Krenning EP, et al. Clinically nonfunctioning pituitary adenoma and octreotide response to long term high dose treatment, and studies in vitro. *J Clin Endocrinol Metab* 1992;75:1310-1317.

[50] van Royen EA, Verhoeff NP, Meylaerts SA, Miedema AR. Indium-111-DTPA-octreotide uptake measured in normal and abnormal pituitary glands. *J Nucl Med* 1996;37:1449-1451.

[51] Schmidt M, Scheidhauer K, Luyken C, Voth E, Hildebrandt G, Klug N, et al. Somatostatin receptor imaging in intracranial tumours. *Eur J Nucl Med* 1998;25:675-686.

[52] Curtò L, Ruggeri RM, Ferone D, Pivonello R, Squadrito S, Campennì A, et al. Lack of Somatostatin analogs effectiveness in gonadotropin-secreting pituitary adenomas. *The Endocrinologist* 2006;16:208-213.

[53] Acosta-Gomez MJ, Muros MA, Llamas-Elvira JM, Ramirez A, Ortega S, Sabatel G, et al. The role of somatostatin receptor scintigraphy in patients with pituitary adenoma or post-surgical recurrent tumours. *Br J Radiol* 2005;78:110-115.

[54] Lindsay JR, Nieman LK. Cushing's Disease: Medical Management. In Swearingen B, Biller BMK (editors), Contemporary Endocrinology: Diagnosis and Management of Pituitary Disorders. *Humana Press,* Totowa, NJ 2008, pp 223-236.

[55] Lauriero F, Pierangeli E, Rubini G, Resta M, D'Addabbo A. Pituitary adenomas: the role of ^{111}In-DTPA-octreotide SPET in the detection of minimal post-surgical residues. *Nucl Med Commun* 1998;19:1127-1134.

[56] Steiner E, Knosp E, Herold CJ, Kramer J, Stiglbauer R, Staniszewski K, et al. Pituitary adenomas: Findings of postoperative MR imaging. *Radiology* 1992;185:521-527.

[57] Lamberts SW, Hofland LJ, de Herder WW, Kwekkeboom DJ, Reubi JC, Krenning EP. Octreotide and related somatostatin analogs in the diagnosis and treatment of pituitary disease and somatostatin receptor scintigraphy. Front Neuroendocrinol 1993;14:27-55.

[58] Law WP, Fiumara F, Fong W, Macfarlane DJ. The 'double pituitary hot spot' sign of skull base meningioma on gallium-68-labelled somatostatin analogue PET. *J Med Imaging Radiat Oncol* 2013;57:680-683.

[59] Luyken C, Hildebrandt G, Krisch B, Scheidhauer K, Klug N. Clinical relevance of somatostatin receptor scintigraphy in patients with skull base tumours. *Acta Neurochir Suppl* 1996;65:102-104.

[60] Isidori AM, Kaltsas GA, Pozza C, Frajese V, Newell-Price J, Reznek RH, et al. The ectopic ACTH syndrome: clinical features, diagnosis, management and long-term follow-up. *J Clin Endocrinol Metab* 2006;91:371-377.

[61] Aniszewski JP, Young WF Jr, Thompson GB, Grant CS, van Heerden JA. Cushing syndrome due to ectopic adrenocorticotropic hormone secretion. *World J Surg* 2001;25:934-940.

[62] Ilias I, Torpy DJ, Pacak K, Mullen N, Wesley RA, Nieman LK. Cushing's syndrome due to ectopic corticotropin secretion: twenty years' experience at the National Institutes of Health. *J Clin Endocrinol Metab* 2005;90:4955-4962.

[63] de Herder WW, Krenning EP, Malchoff CD, Hofland LJ, Reubi JC, Kwekkeboom DJ, et al. Somatostatin receptor scintigraphy: its value in tumor localization in patientswith Cushing's syndrome caused by ectopic corticotropin or corticotropin-releasing hormone secretion. *Am J Med* 1994;96:305-312.

[64] Weiss M, Yellin A, Huszar M, Eisenstein Z, Bar-Ziv J, Krausz Y. Localization of adrenocorticotropic hormone-secreting bronchial carcinoid tumor by somatostatin-receptor scintigraphy. *Ann Intern Med* 1994;121:198-199.

[65] Phlipponneau M, NocaudieM, Epelbaum J, deKeyzer Y, Lalau JD, Marchandise X, et al. Somatostatin analogs for the localization and preoperative treatment of an adrenocorticotropin-secreting bronchial carcinoid tumor. *J Clin Endocrinol Metab* 1994;78:20-24.

[66] Lefebvre H, Jegou S, Leroux P, Dero M, Vaudry H, Kuhn JM. Characterization of the somatostatin receptor subtype in a bronchial carcinoid tumor responsible for Cushing's syndrome. *J Clin Endocrinol Metab* 1995;80:1423-1428.

[67] Matte J, Roufosse F, Rocmans P, Schoutens A, Jacobovitz D, Mockel J. Ectopic Cushing's syndrome and pulmonary carcinoid tumour identified by [111In-DTPA-D-Phe1]octreotide. *Postgrad Med J* 1998;74:108-110.

[68] Bakalakos EA, Cawley K, O'Dorisio TM, Heck C, Schirmer WJ. Localization of ectopic corticotropin-producing carcinoid tumor with use of indium-111 pentetreotide scintigraphy. *Endocr Pract* 1998;4:378-381.

[69] Tsagarakis S, Christoforaki M, Giannopoulou H, Rondogianni F, Housianakou I, Malagari C, et al. A reappraisal of the utility of somatostatin receptor scintigraphy in patients with ectopic adrenocorticotropin Cushing's syndrome. *J Clin Endocrinol Metab* 2003;88:4754-4758.

[70] Tremble JM, Buxton-Thomas M, Hopkins D, Kane P, Bailey D, Harris PE. Cushing's syndrome associated with a chemodectoma and a carcinoid tumour. *Clin Endocrinol* (Oxf) 2000;52:789-793.

[71] Tabarin A, Valli N, Chanson P, Bachelot Y, Rohmer V, Bex-Bachellerie V, et al. Usefulness of somatostatin receptor scintigraphy in patients with occult ectopic adrenocorticotropin syndrome. *J Clin Endocrinol Metab* 1999;84:1193-1202.

[72] de Herder WW, Lamberts SW. Octapeptide somatostatin analogue therapy of Cushing's syndrome. *Postgrad Med J* 1999;75:65-66.

[73] Jansson JO, Svensson J, Bengtsson BA, Frohman LA, Ahlman H, Wangberg B, et al. Acromegaly and Cushing's syndrome due to ectopic production of GHRH and ACTH by a thymic carcinoid tumour: in vitro responses to GHRH and GHRP-6. *Clin Endocrinol* (Oxf) 1998;48:243-250.

[74] Pacak K, Ilias I, Chen CC, Carrasquillo JA, Whatley M, Nieman LK. The role of [^{18}F]fluorodeoxyglucose positron emission tomography and [^{111}In]-diethylenetriaminepentaacetate-D-Phe-pentetreotide scintigraphy in the localization of

ectopic adrenocorticotropin-secreting tumors causing Cushing's syndrome. *J Clin Endocrinol Metab* 2004;89:2214-2221.

[75] Ilias I, Torpy DJ, Pacak K, Mullen N, Wesley RA, Nieman LK. Cushing's syndrome due to ectopic corticotropin secretion: twenty years' experience at the National Institutes of Health. *J Clin Endocrinol Metab* 2005;90:4955-4962.

[76] Zemskova MS, Gundabolu B, Sinaii N, Chen CC, Carrasquillo JA, Whatley M, et al. Utility of various functional and anatomic imaging modalities for detection of ectopic adrenocorticotropin-secreting tumors. *J Clin Endocrinol Metab* 2010;95:1207-1219.

[77] More J, Young J, Reznik Y, Raverot G, Borson-Chazot F, Rohmer V, et al. Ectopic ACTH syndrome in children and adolescents. *J Clin Endocrinol Metab* 2011;96:1213-1222.

[78] Ghazi AA, Amirbaigloo A, Abbasi Dezfooli A, Saadat AA, Ghazi S, Pirafkari M, et al. Ectopic acromegaly due to growth hormone releasing hormone. *Endocrine* 2013;43:293-302.

[79] Morel O, Giraud P, Bernier MO, Le Jeune JJ, Rohmer V, Jallet P. Ectopicacromegaly: localization of the pituitary growth hormone-releasing hormone producing tumor by In-111 pentetreotide scintigraphy and report of two cases. *Clin Nucl Med* 2004;29:841-843.

[80] Ramírez C, Hernández-Ramirez LC, Espinosa-de-los-Monteros AL, Franco JM, Guinto G, Mercado M. Ectopic acromegaly due to a GH-secreting pituitary adenoma in the sphenoid sinus: a case report and review of the literature. *BMC Res Notes* 2013;12,6:411.

[81] Garby L, Caron P, Claustrat F, Chanson P, Tabarin A, Rohmer V, et al. Clinical characteristics and outcome of acromegaly induced by ectopic secretion of growth hormone-releasing hormone (GHRH): a French nationwide series of 21 cases. *J Clin Endocrinol Metab* 2012;97:2093-2104.

[82] Biermasz NR, Smit JW, Pereira AM, Frölich M, Romijn JA, Roelfsema F. Acromegaly caused by growth hormone-releasing hormone-producing tumors: long-term observational studies in three patients. *Pituitary* 2007;10:237-249.

[83] Butler PW, Cochran CS, Merino MJ, Nguyen DM, Schrump DS, Gorden P. Ectopic growth hormone-releasing hormone secretion by a bronchial carcinoid tumor: clinical experience following tumor resection and long-acting octreotide therapy. *Pituitary* 2012;15:260-265.

[84] Greenman Y, Woolf P, Coniglio J, O'Mara R, Pei L, Said JW, et al. Remission of acromegaly caused by pituitary carcinoma after surgical excision of growth hormone-secreting metastasis detected by 111-indium pentetreotide scan. *J Clin Endocrinol Metab* 1996;81:1628-1633.

[85] Song M, Wang H, Song L, Tian H, Ge Q, Li J, et al. Ectopic TSH-secreting pituitary tumor: a case report and review of prior cases. *BMC Cancer* 2014,14:544. doi: 10.1186/1471-2407-14-544.

[86] Pugnale N, Waridel F, Bouzourène H, Boubaker A, Pugnale M, Gaillard RC, et al. Pharyngeal pituitary non-functioning adenoma with normal intra-sellar gland: massive tumor shrinkage on octreotide therapy. *Eur J Endocrino*l 2003;148:357-364.

[87] Maxwell JE, Howe JR. Imaging in neuroendocrine tumors: an update for the clinician. *Int J Endo Oncol* 2015;2:159-168.

[88] Lu SJ, Gnanasegaran G, Buscombe J, Navalkissoor S. Single photon emission computed tomography/computed tomography in the evaluation of neuroendocrine tumours: a review of the literature. *Nucl Med Commun* 2013;34:98-107.
[89] Schillaci O, Filippi L, Manni C, Santoni R. Single-photon emission computed tomography/computed tomography in brain tumors. *Semin Nucl Med* 2007;37:34-47.
[90] Kwekkeboom DJ, Krenning EP, Scheidhauer K, Lewington V, Lebtahi R, Grossman A, et al. ENETS Conse nsus Guidelines for the Standards of Care in Neuroendocrine Tumors: somatostatin receptor imaging with (111)In-pentetreotide. *Neuroendocrinology* 2009;90:184-189.
[91] Balon HR, Brown TL, Goldsmith SJ, Silberstein EB, Krenning EP, Lang O, et al. The SNM practice guideline for somatostatin receptor scintigraphy 2.0. *J Nucl Med Technol* 2011;39:317-324.
[92] Heiss WD, Herholz K. Brain receptor imaging. *J Nucl Med* 2006;4:302-312.
[93] Van Laere K, Varrone A, Booij J, Vander Borght T, Nobili F, Kapucu OL, et al. EANM procedure guidelines for brain neurotransmission SPECT/PET using dopamine D2 receptor ligands, version 2. *Eur J Nucl Med Mol Imaging.* 2010;37:434-442.
[94] de Herder WW, Reijs AEM, Feelders RA, van Aken MO, Krenning EP, van der Lely AJ, et al. Diagnostic imaging of dopamine receptors in pituitary adenomas. *Eur J Endocrinol* 2007;156:S53-S56.
[95] Pivonello R, Matrone C, Filippella M, Cavallo LM, Di Somma C, Cappabianca P, et al. Dopamine receptor expression and function in clinically nonfunctioning pituitary tumors: comparison with the effectiveness of cabergoline treatment. *J Clin Endocrinol Metab* 2004;89:1674-1683.
[96] Pivonello R, Ferone D, de Herder WW, Kros JM, De Caro ML, Arvigo M, et al. Dopamine receptor expression and function in corticotroph pituitary tumors. *J Clin Endocrinol Metab* 2004;89:2452-2462.
[97] Bevan JS, Burke CW. Non-functioning pituitary adenomas do not regress during bromocriptine therapy but possess membranebound dopamine receptors which bind bromocriptine. *Clin Endocrinol* 1986;25:561-572.
[98] Koga M, Nakao H, Arao M, Sato B, Noma K, Morimoto Y, et al. Demonstration of specific dopamine receptors on human pituitary adenomas. *Acta Endocrinol* 1987;114:595-602.
[99] Ferone D, Lastoria S, Colao A, Varrella P, Cerbone G, Acampa W, et al. Correlation of scintigraphic results using ^{123}I-methoxybenzamide with hormone levels and tumor size response to quinagolide in patients with pituitary adenomas. *J Clin Endocrinol Metab* 1998;83:248-252.
[100] de Herder WW, Reijs AE, Kwekkeboom DJ, Hofland LJ, Nobels FR, Oei HY, et al. In vivo imaging of pituitary tumours using a radiolabelled dopamine D2 receptor radioligand. *Clin Endocrinol* 1996;45:755-767.
[101] Ichise M, Ballinger JR. SPECT imaging of dopamine receptors. *J Nucl Med* 1996;37:1591-1595.
[102] Pirker W, Riedl M, Luger A, Czech T, Rossler K, Asenbaum S, et al. Dopamine D2 receptor imaging in pituitary adenomas using iodine-123-epidepride and SPECT. *J Nucl Med* 1996;37:1931-1937.
[103] de Herder WW, Reijs AEM, de Swart J, Kaandorp Y, Lamberts SWJ, Krenning EP, et al. Comparison of iodine-123 epidepride and iodine-123 IBZM for dopamine D2

receptor imaging in clinically non-functioning pituitary macroadenomas and macroprolactinomas. *Eur J Nucl Med* 1999;26:46-50.

[104] Leslie WD, Abrams DN, Greenberg CR, Hobson D. Comparison of iodine-123-epidepride and iodine-123-IBZM for dopamine D2 receptor imaging. *J Nucl Med* 1996;37:1589-1591.

[105] Colao A, Ferone D, Lastoria S, Cerbone G, Di Sarno A, Di Somma C, et al. Hormone levels and tumour size response to quinagolide and cabergoline in patients with prolactin-secreting and clinically non-functioning pituitary adenomas: predictive value of pituitary scintigraphy with ^{123}I-methoxybenzamide. *Clin Endocrinol* (Oxf) 2000;52:437-445.

[106] Panza N, Rambaldi PF, Battista C, Ambrosio G, Cascini GL, Schilliro F, et al. Receptor imaging with ^{111}In-pentreotide and ^{123}I-methoxybenzamide, and inhibition tests with octreotide and bromocriptine of mixed growth hormone/prolactin-secreting pituitary tumors. *Biomed Pharmacother* 1999;53:319-322.

[107] Ferone D, Pivonello R, Lastoria S, Faggiano A, del Basso De Caro ML, Cappabianca P, et al. In vivo and in vitro effects of octreotide, quinagolide and cabergoline in four hyperprolactinaemic acromegalics: Correlation with somatostatin and dopamine D2 receptor scintigraphy. *Clin Endocrinol* 2001;54:469-477.

[108] de Herder WW, Reijs AEM, Feelders RA, van Aken MO, Krenning EP, Tanghe HL, et al. Dopamine agonist therapy of clinically non-functioning pituitary macroadenomas. Is there a role for ^{123}I-epidepride dopamine D2 receptor imaging? *Eur J Endocrinol* 2006;155:1–8.

[109] Petrossians P, de Herder W, Kwekkeboom D, Lamberigts G, Stevenaert A, Beckers A. Malignant prolactinoma discovered by D2 receptor imaging. *J Clin Endocrinol Metab* 2000;85:398-401.

[110] Ambrosini V, Campana D, Tomassetti P, Fanti S. Ga-labelled peptides for diagnosis of gastroenteropancreatic NET. *Eur J Nucl Med Mol Imaging* 2012;39:s52-s60.

[111] Buchmann I, Henze M, Engelbrecht S, Eisenhut M, Runz A, Schäfer M, et al. Comparison of ^{68}Ga-DOTATOC PET and ^{111}In-DTPAOC (Octreoscan) SPECT in patients with neuroendocrine tumours. *Eur J Nucl Med Mol Imaging* 2007;34:1617-1626.

[112] Etchebehere EC, de Oliveira Santos A, Gumz B, Vicente A, Hoff PG, Corradi G, et al. ^{68}Ga-DOTATATE PET/CT, ^{99m}Tc-HYNIC-octreotide SPECT/CT, and whole-body MR imaging in detection of neuroendocrine tumors: a prospective trial. *J Nucl Med.* 2014;55:1598-1604.

[113] Kuyumcu S, Ozkan ZG, Sanli Y, Yilmaz E, Mudun A, Adalet I, et al. Physiological and tumoral uptake of (68)Ga-DOTATATE: standardized uptake values and challenges in interpretation. *Ann Nucl Med* 2013;27:538-545.

[114] Kunikowska J, Krolicki L, Pawlak D, Zerizer I, Mikołajczak R. Semiquantitative analysis and characterization of physiological biodistribution of (68)Ga-DOTATATE PET/CT. *Clin Nucl Med* 2012;37:1052-1057.

[115] Shastry M, Kayani I, Wild D, Caplin M, Visvikis D, Gacinovic S, et al. Distribution pattern of ^{68} Ga-DOTATATE in disease-free patients. *Nucl Med Commun* 2010;31:1025-1032.

[116] Veit JA, Boehm B, Luster M, Scheuerle A, Rotter N, Rettinger G, et al. Detection of paranasal ectopic adrenocorticotropic hormone-secreting pituitary adenoma by Ga-68-

DOTANOC positron-emission tomography-computed tomography. *Laryngoscope* 2013;123:1132-1135.

[117] Sala E, Ferrante E, Verrua E, Malchiodi E, Mantovani G, Filopanti M, et al. Growth hormone-releasing hormone-producing pancreatic neuroendocrine tumor in a multiple endocrine neoplasia type 1 family with an uncommon phenotype. *Eur J Gastroenterol Hepatol* 2013;25:858-862.

[118] Naswa N, Das CJ, Sharma P, Karunanithi S, Bal C, Kumar R. Ectopic pituitary adenoma with empty sella in the setting of MEN-1 syndrome: detection with ^{68}Ga-DOTANOC PET/CT. *Jpn J Radiol* 2012;30:783-786.

[119] Novruzov F, Aliyev JA, Jaunmuktane Z, Bomanji JB, Kayani I. The use of ^{68}Ga DOTATATE PET/CT for diagnostic assessment and monitoring of ^{177}Lu DOTATATE therapy in pituitary carcinoma. *Clin Nucl Med* 2015;40:47-49.

[120] d'Amico A, Stąpór-Fudzińska M, Tarnawski R. CyberKnife radiosurgery planning of a secreting pituitary adenoma performed with ^{68}Ga DOTATATE PET and MRI. *Clin Nucl Med* 2014 Dec;39:1043-1044.

[121] Eriksson B, Orlefors H, Oberg K, Sundin A, Bergstrom M, Langstrom B. Developments in PET for the detection of endocrine tumours. *Best Pract Res Clin Endocrinol Metab* 2005;19:311-324.

[122] Binderup T, Knigge U, Loft A, Mortensen J, Pfeifer A, Federspiel B, et al. Functional imaging of neuroendocrine tumors: a head-to-head comparison of somatostatin receptor scintigraphy, ^{123}I-MIBG scintigraphy, and ^{18}F-FDG PET. *J Nucl Med* 2010;51:704-712.

[123] Ryu SI, Tafti BA, Skirboll SL. Pituitary adenomas can appear as hypermetabolic lesions in F-FDG PET imaging. *J Neuroimaging* 2010;20:393-396.

[124] Seok H, Lee EY, Choe EY, Yang WI, Kim JY, Shin DY, et al. Analysis of ^{18}F-fluorodeoxyglucose positron emission tomography findings in patients with pituitary lesions. *Korean J Intern Med* 2013;28:81-88.

[125] Alzahrani AS, Farhat R, Al-Arifi A, Al-Kahtani N, Kanaan I, Abouzied M. The diagnostic value of fused positron emission tomography/computed tomography in the localization of adrenocorticotropin-secreting pituitary adenoma in Cushing's disease. *Pituitary* 2009;12:309-314.

[126] De Souza B, Brunetti A, Fulham MJ, Brooks RA, DeMichele D, Cook P, et al. Pituitary microadenomas: a PET study. *Radiology* 1990;177:39-44.

[127] Zhao X, Xiao J, Xing B, Wang R, Zhu Z, Li F. Comparison of ^{68}Ga DOTATATE to ^{18}F-FDG uptake is useful in the differentiation of residual or recurrent pituitary adenoma from the remaining pituitary tissue after transsphenoidal adenomectomy. *Clin Nucl Med* 2014;39:605-608.

[128] Tang BNT, Levivier M, Heureux M, Wikler D, Massager N, Devriendt D, et al. ^{11}C-methionine PET for the diagnosis and managementof recurrent pituitary adenomas. *Eur J Nucl Med Mol Imaging* 2006;33:169-178.

[129] Muhr C. Positron emission tomography in acromegaly and other pituitary adenoma patients. *Neuroendocrinology* 2006;83:205-210.

[130] Ikeda H, Abe T, Watanabe K. Usefulness of composite methionine-positron emission tomography/3.0-tesla magnetic resonance imaging to detect the localization and extent of early-stage Cushing adenoma. *J Neurosurg* 2010;112:750-755.

[131] Bergström M, Muhr C, Lundberg PO, Langstrom B. PET as a tool in the clinical evaluation of pituitary adenomas. *J Nucl Med* 1991;32:610-615.

[132] Rufini V, Calcagni ML, Baum RP. Imaging of Neuroendocrine Tumors. *Semin Nucl Med* 2006;36:228-247.

[133] Ducry J, Gomez F, Prior JO, Boubaker A, Matter M, Monti M, et al. Mid-gut ACTH-secreting neuroendocrine tumor unmasked with (18)F-dihydroxyphenylalanine-positron emission tomography. *Endocrinol Diabetes Metab Case Rep* 2015;2015:140104. doi: 10.1530/EDM-14-0104.

[134] Anthony LB, Woltering EA, Espenan GD, Cronin MD, Maloney TJ, McCarthy KE. Indium-111-pentetreotide prolongs survival in gastroenteropancreatic malignancies. *Semin Nucl Med* 2002;32:123-132.

[135] Kwekkeboom DJ, Mueller-Brand J, Paganelli G, Anthony LB, Pauwels S, Kvols LK, et al. Overview of results of peptide receptor radionuclide therapy with 3 radiolabeled somatostatin analogs. *J Nucl Med* 2005;46(Suppl 1):S62-S66.

[136] Zaknun JJ, Bodei L, Mueller-Brand J, Pavel ME, Baum RP, Hörsch D, et al. The joint IAEA, EANM, and SNMMI practical guidance on peptide receptor radionuclide therapy (PRRNT) in neuroendocrine tumours. *Eur J Nucl Med Mol Imaging* 2013;40:800-816.

[137] Baldari S, Ferraù F, Alafaci C, Herberg A, Granata F, Militano V, et al. First demonstration of the effectiveness of peptide receptor radionuclide therapy (PRRT) with ^{111}In-DTPA-octreotide in a giant PRL-secreting pituitary adenoma resistant to conventional treatment. *Pituitary* 2012;15(Suppl 1):S57-S60.

[138] De Jong M, Breeman WA, Bernard BF, Bakker WH, Schaar M, van Gameren A, et al. [^{177}Lu-DOTA^0,Tyr^3] octreotate for somatostatin receptor-targeted radionuclide therapy. *Int J Cancer* 2001;92:628-633.

[139] Imhof A, Brunner P, Marincek N, Briel M, Schindler C, Rasch H, et al. Response, survival, and long-term toxicity after therapy with the radiolabeled somatostatin analogue [^{90}Y-DOTA]-TOC in metastasized neuroendocrine cancers. *J Clin Oncol* 2011;29:2416-2423.

[140] Kwekkeboom DJ, Kam BL, van Essen M, Teunissen JJ, van Eijck CH, Valkema R, et al. Somatostatin-receptor-based imaging and therapy of gastroenteropancreatic neuroendocrine tumors. *Endocr Relat Cancer* 2010;17:R53-R73.

[141] Kam BLR, Teunissen JJM, Krenning EP, de Herder WW, Khan S, van Vliet EI, et al. Lutetium-labelled peptides for therapy of neuroendocrine tumours. *Eur J Nucl Med Mol Imaging* 2012;39(Suppl 1):103-112.

[142] Bodei L, Cremonesi M, Zoboli S, Grana C, Bartolomei M, Rocca P, et al. Receptor-mediated radionuclide therapy with ^{90}Y-DOTATOC in association with amino acid infusion: a phase I study. *Eur J Nucl Med Mol Imaging* 2003;30:207-216.

[143] Chinol M, Bodei L, Cremonesi M, Paganelli G. Receptor-mediated radiotherapy with Y-DOTA-DPhe-Tyr-octreotide: the experience of the European Institute of Oncology Group. *Semin Nucl Med* 2002;32:141-147.

[144] Komor J, Reubi JC, Christ ER. Peptide receptor radionuclide therapy in a patient with disabling non-functioning pituitary adenoma. *Pituitary* 2014;17:227-231.

[145] Goglia U, Ferone D, Sidoti M, Spaziante R, Dadati P, Ravetti JL, et al. Treatment of a pituitary metastasis from a neuroendocrine tumour: case report and literature review. *Pituitary* 2008;11:93-102.

[146] Maclean J, Aldridge M, Bomanji J, Short S, Fersht N. Peptide receptor radionuclide therapy for aggressive atypical pituitary adenoma/carcinoma: variable clinical response in preliminary evaluation. *Pituitary* 2014;17:530-538.

[147] Teunissen JJ, Krenning EP, de Jong FH, de Rijke YB, Feelders RA, van Aken MO, et al. Effects of therapy with [^{177}Lu-DOTA^{0},Tyr^{3}]octreotate on endocrine function. *Eur J Nucl Med Mol Imaging* 2009;36:1758-1766.

In: Pituitary Adenoma
Editor: Dimitrios N. Kanakis

ISBN: 978-1-63484-985-2

Chapter 10

TREATMENT OF PITUITARY ADENOMAS: AN INTEGRATED APPROACH

Olga Karapanou, MD,
and Stylianos Tsagarakis*, MD, PhD, FRCP
Department of Endocrinology, Diabetes and Metabolism,
"Evaggelismos" Hospital, Athens, Greece

ABSTRACT

Treatment of pituitary adenomas aims at correcting hormone hypersecretion, restoring pituitary function and debulking space-occupying neoplasms. Treatment options are surgery, irradiation and medications, where surgery performed via transsphenoidal approach is the procedure of choice, with the exception of prolactinomas that respond well to dopamine agonists both in terms of hormone secretion and tumor regression as well. Surgical success rate lies upon tumor size and invasiveness and neurosurgeon's experience as well, performed by an experienced neurosurgeon, surgery is curative in half of the macroadenomas and approximately 80% of microadenomas with low morbidity and mortality.

Medical treatment is disease specific. As already mentioned dopamine agonists normalize prolactin levels and decrease tumor size in almost all patients with symptomatic micro or macroprolactinomas. In acromegalic patients somatostatin analogues targeting 2 and 5 somatostatin receptor subtypes (octreotide and lanreotide) normalize IGF1 levels in approximately 55% of patients and may be used as monotherapy or in combination with dopamine agonists especially in cases of mixed GH-/PRL-hypersecretion. Pegvisomant, the GH-receptor antagonist is reserved for uncontrolled patients where remission is achieved in about 2/3 of them. Pasireotide, a novel somatostatin analogue multireceptor ligand has recently been developed as tumor-directed therapy for Cushing's disease, but so far experience is limited. To date adrenal steroidogenesis inhibitors (i.e., ketoconazole, metyrapone) have commonly been used in order to restore hypercortizolism.

* Corresponding author: Stylianos Tsagarakis, MD, PhD, FRCP, Department of Endocrinology, Diabetes and Metabolism"Evaggelismos" Hospital, 45-47 Ipsilantou St. 10676 Athens, Greece. E-mail: stsagara@otenet.gr.

Irradiation is reserved as third line treatment for selected patients after failure of surgery or medical treatment, since remission is delayed for several years at the expense of hypopituitarism and other complications such as radionecrosis, cerebrovascular disease or even second tumor formation. There are two main types of radiation therapy, conventional fractionated radiation therapy and stereotactic radiosurgery including several modalities, such as Gamma Knife, CyberKnife, and a linear accelerator, which delivers high-energy photons. The advantage of the latter type is that narrow beams of radiation are delivered with stereotactic accuracy on the target lesion in order to minimize injury to surrounding tissues, and mean time to biochemical remission is shorter compared to conventional radiation. Therefore, there has been a trend towards the use of radiosurgery unless there is substantial residual tumor burden or close proximity to the optic chiasm.

Keywords: medical treatment, transsphenoidal resection, radiation therapy, somatostatin analogues, dopamine agonists

1. INTRODUCTION

Treatment of pituitary tumors depending on size and secretory status is a multidisciplinary approach that involves medications, surgery, radiotherapy and substitution therapy if required. Advances in the knowledge of molecular mechanisms and in the field of microsurgery over the years resulted in a trend favoring surgery and medical treatment and limiting the use of radiation therapy. Consequently, except for prolactinomas responding well to medical treatment, surgery remains the treatment of choice for GH-secreting, ACTH-secreting and selected cases of non-functioning pituitary adenomas, as described below. The rationale for surgery is biochemical cure, restoration of normal pituitary function and decompression of the surrounding neural structures [1]. The favored surgical approach is via the transsphenoidal route, while the transcranial approach is reserved for huge tumors with suprasellar extension. Surgical techniques are described in subsequent capitels of this book. The potential advantage of the endoscope versus microscope is the panoramic view of the operative field providing visualization of the suprasellar compartment and carvenous sinus walls, unlike the microscope which is limited by line of sight. However, there is no definitive evidence of superiority of the endoscopic versus the microscopic approach with regard to short- and long-term remission rates, recurrence, or complications [2, 3]. High-volume medical centers with dedicated pituitary surgeons who perform 50 or more transsphenoidal procedures per year yield the best surgical outcomes with low morbidity and mortality [4, 5]. A well-coordinated team approach-anchored by an endocrinologist and an experienced neurosurgeon and assisted by a dedicated neuroradiologist may offer optimal treatment outcomes [6]. Post-operative management is more or less the same, while preparation for surgery, remission criteria and success rates depend on the type of the clinically functioning adenoma and are presented below.

1.1. Postoperative Course

Postoperative management should include monitoring for electrolyte abnormalities, including diabetes insipidus and syndrome of inappropriate secretion of antidiuretic hormone, for up to 2 weeks. In the postoperative setting, especially for GH-secreting adenomas the presence of increased diuresis may reflect obligate natriuresis after a rapid reduction in GH and IGF1 values. Hyponatremia due to the syndrome of inappropriate secretion of antidiuretic hormone may manifest 5 to 14 days postoperatively in 5% to 10% of the patients after any transsphenoidal procedure. Mild cases respond to fluid restriction, but severe cases may necessitate intravenous administration of hypertonic saline [7, 8]. Diabetes insipidus (DI) is a common transient event in about 20% of patients who undergo a transsphenoidal procedure, necessitating at least one treatment of desmopressin in about 10% and long-term treatment in 2% to 7% of all patients undergoing transsphenoidal procedures. There may be a higher association of diabetes insipidus with intraoperative cerebrospinal fluid (CSF) leaks [9]. Typical triphasic response induced by pituitary stalk sectioning is characterized by a first phase of diabetes insipidus occurring in immediate postoperative period up to day 6, a second phase of antidiuresis occurring from day 7 to day 12, followed by a third phase of reoccurrence of diabetes insipidus [10, 11]. The first phase is thought to be caused by axon shock, the second one is due to unregulated release of vasopressin from the store of hormone in the degenerating axons of the posterior pituitary. Excess administration of fluids in this phase will produce hyponatremia and syndrome of inappropriate antidiuretic hormone (SIADH). Hyponatremia's manifestations include headaches, nausea, vomiting and seldom seizures [12]. As degenerated neurons are depleted of vasopressin, the third phase of DI is installed. Of note, the second phase of the triphasic response (i.e., uncontrolled release of vasopressin due to axon trauma) may occur without preceding or subsequent DI. This syndrome of transient hyponatremia has been referred to as isolated second phase and has been reported in 10-25% of patients after pituitary surgery [8].

Adrenal function must be evaluated in the immediate postoperative period and replaced as appropriate. The rest of pituitary hormone testing, including the thyroid and gonadal axes, should be performed at 6 to 12 weeks postoperatively, in order to assess pituitary function and the need for hormone replacement therapy [13].

2. Molecular Basis for Medical Treatment

2.1. Dopamine Agonists

The introduction of dopamine agonists changed dramatically the treatment of pituitary tumors Dopamine is the predominant catecholamine neurotransmitter in the human central nervous system but also serves as a modulator of cardiovascular and renal function, gastrointestinal (GI) motility [14]. Dopamine agonists (DA) exert their functions via binding to dopamine receptors [14]. Dopamine receptors are G-protein coupled receptors acting via adenyl cyclase modulation. There are 5 receptor subtypes divided into two categories: D1-like (D1 and D5) and D2-like (D2, D3 and D4). D1-like have mainly stimulatory, while D2-like inhibitory properties at intracellular cAMP level [14]. Dopamine receptors are expressed in most cell types of the anterior pituitary gland including GH-secreting, prolactin-secreting, ACTH-secreting and clinically nonfunctioning tumors [15]. Dopamine agonists are the older drugs, the introduction of which in the mid-1970s dramatically changed the treatment of pituitary tumors [16]. All dopamine agonists except for quinagolide are ergot alkaloids. The most commonly used are bromocriptine and cabergoline, while use of the older lisuride, pergolide, quinagolide or metergoline has almost nowadays been abandoned. Bromocriptine is a lysergic acid derivative with a bromine substitution at position [17]. It is a strong dopamine agonist that decreases prolactin synthesis, DNA synthesis, and the overall size of the prolactinoma. Due to its short half-life it requires twice daily administration. Tolerance is better when one starts with the lowest possible dose of 1.25 mg daily and increases the dose gradually to 1.25 mg each week, until prolactin levels are normal or a dose of 2.5 mg twice daily is reached, which is effective in 66% of cases [18]. Another alternative to oral administration is vaginal usage of the same drug, which is well tolerated and avoids the liver first pass metabolism [19]. Cabergoline shares many characteristics and adverse events of bromocriptine but has a very long half-life allowing weekly dosing. It is more effective in suppressing prolactin levels and reducing tumor size [20]. The low rate of side effects and the weekly dosage make cabergoline a better choice for initial treatment. It can also be given vaginally if nausea occurs when taken orally [21]. A weekly dose of 1 mg is usually adequate for hyperprolactinemia. Though both drugs have been shown to be safe in pregnancy, the number of reports studying bromocriptine in pregnancy far exceeds that of cabergoline. Between the two dopamine agonists, bromocriptine and cabergoline, the latter is more effective and has fewer side-effects [22].

2.2. Somatostatin Analogues

Somatostatin is an inhibitory hormone widely distributed throughout the entire body, mostly abundant in the central nervous system, gastrointestinal tract and pancreas. In central nervous system (CNS), somatostatin acts as an inhibitor of the release of growth hormone (GH) and thyroid-stimulating hormone (TSH). In the gastrointestinal (GI) tract, it inhibits the release of several GI hormones i.e., insulin, glucagon, gastrin, cholecystokinin, vasoactive intestinal peptide (VIP) and secretin and exocrine gastric acid, pepsin, pancreatic enzymes, bile and intestinal fluids secretions as well [23]. Somatostatin exists in two molecular forms, somatostatin-14 and somatostatin-28 and mediates its biological effects through activation of transmembrane G-protein-coupled somatostatin receptors. To date, 5 dinstinct somatostatin receptors (sst1-5) have been identified [24]. Normal tissue distribution of ssts varies: human anterior pituitary expresses all 5 subtypes [25]. Differential expression of ssts in certain neuroendocrine tumors favors the application of somatostatin receptor ligands-based therapies, for example GH adenomas express sst2 and to a lesser extent sst5 while ACTH adenomas express sst5 [24]. Signaling pathways coupled to somatostatin receptor activation include inhibition of adenyl cyclase and activation of phosphotyrosine phosphatase (PTP) activity. Certain somatostatin receptor subtypes couple to inward-rectifying K+ channels (sst2, 3, 4, 5), to voltage dependent Ca^{2+} channels (sst1, sst2), to a Na+/H+ exchanger (sst1), as well as to phospholipase C (sst2, sst5) and phospholipase A2 (sst4) [26]. Anti-secretory activity is exerted via inhibition of adenyl cyclase and the influx of Ca^{++}, whereas antiproliferative properties include activation of PTP. In addition, indirect anti-proliferative activity includes inhibition of angiogenesis and modulation of the immune system [27].

Native somatostatin has a very short half-life of 2-3min, as it is rapidly degraded by circulating blood peptidases. In order to increase resistance to peptidases and thereby allow systemic delivery by virtue of longer circulation times, several synthetic somatostatin analogues have been developed with varying affinities for the different sst subtypes. The most widely used is an 8-amino acid peptide, octreotide (Sandostatin®) with a prolonged half life of 90-120min and selective affinity for sst2 and to a lesser extent for sst5 receptors, which is 40-fold more potent in inhibiting GH secretion from GH-secreting pituitary adenomas [24, 28, 29]. Due to its limited half-life a 3-time daily injection was needed (100 μg tid titrating up to 1.5 mg daily), but this regimen was gradually replaced by long-acting formulations i.e., octreotide LAR [30]. and depot lanreotide (Somatulin Autogel) [31]. In the former formulation octreotide is delivered by polymeric microspheres, concentration rises the first day after injection, then declines in the following 2-6 days and reaches a plateau phase during days 11-40. Steady-state concentrations are usually obtained after 2-3 injections. The usual starting dose is 20mg monthly, titrated up to 40 mg monthly depending on clinical and biochemical response [32]. In the latter formulation lanreotide is delivered as an aqueous small volume mixture of 60, 90 or 120 mg, in prefilled syringes for deep subcutaneous administration. The pharmacokinetic profile of lanreotide autogel shows peak concentrations on day 1, with a subsequent elimination half-life of 25 days [31].

Formerly referred as SOM230, pasireotide diaspartate (SigniforTM, Novartis Pharmaceuticals) is a cyclic hexapeptide with in vitro binding affinity 40-, 30-, and 5-fold higher for sst5, sst1, and sst3, respectively, and 2-fold lower for sst2 [33]. As depicted in (Table. 1). Pasireotide exists as a subcutaneous formulation and as long-acting one (LAR) (20, 40 and 60mg given intramuscularly once every 28 d). The effective elimination T1/2 of pasireotide (approximately 7−11 h) is longer than that of octreotide, thus subcutaneous pasireotide is suitable for a twice-daily (bid) dosing regimen [34].

Table 1. Binding affinities (mean ±SEM of IC50 values expressed as nmol/L) of somatostatin-14, pasireotide, octreotide and lanreotide to the five human somatostatin receptors (ssts)

Compound	Sst1	Sst2	Sst3	Sst4	Sst5
Somato statin-14	0.93 ± 0.12	0.15 ± 0.2	0.56 ± 0.17	1.50 ± 0.4	0.29 ± 0.4
Pasireotide	9.3 ± 0.1	1.0±0.1	1.5±0.3	>1,000	0.16 ± 0.01
Octreotide	280 ± 80	0.38 ± 0.08	7.1 ± 1.4	>1,000	6.3 ± 1.0
Lanreotide	180 ± 20	0.54 ± 0.08	14 ± 9	230 ± 40	17 ± 5

3. Pituitary Radiation Therapy

The techniques of pituitary irradiation have improved over the years in order to avoid radiation exposure of surrounding tissues. There are two main types of pituitary radiation therapy, conventional radiation therapy and stereotactic radiosurgery. Conventional radiotherapy is administered by a linear accelerator (4-8 MeV) commonly from 2 to 3 portals in a total dose of 40-50 Gy fractionated in at least 20 sessions over a 5- to 6- week period

[35]. Stereotactic radiosurgery includes Gamma knife, Cyberknife and a linear accelerator which delivers high-energy photons. Some centers use proton particles for stereotactic radiosurgery [36]. Candidates for stereotactic radiosurgery are well-visualized small adenoma remnants showing evidence of growth at repeat MRI, with suspicious invasive characteristics close to the cavernous sinus and far from the optic chiasm.

4. Specific Disease Treatment

4.1. GH-Secreting Pituitary Adenomas (Acromegaly)

Surgery is the primary treatment for most patients, especially in case of optic chiasm compression. Even in patients with parasellar disease and low likelihood of surgical cure, surgical debulking may be considered in order to enhance response to medical treatment [37, 38, 39]. Therapeutic goals include age-normalized IGF1 and a random GH value less than 1 ng/ml while maintaining the same GH and IGF1 assay in the same patient throughout management [40]. Surgical adjuncts to improve outcome depend on surgeon and available resources and include intraoperative MRI [41], neuronavigation [42] and intraoperative GH determination [43]. Surgical remission predictive markers include Knosp grade, defining cavernous sinus invasion and preoperative GH and IGF1 levels [44]. Knosp grade 0-2 tumors are associated with higher remission rates compared to Knosp grade 3-4 tumors, also, the higher the preoperative GH and IGF1 levels the lower the surgical remission rates [2]. The most common perioperative complications are sinonasal ones, followed by postoperative CSF leak, while carotid injury and meningitis are quite rare [45, 46]. The prevalence of postoperative complications is inversely related to the experience of neurosurgeon [47] New-onset pituitary dysfunction has been reported in less than 10% [48].

a. Surgical Outcome Assessment

The role of an early postoperative value may be limited because an elevated value may reflect GH stress with normal somatotroph GH production [48]. However, on postoperative day 1, a fasting GH less than 2 μg/l correlates with long-term remission [48]. The decline in IGF1 is more delayed compared with GH, likely due to differential half-life of IGF-binding proteins. Thus, an IGF1 level and a random GH should be measured at 12 weeks or later. In patients with random GH greater than 1 μg/l, a nadir GH after glucose load (75 gr per os) should be measured. A nadir GH value less than 1ng/ml may be used to define disease control postoperatively, although use of a lower nadir GH of less than 0.4ng/ml has been suggested as a better predictor of long-term cure [49, 50]. If serum IGF1 level is elevated at 12 weeks, repeated testing in 9 to 12 weeks should be considered to determine whether there may be delayed biochemical normalization, before proceeding with potential surgical reexploration, medical therapy, or radiation therapy [13]. Repeat surgery is indicated if there is residual tumor that is surgically accessible with curative potential or in case there are persistent mass effects upon the optic chiasm [51].

b. Time for Imaging Studies

An imaging study in order to assess residual tumor and adjacent structures is performed at least 12 weeks after surgery to allow for involution of gel foam and fat packing [52]. MRI is the imaging modality of choice followed by CT scan when the MRI is contraindicated or unavailable [40].

c. Medical Therapy

Medical therapy is often indicated as adjuvant therapy and there are three classes of drugs, somatostatin analogs (SSAs) and dopamine agonists (DAs) both target the adenoma. The third class is the GH receptor antagonist (growth hormone releasing hormone, GHRH) pegvisomant which bypasses the tumor and prevents GH function systematically. Choice is based upon disease activity, presence of co-morbidity and cost. Usually medical therapy endpoints are similar to surgical response including age- and sex-normalized IGF1 and GH < 1μg/l. The GH response to glucose suppression has not been found to be useful for assessing biochemical control [53]. Of note, GH levels should not be measured if pegvisomant is administered because GH levels will increase on this therapy due to the lack of GH feedback autoinhibition, thus these values will have no relevance with regard to efficacy and dosing.

- Somatostatin analogues

Somatostatin analogues are effective in normalizing GH and IGF1 levels in 50-70% of patients, while octreotide LAR and lanreotide Autogel have similar efficacy profiles [40]. Apart from biochemical control somatostatin analogues have been shown to induce tumor shrinkage especially if given as first-line treatment [54, 55], although their antisecretory and antiproliferative effect may be dissociated [56]. A recent meta-analysis including 41 studies demonstrated that significant tumor shrinkage is achieved in almost 2/3 of patients, especially if given as first-line therapy, while tumor shrinkage was positively correlated with biochemical control [57]. Similar response rates have been shown in the prospective PRIMARY study, 62.9% of treatment-naïve patients exhibited significant tumor shrinkage after administration of lanreotide Autogel 120 mg for 48 weeks [58]. Although somatostatin's antitumoral effect is unequivocal, the role of preoperative somatostatin analogues in terms of improved surgical cure rates is rather conflicting. According to Losa et al. preoperative treatment with long-acting somatostatin analogues does not improve surgical success rates [59]. Mao et al. have shown the opposite but in fewer number of patients [60].

In conclusion, current clinical practice guidelines suggest a preoperative treatment with somatostatin analogues for a 3-month period in case of invasive macroadenomas when the overall surgical remission rate is below 50% [61]. Smaller tumors with lower baseline GH and IGF1 levels are more likely to respond [62, 63]. Densely granulated tumors are more somatostatin analogue responsive than the more common sparsely granulated ones [64]. Hypointense T2-weighted tumor MRI images which correlate with dense tumor granularity represent another feature predictive of response to somatostatin analogues [64]. On the contrary, resistance to somatostatin analogue therapy has been observed in patients carrying an aryl hydrocarbon receptor interacting protein (AIP) mutation. Of note, these adenomas are usually sparsely granulated. Even a low AIP expression in the adenoma is associated with resistance to somatostatin analogues and this interaction might explain some cases of adenomas exhibiting resistance to somatostatin analogue therapy despite high sst2 expression [65]. Acute GH response to a subcutaneous octreotide injection is not helpful in determining somatostatin analogue response [66].

Octreotide LAR and lanreotide Autogel have similar side effect profiles [67, 68]. Common side effects are gastrointestinal upset, malabsorption, constipation, gallbladder disease (gallbladder sludge or gallstone formation), hair loss, and bradycardia [69]. There is relatively low risk of moderate impairment in glucose tolerance or even overt diabetes due to decreased insulin levels, in such case, dose lowering, addition of glucose-lowering agents or substitution with pegvisomant which improves insulin sensitivity may be considered [70].

Regarding pasireotide, in a randomised clinical phase II trial on 60 patients with acromegaly, 27% of the patients were found to display a biochemical response after 3 months of pasireotide treatment defined as GH < 2.5 ng/ml and IGF1 normalization [71]. A head-to-head prospective study of 385 medically naïve patients, randomized either to pasireotide LAR or octreotide LAR, demonstrated that biochemical control was achieved by significantly more pasireotide LAR patients than octreotide LAR patients, specifically pasireotide was more effective than octreotide LAR at inhibiting IGF1 and equally effective at inhibiting GH. This may be due to the higher affinity and functional activity of pasireotide at hepatic sst1, sst3 and sst4 receptors [72].

Similarly to somatostatin analogues, pasireotide's major adverse event is diabetes mellitus via not only reduced insulin secretion but also reduced glycagon-like peptide (GLP-1) and glucose-dependent insulinotropic polypeptide. Diabetes should be managed initially with metformin, and staged treatment intensification with a dipeptyl-peptidase 4 inhibitor switching to a GLP-1 receptor agonist or insulin when necessary [73, 74].

- GH-receptor antagonist (pegvisomant)

Pegvisomant is a recombinant GH-receptor antagonist. GH acts via binding to 2 distinct GH-receptor dimmers, pegvisomant abrogates functional dimerization and subsequent intracellular signaling (Figure 1) resulting in dose-dependent reduction and normalization of serum IGF1 levels in up to 95% of patients [75]. On the contrary, due to the interrupted negative feedback mechanism from diminished IGF1 levels GH levels increase, thus GH measurement is unreliable in terms of monitoring biochemical response [76]. Pegvisomant is administered subcutaneously as 10, 15 or 20mg daily injections. Mean daily pegvisomant dose required for IGF1 normalization is 17.4mg, although some patients may need higher doses up to 40mg daily [77]. Co-administration of pegvisomant as once or twice a week dosing with somatostatin analogues normalizes IGF1 levels in over 90% of patients, improves quality of life and decreases tumor size in approximately 20% of patients [78]. During pegvisomant therapy glucose homeostasis is improved, therefore it might be useful for patients with impaired glucose tolerance or overt diabetes [67].

Due to its mechanism of action and subsequent increase in GH levels, pegvisomant is deprived of antiproliferative effects and tumor growth has been reported in 3-5% of patients [76, 79]. Therefore, clinicians should have in mind that pegvisomant is not an option for aggressive tumors abutting the optic chiasm [79]. MRI imaging should be performed at 6-month intervals during the first year of treatment and annually thereafter [13]. Another adverse event is abnormal liver function tests. According to the German Pegvisomant Observational Study, transaminase levels greater than 3 times normal were noted in 5.2% of patients. Although abnormal liver function tests are usually asymptomatic, transient and self-limited, liver function tests should be regularly monitored in patients receiving pegvisomant treatment [80]. Other uncommon side-effects are local allergic reactions and local lipohypertrophy [81].

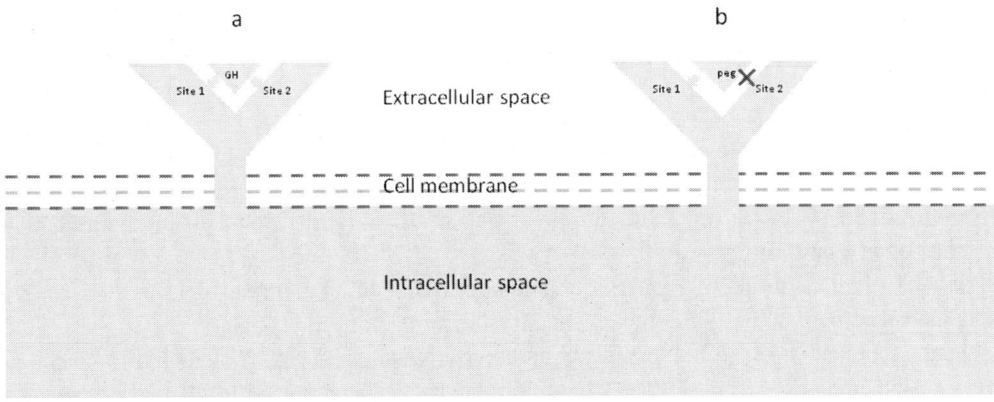

Figure 1. Binding of growth hormone receptor to its natural ligand (a) and pegvisomant (b).

- Dopamine agonists

Dopamine agonists were the only medical treatment available for acromegaly until 1980s. In contrast to the management of prolactinomas, higher doses of cabergoline (up to 7 mg weekly) may be needed for acromegaly control [82]. Cabergoline may be used in patients with modest elevations of IGF1 levels and mild symptoms of GH excess or as add-on therapy in patients not reaching biochemical control under somatostatin analogues and in cases of mixed-adenomas with GH and prolactin co-secretion. GH, prolactin and IGF1 levels should be repeated 4-6 weeks after cabergoline initiation or dose change [40]. Common side-effects of dopamine agonists are gastrointestinal upset, nasal congestion, headache, depression, orthostatic hypotension and faintness. Moreover, when administered in doses more than 3 mg daily, in patients with Parkinson disease, cabergoline has been associated with echocardiographically identified valvular abnormalities [83].

d. Radiation Therapy (RT)

Given the availability of effective medical treatment after unsuccessful 1`pituitary surgery, pituitary irradiation in acromegaly is nowadays considered as third-line treatment [40]. Both modes of radiation therapy, conventional fractionated radiation therapy and stereotactic radiosurgery are used for patients with acromegaly. Gamma knife radiosurgery is usually delivered by a cobalt-60 gamma radiation source [84, 85]. Serum GH levels decline by approximately 50% during the first 2 years after radiotherapy and 75% during 5 years [86, 87]. During the long latency period, medical therapy is required that periodically needs to be withheld for 1-3 months for the assessment of disease activity [88]. Conventional RT achieves tumor control in more than 90% and 85% of patients with acromegaly at 10 and 20 years, respectively, and a decrease in tumor volume is expected in about 50% of patients [89,

90]. Following radiation therapy, hypopituitarism gradually develops and approximately 50% of patients require replacement therapy [91].

e. Acromegaly Outcome Predictors

Overall, disease aggressiveness and outcome depend on clinical, radiological and histopathological features. As recently proposed by Cuevas-Ramos et al. [92] tumor size (micro- or macroadenomas), invasiveness (carvenous sinus invasion and internal carotid encasement revealed by MRI) and granulation type (dense or sparse) are reliable markers for patients' classification to three dinstinct acromegaly types.

Type 1 is characterized by the most favorable outcome and comprises densely granulated nonaggressive micro- and macroadenomas extending to sphenoid sinus more frequently than carvenous sinus extension (concave tumor image) and expressing abundant immunoreactive p21 and somatostatin receptor 2.

Type 2 predicts an intermediate biochemical outcome and comprises densely or sparsely granulated macroadenomas without significant extension (flat tumor image).

Type 3 is characterized by sparsely granulated invasive macroadenomas expressing low p21 and somatostatin receptor 2 and commonly compressing the optic chiasm (peanut or round shaped by MRI). Despite multimodality treatment, biochemical outcome is rather adverse.

4.2. ACTH-secreting Pituitary Adenomas

a. Surgical Treatment

Optimal treatment is selective adenomectomy, performed by an experienced neurosurgeon. In patients with microadenomas, remission rates of 65-90% have been demonstrated, with recurrence rates at 5 years (5-10%) and at 10 years (10-20%) [93], with young age (25 years or younger) being a significant risk factor for relapse [94]. Surgical cure rates in patients with macroadenomas are somewhat lower, with remission occurring in <65% of patients and relapse rates of 12-45% at 16 years.

Recurrence also occurs sooner than in those with a microadenoma (mean of 16 *vs.* 49 months) [95, 96]. Favorable prognostic factors associated with successful adenomectomy include detection of the microadenoma by magnetic resonance imaging (MRI), a well-defined tumor that is not invading either the basal dura or cavernous sinus, histological confirmation of an ACTH-secreting tumor, low postoperative serum cortisol levels, and long-lasting post-operative adrenal insufficiency [97, 98, 99]. If sellar exploration fails to localize a pituitary microadenoma, total or partial hypophysectomy may be indicated, with lower remission rates (approaching 70%) than selective adenomectomy and a higher rate of complications and hypopituitarism [100, 101]. Postsurgical recurrence of Cushing's disease (CD) may be higher than that associated with other types of pituitary tumors [93]. Adverse events relating to transsphenoidal surgery vary with various complications reported, including diabetes insipidus (either temporary or permanent), hypogonadism, hypothyroidism, cerebrospinal fluid (CSF) rhinorrhea, severe growth hormone deficiency, bleeding, and meningitis [96, 102].

b. Surgical Outcome Assessment

In ACTH-dependent Cushing's syndrome we aim at the restoration of hypercortisolism and reversal of clinical features with minimal morbidity. Tumor resection leads to corticosteroid deficiency because the remaining normal corticotroph cells have been suppressed by long-standing hypercortisolism. As a result, hypocortisolism provides an index of surgical success. However, patients with minimal preoperative hypercortisolism, because of medical treatment or mild disease, may be eucortisolemic and not require additional therapy. Thus, the decision to treat a patient with cortisol-lowering medications before surgery should be undertaken with the realization that the ability to assess cure may be compromised. Glucocorticoid withdrawal symptoms i.e., nausea, fatigue, joint pains should be anticipated in all patients after successful transphenoidal resection and treated with glucocorticoid replacement therapy until the axis recovers. Remission should be assessed by measuring morning serum cortisol during the first postoperative week by withholding treatment with glucocorticoids the previous evening. If glucocorticoid treatment is withheld, it is essential that the patient is monitored closely for signs of hypoadrenalism, preferably in-hospital [93]. Because glucocorticoids may suppress any remaining tumor tissue and mask persistent disease, their use should be avoided, or the dosage minimized, when cure is assessed. A morning serum cortisol level of less than 2 μg/dl (~50 nmol/liter) is associated with remission and a 10-year recurrence rate of approximately 10% [103, 104, 105]. A persistent serum cortisol level above 5μg/dl (~140 nmol/liter) for up to 6 weeks requires further evaluation. If persistent hypercortisolism is excluded, the recurrence rate is higher in these patients than in those with lower values. When serum cortisol levels are between 2 and 5 μg/dl, the patient can be considered in remission and can be observed without additional treatment for Cushing's disease, as the recurrence rate appears to be no greater than that seen in patients with serum cortisol levels less than 2μg/dl [105, 106, 107, 108]. Taking into account that cortisol levels may fall more gradually, it is important to ensure that the cortisol level has reached a nadir before considering further therapy. Measurement of urinary free cortisol (UFC) can provide additional useful information when the serum cortisol level is equivocal. UFC values below 20 μg/24 h (55 nmol/24 h) suggest remission, whereas values in the normal range (20-100 μg/24 h, 55-276 nmol/24 h) are equivocal. Values above the normal range indicate persistent tumor [93]. Again assessment of thyroid, gonadal axis, water balance and timing of imaging should be scheduled as already described in GH-secreting adenomas.

c. Management of Persistent Disease after Transsphenoidal Surgery

If transsphenoidal resection is not curative, second-line therapeutic options include repeat pituitary surgery, radiotherapy or bilateral adrenalectomy.

d. Repeat Surgery for Persistent or Recurrent Disease

Repeat pituitary surgery may be undertaken if disease persists after initial surgery, although there is an overall lower rate of success than that seen after the first operation [108, 109, 110]. The ideal time for repeat surgery is as soon as persistent, recurrent disease is evident. A delay of 4-6 weeks may be required to confirm the need for reoperating, because of continued partial improvement in cortisol levels after the initial surgery. Repeat surgery has shown to be curative in approximately 50% with higher success rates in case the tumor is radiologically evident [108, 109, 110]. In case repeat surgery is unsuccessful, the choice between bilateral adrenalectomy and pituitary radiotherapy needs to be individualized, according to pituitary status after pituitary surgery as well as the capacity of the patient to tolerate medical therapy while awaiting the effects of radiotherapy. Bilateral adrenalectomy may be indicated in patients with persistent hypercortisolism, despite treatment with adrenal enzyme inhibitors or with intolerance to these agents or as an alternative to long-term medical treatment after pituitary radiotherapy, and in women who wish to maintain fertility without the need for ovulation induction.

e. Bilateral Adrenalectomy

Bilateral adrenalectomy is a definitive treatment that provides immediate control of hypercortisolism, at the expense of permanent hypoadrenalism requiring lifelong supplementation with glucocorticoids and mineralocorticoids. The morbidity of this procedure can be minimized by the use of endoscopic approaches [111, 112, 113]. Patients require regular MRI scans and assessment of plasma ACTH levels, to ascertain whether there is corticotroph tumor progression because of the risk of developing Nelson's syndrome [114, 115].

f. Pituitary Radiotherapy

Depending on local availability, pituitary radiotherapy can be performed in different ways, either by conventional fractionated radiotherapy or by stereotactic radiosurgery (Gamma knife or proton beam therapy). Radiation therapy can eliminate tumors invading the dura or cavernous sinus, both of which are frequent causes of surgical failure, which repeat surgery cannot do. Control of hypercortisolemia is achieved in approximately 50% of patients at 2 years [116, 117, 118], although success increases further with time. There is no clear evidence that stereotactic radiosurgery accelerates the time to disease control. Long-term follow-up is necessary and while waiting for the radiotherapy outcome, patients are on medical treatment, usually with inhibitors of steroidogenesis, which should periodically be withheld to assess remission. The risk of second tumor formation after pituitary radiation is considered to be in the range of 1-2% [119], but this may not be due to the radiotherapy *per se*. The main complication is failure of some pituitary functions which is expected in up to 50% of patients. There is no clear evidence that targeted stereotactic radiosurgery minimizes this adverse effect. There is also a potential risk of cerebrovascular complications, although these are probably minimized with modern radiotherapy techniques [120, 121].

g. Medical Therapy

Medical therapy may be used to lower circulating cortisol levels prior to surgery and improve patient's preoperative state, and also as adjunctive therapy after pituitary irradiation and/or unsuccessful surgery [93]. Medical therapy for Cushing's disease can be targeted at different levels, pituitary-directed, adrenal-blocking and glucocorticoid antagonizing drugs and should be tailored in each individual patient (Figure 2) [122].

- Pituitary-directed therapy

Somatostatin analogues: As already mentioned, somatostatin exerts its actions via activation of somatostatin receptors, of which all but sst4 are expressed in pituitary adenomas.

Corticotroph-pituitary adenomas predominantly express sst5 and to a lesser extent sst2 [123, 124, 125]. The reason for that differential expression of somatostatin receptors is the suppressive effect of the high circulating cortisol levels on sst2 concentration, on the contrary sst5 expression is less sensitive [126]. Thus, the target in Cushing's disease is sst5, with a potential of sst2 up-regulation with further cortisol levels lowering. On that basis, the novel somatostatin receptor multi-ligand pasireotide (SOM230) has been tested as the most appropriate therapy in terms of inhibiting ACTH secretion by corticotroph adenomas. Recently, in a double-blinded multicenter phase 3 study of 162 patients with Cushing's disease, randomly assigned to receive subcutaneous pasireotide at a dose of 600 μg (82 patients) or 900 μg (80 patients) twice daily, it was shown that UFC normalization was achieved in 15 and 26% of patients respectively at 6 months [127]. An important observation of the study is that responders could be identified within 2 months of treatment. In an extension phase of the study, a further improvement in signs and symptoms was observed from the 12- to 24-month treatment period, accompanied by sustained reductions in UFC, plasma ACTH and serum cortisol [128]. Hyperglycemia was the major reported adverse event mediated through pasireotide inhibition of incretin secretion [129]. Pasireotide has been recently approved in Europe for the therapy of patients with Cushing's disease who are poor surgical candidates or after unsuccessful surgery.

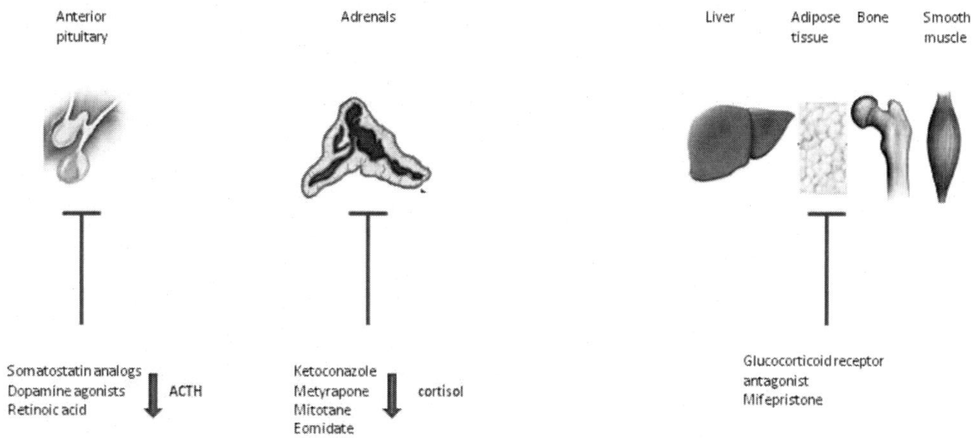

Figure 2. Medical therapy for Cushing's disease.

Dopamine agonists: Corticotroph adenomas predominantly express D2 as demonstrated by in situ hybridization studies, RTPCR, and immunohistochemistry [130, 131], while a recent study showed co-expression of D2 and sst5 in approximately 60% of corticotroph adenomas [123]. Few small prospective studies of cabergoline treatment demonstrated normalization of UFC or serum cortisol levels was achieved in only 25-35% within predefined time-frames of 3-6 months [132, 133], although in the long-term follow-up escape from therapeutic response has been recorded [133, 134, 135]. Moreover, with high doses of cabergoline, there is risk of fibrosis of cardiac valves due to the activation of serotonin receptor 2B on valvular fibroblasts [83, 136].

Other pituitary-directed treatment modalities: Recently, in a prospective, multicenter study, 7 patients with CD were treated with 10mg up to 80mg retinoic acid daily for 6-12 months. Normalization of UFC was observed in 3 patients, and only mild adverse effects were reported [137, 138, 139]. The serotonin antagonist cyproheptadine, as an inhibitor of hypothalamic corticotropin releasing hormone (CRH) and vasopressin secretion as well as the γ-aminobutyric acid uptake inhibitor sodium valproate and PPAR-γ agonists have been tested with very limited efficacy in Cushing's disease [140, 141, 142].

- Adrenal-blocking agents

Although originally developed as antifungal agent, ketoconazole is one of the most widely used adrenal-blocking agents. Inhibitory effect is exerted on multiple steroidogenic enzymes such as 11β-hydroxylase, 17-hydroxylase and 18-hydroxylase [143, 144]. Starting dose is 200-400 mg daily titrated up to 1200mg daily until biochemical remission is usually achieved within 3 months, and this is the time frame to evaluate efficacy of ketoconazole treatment. Under ketoconazole half of the patients achieve biochemical remission [145]. Major adverse events of this agent are hepatotoxicity, gastrointestinal complaints and hypogonadism in men. Given that proton pump inhibitors reduce the bioavailability of ketoconazole, ketoconazole should not be used in combination with these drugs [146].

Metyrapone: Cortisol has a fast-acting, strong cortisol lowering effect by inhibition of 11β-hydroxylase. Daily dose used varies between 500 and 6000mg [147] and biochemical control is achieved in 75% of patients [148]. Adverse events include acne, hirsutism, hypokalemia and hypertension due to the loss of feedback ACTH inhibition, resulting in overstimulation of adrenal androgen and mineralocorticoid precursor (e.g., desoxycorticosterone) production.

Mitotane: Mitotane is an adrenolytic drug that inhibits mitochondrial side chain cleavage enzyme (CYP11A1), 11β-hydroxylase (CYP11B1) and 18-hydroxylase (CYP11B2). This drug is primarily used as both cortisol-lowering and antitumoral for the treatment of patients with adrenocortical carcinoma [149]. Mitotane stimulates CYP3A4 expression and increases cortisol metabolism, thus corticosteroid replacement doses need to be increased to avoid adrenal crisis [150]. Nowadays mitotane is also used for Cushing's disease achieving remission rates up to 83%, [151] with lower doses than those used for adrenocortical carcinoma. However, its use is limited in Cushing's disease due to considerable gastrointestinal, neurological and hepatic side effects [152]. Finally, because of the stimulatory effect of mitotane on cortisol binding globulin levels [153], serum cortisol is not a reliable marker for the follow-up of patients treated with the drug [154].

Etomidate: The anesthetic drug etomidate inhibits 17-hydroxylase (CYP17) and 11 β-hydroxylase. This drug is fast-acting and can be used parenterally in doses between 0.03 and 0.3 mg/kg/h in patients with acute and/or life-threatening Cushing's syndrome (CS) [155].

Novel adrenal-blocking agents: LCI699 is a potent inhibitor of 11 β-hydroxylase and 18-hydroxylase [156, 157]. In a preliminary open-labeled study, 11 patients with mild to severe CD received oral LCI699 for 10 weeks. UFC normalization was achieved in 10 of 11 patients on day 70 at a median dose between 5 and 10 mg twice a day. Adverse events were gastrointestinal ones and drug-related hypokalemia [158].

- Glucocorticoid receptor antagonists

To date, the only glucocorticoid receptor antagonist available for clinical use is mifepristone, which is also widely known as contraceptive pill due to its antiprogestin activity. Mifepristone demonstrates 18-fold higher affinity for the glucocorticoid receptor than cortisol [159] and has proven to be highly effective in patients with Cushing's disease [158]. Mifepristone is approved in the US to control hyperglycemia in adults with endogenous CS, who have type 2 diabetes or glucose intolerance and who have remained unresponsive to previous surgery or are not eligible for surgery. However, several drawbacks make it an unfavorable medical treatment option, lack of biochemical monitoring data during treatment, meaning that over-treatment can result in adrenal insufficiency, risk of worsening hypokalemia and hypertension and in females endometrial hyperplasia. For these reasons, mifepristone is saved for severe complications of hypercortisolism, for those patients that are not candidates for surgery and those waiting for the maximum efficacy of radiotherapy [158].

h. Combination Medical Treatment

Medical treatment combination allows for lower doses and thus less adverse events. Moreover, biochemical remission may be rapidly achieved in order to reverse morbidity and mortality. Drug combination i.e., sst5 and D2-targeting drugs may also have potentiating effects on ACTH secretion by the corticotroph adenoma. Pasireotide (300 μg/d which could be increased to 750 μg/d) can be combined with cabergoline 1.5mg every other day, if urinary free cortisol is not normal after 1 month of pasireotide monotherapy. Ketoconazole 600 mg/d may be added to pasireotide and cabergoline, if after another month of combination treatment UFC is still elevated [160]. Another potential advantage is the up-regulation of sst2 expession as a result of the normalization of cortisol production. As a result pasireotide efficacy could be enhanced and sequential treatment with sst2 analogues could be attempted [161].

5. PROLACTINOMAS

Dopamine agonists are considered the treatment of choice for symptomatic prolactin-secreting micro or macroadenomas, since they normalize prolactin levels, reduce tumor size and restore gonadal function. Specifically, a systematic review commissioned by the Endocrine Society to evaluate the treatment effects of dopamine agonists in patients with hyperprolactinemia [162]. demonstrated in proportions (median, range) of patients with improved outcomes, reduction in tumor size (62%, 20-100%), resolution of visual field defects (67%, 33-100%), resolution of amenorrhea (78%, 40-100%), resolution of infertility (53%, 10-100%), improvement of sexual function (67%, 6-100%), resolution of galactorrhea (86%, 33-100%) and normalization of prolactin level (68%, 40-100%). Cabergoline is preferable compared to other dopamine agonists, since it has higher efficacy in normalizing prolactin levels, as well as a higher frequency of pituitary tumor shrinkage. A probable explanation is that cabergoline has a higher affinity for dopamine receptor binding sites. Results of a multicenter study indicate that bromocriptine decreases pituitary tumor size by approximately 50% in two thirds of patients, compared with a 90% decrease with cabergoline [163]. Moreover, compliance is better with cabergoline due to the lower incidence of unpleasant side effects i.e., orthostasis, nausea and headaches [164]. Overall, control of hyperprolactinemia requires doses of cabergoline ranging from 0.25 to 3 mg/wk, however, occasional patients may require doses up to 11 mg/wk [165, 166, 167]. Although treatment in case of macroprolactinomas is unequivocal, management of microprolactinomas varies. First of all, therapy of asymptomatic patients harboring microprolactinomas is not indicated [162]. For hypogonadal amenorrhoic premenopausal women who are not desirous of pregnancy, oral contraceptives is an acceptable alternative to dopamine agonists, less expensive and with fewer side effects [162, 168]. However, the effect of oral estrogen therapy on the growth of microadenomas has not been examined through randomized controlled trials.

5.1. Follow-up of Patients with Prolactinomas

In patients who begin dopamine agonist therapy, follow-up includes: 1) periodic prolactin measurement starting 1 month after therapy, to guide treatment intensification to achieve normal prolactin level and reversal of hypogonadism, 2) repeat MRI in 1 yr (or in 3 months in patients with macroprolactinoma, if prolactin levels continue to rise while patient is receiving dopaminergic agents, or if new symptoms, e.g., galactorrhea, visual disturbances, headaches, or other hormonal disorders, occur), 3) visual field examinations in patients with macroadenomas at risk of impinging the optic chiasm, and 4) assessment and management of comorbidities, e.g., sex steroid-dependent bone loss, persistent galactorrhea in the face of normalized prolactin levels, and pituitary trophic hormone reserve [162]. Provided that the patient is on careful clinical and biochemical follow-up, therapy may be tapered and perhaps discontinued in patients who have been treated with dopamine agonists for at least 2 years, who no longer have elevated serum prolactin, and who have no visible tumor remnant on MRI [167]. The risk of recurrence after withdrawal ranges from 26 to 69% [169, 170] and all studies have shown that recurrence is predicted by prolactin levels at diagnosis and by tumor size. Recurrences are most likely to occur in the year after withdrawal, and in one study the risk of recurrence was 18% per millimeter of tumor mass [170]. Withdrawal of therapy has been associated with no evidence of tumor growth, but up to 28% of such patients may develop hypogonadism [170]. Suggesting the need for long-term surveillance and treatment of these patients. For patients who after 2 years of therapy have achieved normal prolactin levels and no visible tumor remnant and for whom dopamine agonists have been tapered or discontinued, follow-up includes:

1. measurement of serum prolactin levels every 3 months for the first year and then annually thereafter, and
2. MRI, if prolactin increases above normal levels [171]. In women with microprolactinomas, it may be possible to discontinue dopaminergic therapy when menopause occurs. Surveillance for increasing size of the pituitary tumor should continue on a periodic basis

5.2. Management of Resistant or Malignant Prolactinoma

Dopamine agonist resistance is defined by a failure to achieve a normal prolactin level on maximally tolerated doses of dopamine agonist and a failure to achieve a 50% reduction in tumor size [172]. Furthermore, failure to restore fertility in patients receiving standard doses of dopamine agonist may also reflect resistance to treatment. Some patients may have discordant responses, i.e., reduction in tumor size without normalization of prolactin levels and vice versa, and others may be partially resistant and require higher than typical doses of dopamine agonists to achieve a response. Dopamine agonist resistance differs from intolerance, where side effects of the agonists preclude their use. The mechanism of dopamine agonist resistance is not completely understood. There is a decreased number of D2 receptors expressed on resistant prolactinomas [173, 174]. Dopamine receptor binding is normal, and no dopamine receptor mutation has been identified in prolactinomas. D2 receptor isoform ratios may differ, and molecular alterations may occur downstream of the D2 receptor. It is likely, therefore, that different mechanisms underly dopamine agonist resistance in prolactinomas. Microadenomas are less resistant to dopamine agonists than are macroadenomas. Ten percent of patients with microadenomas and 18% of patients with macroadenomas do not achieve normal prolactin levels on cabergoline [165, 166]. Increasing the cabergoline dose to as much as 11 mg/wk has been necessary in a few patients to overcome resistance. Although high doses of cabergoline may be necessary to overcome resistance, caution must be exhibited with protracted use of high-doses because of the potential risk of cardiac valvular disease. Dose increases should be stepwise and guided by prolactin levels. In patients who require very high doses for prolonged periods, echocardiography may be necessary to assess valvular abnormalities. Although the precise dose and duration cannot be identified at this time, patients receiving typical doses of cabergoline (1-2 mg/wk) likely will not require regular echocardiographic screening. Another approach to overcome resistance is the switch from cabergoline to bromocriptine, since approximately 10% of patients are resistant to the former. Finally clinicians should offer transsphenoidal surgery to symptomatic patients with prolactinomas who cannot tolerate high doses of cabergoline or who are not responsive to dopamine agonist therapy. For those patients who fail surgical treatment or who harbor aggressive or malignant prolactinomas there is a place for radiation therapy [162].

A prolactinoma is considered malignant when metastases within or outside the central nervous system are detected [175, 176]. Surgery may be necessary to diminish the compressive effects of the lesion. Several case reports suggest the effective use of temozolomide, an alkylating agent [177, 178]. Temozolomide has been shown to reduce prolactin levels and control tumor growth if tumor specimens do not express O^6-methylguanine-DNA methyltransferase (MGMT) [178, 179, 180].

5.3. Prolactinoma and Pregnancy

In women with prolactinomas, dopamine agonists should be discontinued once they become pregnant, except for those with aggressive macroadenomas not previously irradiated or surgically treated, having 31% risk of tumor growth during pregnancy [181]. Microadenomas rarely grow during pregnancy. In a review of studies that included 457 pregnant women harboring microadenomas, 2.6% developed symptomatic tumor growth [181]. Thus, the recommended approach is discontinuation of dopamine agonists and clinical examination of the patients during each trimester. Serum prolactin measurements are meaningless during pregnancy since estrogen stimulate lactotroph hyperplasia [182] and prolactin levels increase by 10-fold [183] MRI should not be routinely performed, unless there is clinical evidence for tumor growth such as visual field compromise. In that case, visual field assessment and pituitary MRI without the use of gadolinium is mandatory [162]. Extensive experience in over 6000 pregnancies with bromocriptine grants for its safe use [184]. Experience with cabergoline is far less. Subsequently, a growing prolactinoma during pregnancy should be treated with bromocriptine, if the patient cannot tolerate bromocriptine cabergoline may be administered. If dopamine agonist therapy does not decrease tumor size and lead to improved symptoms, surgical resection may be indicated. If the fetus is near term, it may be reasonable to induce delivery before neurosurgical intervention is undertaken.

6. Nonfunctioning Pituitary Adenomas

Nonfunctioning pituitary adenomas do not secrete biologically active pituitary hormones and represent 30% of all pituitary tumors [185]. Most clinically nonfunctioning pituitary adenomas are of gonadotroph origin as determined by immunocytochemical studies [186]. Because of the increased availability and use of magnetic resonance image (MRI), the vast majority of nonfunctioning pituitary adenomas are incidentally diagnosed, [187, 188] about two-thirds of these incidentalomas are microadenomas and the rest macroincidentalomas.

The first choice of therapy is transsphenoidal resection. Absolute indications for surgery include:

1. A visual field deficit due to the lesion or other visual abnormalities, such as ophalmoplegia or neurological compromise.
2. Optic nerve or chiasm compression on MRI.
3. Pituitary apoplexy with visual disturbance.
4. Hypersecreting tumors other than prolactinomas [189].

Relative indications are:

1. Loss of endocrinological function.
2. Clinically significant growth of the incidentaloma.
3. A lesion close to the chiasm in a woman planning to become pregnant.
4. Unremitting headache [189].

6.1. Surgery Outcome in Nonfunctiong Pituitary Adenomas

Tumor may recur even after 10 years post-operatively, making long-term radiological surveillance mandatory.[190] The major predictor of relapse rate is the size of the post-operative remnant, and it is higher for those with extra-sellar tumor remnant (approximately

50% relapse rate) compared with intrasellar tumor remnant (20%). Finally, the younger the patient at surgery, the higher the risk of relapse [190]. Consequently, it may be worth considering irradiation for those patients who have post-operatively a significant tumor remnant and in particular an extrasellar pituitary remnant as a mean of preventing tumor regrowth [191, 192]. Treatment with somatostatin analogues (SSA) and dopamine agonists (DA) induced some beneficial effects on visual field defects and was also followed by tumour shrinkage in a minority of cases. However, due to the lack of randomized, placebo-controlled trials their use is not evidence-based [193].

In patients not meeting criteria for surgery, a conservative follow-up approach is indicated including the following:

6.2. Imaging Studies

MRI scan should be repeated 6 months after the initial scan in case of macroadenoma or in one year in case of microadenoma. In patients whose incidentaloma does not change in size, we suggest repeating the MRI every year for macroincidentalomas and every 1-2 years in microincidentalomas for the following 3 years and gradually less frequently thereafter. In case imaging depicts that adenomas enlarges to abut or compress the optic nerves or chiasm, visual field testing is mandatory [189].

6.3. Endocrine Function Assessment

Clinical and biochemical evaluations for hypopituitarism should be performed 6 months after the initial testing and yearly thereafter, in patients with a pituitary macroincidentaloma, while those with microincidentalomas do not need test for hypopituitarism unless clinical picture or MRI findings change over time [189].

7. TSH-Secreting Pituitary Adenomas

Once diagnosis is made, transsphenoidal resection of the TSH-secreting pituitary adenoma should be persued as first-line treatment. In case surgery is contraindicated or fails, a trial of somatostatin analogues may be attempted, provided that hyperthyroidism is controlled by antithyroid drugs or radioiodine. The rationale for somatostatin analogues as tumor-targeted medical therapy is the abundant expression of sst1, sst2A, sst3 and sst5 mRNAs, predominantly sst2 [194]. Octreotide and lanreotide reduced TSH secretion and normalized FT4 and FT3 levels in 95% of patients harboring pituitary TSH secreting adenomas, while 40% of these patients experienced tumor shrinkage [195]. On the contrary, dopamine agonists have not proven to be effective for TSH-secreting adenomas, because of incomplete suppression or rebound elevation of TSH [196, 197].

8. FSH/LH-Secreting Pituitary Adenomas

These adenomas secrete low levels of FSH, LH or only the biologically inert alpha- or beta-subunits of these hormones. Thus, these tumors are clinically silent and patients commonly present with compressive symptoms such as impaired vision, headache or hypopituitarism. In that case, surgery is considered to be the first choice and in approximately 70% of all cases the patient experiences improvement in visual fields [198]. Recurrence rates range between 6% and 46% [199]. Radiation therapy is used more commonly after transsphenoidal surgery to prevent regrowth of residual gonadotroph adenoma [200]. Exceptionally, functional gonadotropin releasing pituitary adenomas have been described, with clinical manifestations in the form of ovarian hyperstimulation syndrome (OHSS) in premenopausal women and testicular enlargement in men [201]. Although surgery is the cornerstone of therapy, the efficacy of somatostatin analogues has been documented in few cases [201, 202, 203] with resolution of symptoms of hormone hypersecretion. Combined treatment with somatostatin analogues and dopamine agonists has been reported to induce tumor shrinkage as well [201]. Radiotherapy effect on gonadotropinoma mass and secretion, if any, occurs after several years [204].

References

[1] Mortini P, Losa M, Barzaghi R, Boari N, Giovanalli M. Results of transsphenoidal surgery in a large series of patients with pituitary adenoma. *Neurosurgery* 2005; 56:1222-1233.

[2] Jane JA Jr, Starke RM, Elzoghby MA, Reames DL, Payne SC, Thorner MO, et al. Endoscopic Transsphenoidal Surgery for Acromegaly: Remission Using Modern Criteria, Complications, and Predictors of Outcome. *J Clin Endocrinol Metab* 2011;96:1-9.

[3] Starke RM, Raper DM, Payne SC, VanceML, Oldfield EH, Jane JA Jr. Endoscopic vs microsurgical transsphenoidal surgery for acromegaly: outcomes in a concurrent series of patients using modern criteria for remission. *J Clin Endocrinol Metab* 2013; 98:3190-3198.

[4] Ciric I, Ragin A, Baumgartner C, Pierce D. Complications of transsphenoidal surgery: results of a national survey, review of the literature, and personal experience[with discussion]. *Neurosurgery* 1997;40:225-237.

[5] Ahmed S, Elsheikh M, Stratton IM, Page RC, Adams CB, Wass JA. Outcome of transsphenoidal surgery for acromegaly and its relationship to surgical experience. *Clin Endocrinol* (Oxf) 1999;50:561-567.

[6] Atkinson JL, Nippoldt TB. Pituitary neurologic surgery: a unique subspecialty in evolution. *Endocr Pract* 2002;8:356-361.

[7] Kelly DF, Laws ER Jr, Fossett D. Delayed hyponatremia after transsphenoidal surgery for pituitary adenoma: report of nine cases. *J Neurosurg* 1995;83:363-367.

[8] Olson BR, Gumowski J, Rubino D, Oldfield EH. Pathophysiology of hyponatremia after transsphenoidal pituitary surgery. *J Neurosurg* 1997;87:499-507.

[9] Nemergut EC, Zuo Z, Jane JA Jr, Laws ER Jr. Predictors of diabetes insipidus after transsphenoidal surgery: a review of 881 patients. *J Neurosurg* 2005;103:448-454.
[10] Kristof RA, Rother M, Neuloh G, Klingmüller D. Incidence, clinical manifestations, and course of water and electrolyte metabolism disturbances following transsphenoidal pituitary adenoma surgery: a prospective observational study. *J Neurosurg* 2009;111:555-562.
[11] Loh JA, Verbalis JG. Disorders of water and salt metabolism associated with pituitary disease. *Endocrinol Metab Clin North Am* 2008;37:213-234.
[12] Sata A, Hizuka N, Kawamata T, Hori T, Takano K. Hyponatremia after transsphenoidal surgery for hypothalamo-pituitary tumors. *Neuroendocrinology* 2006;83:117-122.
[13] Katznelson L, Atkinson JL, Cook DM, Ezzat SZ, Hamrahian AH, Miller K, et al. American Association of Clinical Endocrinologists medical guidelines for clinical practice for the diagnosis and treatment of acromegaly: a 2011 update. *Endocr Pract* 2011;17(Suppl 4):1-44.
[14] Missale C, Nash SR, Robinson SW, Jaber M, Caron MG. Dopamine receptors: from structure to function. *Physiol Rev* 1998;78:189-225.
[15] Pivonello R, Ferone D, Lombardi G, Colao A, Lamberts SW, Hofland LJ. Novel insights in dopamine receptor physiology. *Eur J Endocrinol* 2007;156(Suppl 1):S13–S21.
[16] Kunzig HJ, Geiger W, Schultz KD, Lose KH. Treatment of galactorrhea-amenorrhea syndrome with 2-Br-alpha-ergocryptin (CB154). Clinical response and pattern of pituitary and steroid hormones before and during therapy. *Arch Gynecol* 1975;218: 85-94.
[17] Vance ML, Evans WS, Thorner MO. Drugs five years later. *Bromocriptine Ann Intern* Med 1984;100:78-91.
[18] Kleinberg DL, Noel GL, Frantz AG. Galactorrhea: a study of 235 cases, including 48 with pituitary tumors. N Engl J Med 1977;296:589-600.
[19] Katz E, Weiss BE, Hassell A, Schran HF, Adashi EY. Increased circulating levels of bromocriptine after vaginal compared to oral administration. *Fertil Steril* 1991;55:882-884.
[20] Di Sarno A, Landi ML, Cappabianca P, Di Salle F, Rossi FW, Pivonello R, et al. Resistance to cabergoline as compered with bromocriptine in hyperprolactinemia: prevalence, clinical definition and therapeutic strategy. *J Clin Endocrinol Metab* 2001; 86:5256-5261.
[21] Motta T, deVincentiis S, Marchini M, Colombo N, D'Alberton A. Vaginal cabergoline in the treatment of hyperprolactinemic patients intolerant to oral dopaminergics. *Fertil Steril* 1996;65:440-442.
[22] Burt MG, Ho KK. Newer options in the management of acromegaly. *Intern Med J* 2006;36:437-444.
[23] Weckbecker G, Lewis I, Albert R, Schmid HA, Hoyer D, Bruns C. Opportunities in somatostatin research: biological, chemical and therapeutic aspects. *Nat Rev Drug Discov* 2003;2:999-1017.
[24] Hofland LJ, Lamberts SW. The pathophysiological consequences of somatostatin receptor internalization and resistance. *Endocr Rev* 2003;24:28-47.

[25] Unger N, Ueberberg B, Schulz S, Saeger W, Mann K, Petersenn S. Differential expression of somatostatin receptor subtype 1-5 proteins in numerous human normal tissues. *Exp Clin Endocrinol Diabetes* 2012;120:482-489.

[26] Patel YC. Somatostatin and its receptor family. *Front Neuroendocrinol* 1999;20:157-198.

[27] Susini C, Buscail L. rationale for the use of somatostatin analogs as antitumor agents. *Ann Oncol* 2006;17:1733-1742.

[28] Anthony L, Freda P. From somatostatin to octreotide LAR: evolution of a somatostatin analogue. *Curr Med Res Opin* 2009;25:2989-2999.

[29] Cozzi R, Attanasio R. Octreotide long-acting repeatable for acromegaly. *Expert Rev Clin Pharmacol* 2012;5:125-143.

[30] Grass P, Marbach P, Bruns C, Lancranjan I. Sandostatin LAR (microencapsulated octreotide acetate) in acromegaly: pharmacokinetic and pharmacodynamic relationships. *Metabolism* 1996;45(8 Suppl1):27-30.

[31] Astruc B, Marbach P, Bouterfa H, Denot C, Safari M, Vitaliti A, et al. Long-acting octreotide and prolonged-release lanreotide formulations have different pharmacokinetic profiles. *J Clin Pharmacol* 2005;45:836-844.

[32] Feelders RA, Hofland LJ, van Aken MO, Neggers SJ, Lamberts SW, de Herder WW, et al. Medical therapy of acromegaly: efficacy and safety of somatostatin analogues. *Drugs* 2009;69:2207-2226.

[33] Bruns C, Lewis I, Briner U, Meno-Tetang G, Weckbecker G. SOM230: a novel somatostatin peptidomimetic with broad somatotropin release inhibiting factor (SRIF) receptor binding and a unique antisecretory profile. *Eur J Endocrinol* 2002;146:707-716.

[34] Golor G, Hu K, Ruffin M, Buchelt A, Bouillaud E, Wang Y, et al. A first-in-man study to evaluate the safety, tolerability, and pharmacokinetics of pasireotide (SOM230), a multireceptor-targeted somatostatin analog, in healthy volunteers. *Drug Des Dev Ther* 2012;6:71-79.

[35] Minniti G, Gilbert DC, Brada M. Modern techniques for pituitary radiotherapy. *Rev Endocr Metab Disord* 2009;10:135-144.

[36] Petit JH, Biller BM, Coen JJ, Swearingen B, Ancukiewicz M, Bussiere M, et al. Proton stereotactic radiosurgery in management of persistent acromegaly. *Endocr Pract* 2007;13:726-734.

[37] Karavitaki N, Turner HE, Adams CB, Cudlip S, Byrne JV, Fazal-Sanderson V, et al. Surgical debulking of pituitary macroadenomas causing acromegaly improves control by lanreotide. *Clin Endocrinol* (Oxf) 2008;68:970-975.

[38] Colao A, Attanasio R, Pivonello R, Cappabianca P, Cavallo LM, Lasio G, et al. Partial surgical removal of growth hormone-secreting pituitary tumors enhances the response to somatostatin analogs in acromegaly. *J Clin Endocrinol Metab* 2006;91:85-92.

[39] Jallad RS, Musolino NR, Salgado LR, Bronstein MD. Treatment of acromegaly: is there still a place for radiotherapy? Pituitary 2007;10:53-59.

[40] Katznelson L, Raws ER Jr, Melmed S, Molitch ME, Murad MH, Utz A, et al. Acromegaly: An endocrine society clinical practice guideline. *J Clin Endocrinol Metab* 2014;99:3933-3951.

[41] Nimsky C, von Keller B, Ganslandt O, Fahlbusch R. Intraoperative high-field magnetic resonance imaging in transsphenoidal surgery of hormonally inactive pituitary macroadenomas.[with discussion] *Neurosurgery* 2006;59:105-114.

[42] Thomale UW, Stover JF, Unterberg AW. The use of neuronavigation in transnasal transsphenoidal pituitary surgery.[with discussion] *Zentralbl Neurochir* 2005;66:126-132.

[43] Valdemarsson S, Ljunggren S, Cervin A, Svensson C, Isaksson A, Nordström CH, et al. Evaluation of surgery for acromegaly: role of intraoperative growth hormone measurement? *Scand J Clin Lab Invest* 2001;61:459-470.

[44] Knosp E, Steiner E, Kitz K, Matula C. Pituitary adenomas with invasion of the carvenous sinus space: a magnetic resonance imaging classification compared with surgical findings. *Neurosurgery* 1993;33:610-617.

[45] Seidman PA, Kofke WA, Policare R, Young M. Anaesthetic complications of acromegaly. *Br J Anaesth* 2000;84:179-182.

[46] Khan ZH, Rasouli MR. Intubation in patients with acromegaly: experience in more than 800 patients. *Eur J Anaesthesiol* 2009;26:354-355.

[47] Barker FG II, Klibanski A, Swearingen B. Transsphenoidal surgery for pituitary tumors in the United States, 1996-2000: mortality, morbidity, and the effects of hospital and surgeon volume. *J Clin Endocrinol Metab* 2003;88:4709-4719.

[48] Krieger MD, Couldwell WT, Weiss MH. Assessment of long-term remission of acromegaly following surgery. *J Neurosurg* 2003;98:719-724.

[49] Freda PU, Post KD, Powell JS, Wardlaw SL. Evaluation of disease status with sensitive measures of growth hormone secretion in 60 postoperative patients with acromegaly. *J Clin Endocrinol Metab* 1998;83:3808-3816.

[50] Giustina A, Chanson P, Bronstein MD, Klibanski A, Lamberts S, Casanueva FF, et al, Acromegaly Consensus Group. A consensus on criteria for cure of acromegaly. *J Clin Endocrinol Metab* 2010;95:3141-3148.

[51] Katznelson L. Approach to the patient with persistent acromegaly after pituitary surgery. *J Clin Endocrinol Metab* 2010;95:4114-4123.

[52] Dina TS, Feaster SH, Laws ER Jr, Davis DO. MR of the pituitary gland postsurgery: serial MR studies following transsphenoidal resection. *Am J Neuroradiol* 1993;14:763-769.

[53] Carmichael JD, Bonert VS, Mirocha JM, Melmed S. The utility of oral glucose tolerance testing for diagnosis and assessment of treatment outcomes in 166 patients with acromegaly. *J Clin Endocrinol Metab* 2009;94:523-527.

[54] Freda PU, Katznelson L, van der Lely AJ, Reyes CM, Zhao S, Rabinowitz D. Long-acting somatostatin analog therapy of acromegaly: a meta-analysis. *J Clin Endocrinol Metab* 2005;90:4465-4473.

[55] Bevan JS. Clinical review: the antitumoral effects of somatostatin analog therapy in acromegaly. *J Clin Endocrinol Metab* 2005;90:1856-1863.

[56] Resmini E, Dadati P, Ravetti JL, Zona G, Spaziante R, Saveanu A, et al. Rapid pituitary tumor shrinkage with dissociation between antiproliferative and antisecretory effects of a long-acting octreotide in an acromegalic patient. *J Clin Endocrinol Metab* 2007;92:1592-1599.

[57] Giustina A, Mazziotti G, Torri V, et al. Meta-analysis on the effects of octreotide on tumor mass in acromegaly. *PLoS One* 2012;7:e36411.

[58] Caron PJ, Bevan JS, Petersenn S, Flanagan D, Tabarin A, Prevost G, et al. Tumor shrinkage with lanreotide Autogel 120 mg as Primary therapy in acromegaly: results of a prospective multicenter clinical trial. *J Clin Endocrinol Metab* 2014;99:1282-1290.

[59] Losa M, Mortini P, Urbaz L, Ribotto P, Castrignano T, Giovanelli M. Presurgical treatment with somatostatin analogs in patients with acromegaly: effects on the remission and complication rates. *J Neurosurg* 2006;104:899-906.

[60] Mao ZG, Zhu YH, Tang HL, Wang DY, Zhou J, He DS, et al. Preoperative lanreotide treatment in acromegalic patients with macroadenomas increases short-term postoperative cure rates: a prospective, randomised trial. *Eur J Endocrinol* 2010;162:661-666.

[61] Jacob JJ, Bevan JS. Should all patients with acromegaly receive somatostatin analogue therapy before surgery and, if so, for how long? *Clin Endocrinol* (Oxf) 2014;81:812-817.

[62] Bhayana S, Booth GL, Asa SL, Kovacs K, Ezzat S. The implication of somatotroph adenoma phenotype to somatostatin analog responsiveness in acromegaly. *J Clin Endocrinol Metab* 2005;90:6290-6295.

[63] Howlett TA, Willis D, Walker G, Wass JA, Trainer PJ. Control of growth hormone and IGF1 in patients with acromegaly in the UK: responses to medical treatment with somatostatin analogues and dopamine agonists. *Clin Endocrinol* (Oxf) 2013;79:689-699.

[64] Kiseljak-Vassiliades K, Shafi S, Kerr JM, Phang TL, Kleinschmidt- DeMasters BK, Wierman ME. Clinical implications of growth hormone-secreting tumor subtypes. *Endocrine* 2012;42:18-28.

[65] Gadelha MR, Kasuki L, Korbonits M. Novel pathway for somatostatin analogs in patients with acromegaly. *Trends in Endocrinology and Metabolism* 2013;24:238-246.

[66] Pokrajac A, Claridge AG, Shakoor SK, Trainer PJ. The octreotide test dose is not a reliable predictor of the subsequent response to somatostatin analogue therapy in patients with acromegaly. *Eur J Endocrinol* 2006;154:267-274.

[67] Ghigo E, Biller BM, Colao A, Kourides IA, Rajicic N, Hutson RK, et al. Comparison of pegvisomant and long-acting octreotide in patients with acromegaly naïve to radiation and medical therapy. *J Endocrinol Invest* 2009; 32:924-933.

[68] Colao A, Auriemma RS, Savastano S, Galdiero M, Grasso LF, Lombardi G, et al. Glucose tolerance and somatostatin analog treatment in acromegaly: a 12-month study. *J Clin Endocrinol Metab* 2009;94:2907-2914.

[69] Zhao S, Rabinowitz D. Long-acting somatostatin analog therapy of acromegaly: a meta-analysis. *J Clin Endocrinol Metab* 2005;90:4465-4473.

[70] Jorgensen JO, Feldt-Rasmussen U, Frystyk J, Chen JW, Kristensen LO, Hagen C, et al. Cotreatment of acromegaly with a somatostatin analog and a growth hormone receptor antagonist. *J Clin Endocrinol Metab* 2005;90:5627-5631.

[71] Petersenn S, Schopohl J, Barkan A, Mohideen P, Colao A, Abs R, et al. Pasireotide (SOM230) demonstrates efficacy and safety in patients with acromegaly: a randomized, multicenter, phase II trial. *J Clin Endocrinol Metab* 2010;95:2781-2789.

[72] Colao A, Bronstein MD, Freda P, Gu F, Shen CC, Gadelha M, et al. Pasireotide versus octreotide in acromegaly: a head-to-head superiority study. *J Clin Endocrinol Metab* 2014;99:791-799.

[73] Henry RR, Ciaraldi TP, Armstrong D, Burke P, Ligueros-Saylan M, Mudaliar S. Hyperglycemia associated with pasireotide: results from a mechanistic study in healthy volunteers. *J Clin Endocrinol Metab* 2013;98:3446-3453.
[74] Colao A, De Block C, Gaztambide MS, Kumar S, Seufert J, Casanueva FF. Managing hyperglycemia in patients with Cushing's disease treated with pasireotide: medical expert recommendations. *Pituitary* 2014;17:180-186.
[75] Trainer PJ, Drake WM, Katznelson L, Freda PU, Herman-Bonert V, van der Lely AJ, et al. Treatment of acromegaly with the growth hormone-receptor antagonist pegvisomant. *N Engl J Med* 2000;342:1171-1177.
[76] van der Lely AJ, Hutson RK, Trainer PJ, Besser GM, Barkan AL, Katznelson L, et al. Long-term treatment of acromegaly with pegvisomant, a growth hormone receptor antagonist. *Lancet* 2001;358:1754-1759.
[77] Higham CE, Chung TT, Lawrance J, Drake WM, Trainer PJ. Long-term experience of pegvisomant therapy as a treatment for acromegaly. *Clin Endocrinol* (Oxf) 2009;71:86-91.
[78] Neggers SJ, van der Lely AJ. Combination treatment with somatostatin analogues and pegvisomant in acromegaly. *Growth Horm IGF Res* 2011;21:129-133.
[79] Frohman LA, Bonert V. Pituitary tumor enlargement in two patients with acromegaly during pegvisomant therapy. *Pituitary* 2007;10:283-289.
[80] Schreiber I, Buchfelder M, Droste M, Forssmann K, Mann K, Saller B, et al, German Pegvisomant Investigators. Treatment of acromegaly with the GH receptor antagonist pegvisomant in clinical practice: safety and efficacy evaluation from the German Pegvisomant Observational Study. *Eur J Endocrinol* 2007;156:75-82.
[81] Bonert VS, Kennedy L, Petersenn S, Barkan A, Carmichael J, Melmed S. Lipodystrophy in patients with acromegaly receiving pegvisomant. *J Clin Endocrinol Metab* 2008;93:3515-3518.
[82] Moyes VJ, Metcalfe KA, Drake WM. Clinical use of cabergoline as primary and adjunctive treatment for acromegaly. *Eur J Endocrinol* 2008;159:541-545.
[83] Schade R, Andelsohn F, Suissa S, Hawerkamp W, Garbe E. Dopamine agonists and the risk of cardiac-valve regurgitation. *N Engl J Med* 2007;356:29-38.
[84] Milker-Zabel S, Debus J, Thilmann C, Schlegel W, Wannenmacher M. Fractionated stereotactically guided radiotherapy and radiosurgery in the treatment of functional and nonfunctional adenomas of the pituitary gland. *Int J Radiat Oncol Biol Phys* 2001;50:1279-1286.
[85] Minniti G, Traish D, Ashley S, Gonsalves A, Brada M. Fractionated stereotactic conformal radiotherapy for secreting and nonsecreting pituitary adenomas. *Clin Endocrinol* (Oxf) 2006;64:542-548.
[86] Wass JA. Radiotherapy in acromegaly: a protagonist's view point. *Clin Endocrinol* (Oxf) 2003;58:128-131.
[87] Biermasz NR, Van Dulken H, Roelfsema F. Postoperative radiotherapy in acromegaly is effective in reducing GH concentration to safe levels. *Clin Endocrinol* (Oxf) 2000;53:321-327.
[88] Minniti G, Jaffrain-Rea ML, Osti M, Esposito V, Santoro A, Solda F, et al. The long-term efficacy of conventional radiotherapy in patients with GH-secreting pituitary adenomas. *Clin Endocrinol* (Oxf) 2005;62:210-216.

[89] Brada M, Rajan B, Traish D, Ashley S, Holmes-Sellors PJ, Nussey S, et al. The long-term efficacy of conservative surgery and radiotherapy in the control of pituitary adenomas. *Clin Endocrinol* (Oxf) 1993;38:571-578.

[90] Langsenlehner T, Stiegler C, Quehenberger F, Feigl GC, Jakse G, Mokry M, et al. Long-term follow-up of patients with pituitary macroadenomas after postoperative radiation therapy: analysis of tumor control and functional outcome. *Strahlenther Onkol* 2007;,183:241-247.

[91] Hannon MJ, Barkan A, Drake WM. The role of radiotherapy in acromegaly. Neuroendocrinology 2015, June 17[Epub ahead of print].

[92] Cuevas-Ramos D, Carmichael JD, Cooper O, Bonert VS, Gertych A, Mamelak AN, et al. A structural and functional acromegaly classification. *J Clin Endocrinol Metab* 2015;100:122-131.

[93] Biller BM, Grossman AB, Stewart PM, Melmed S, Bertagna X, Bertherat J, et al. Treatment of adrenocorticotropin-dependent Cushing's syndrome: a consensus statement. *J Clin Endocrinol Metab* 2008;93:2454-2462.

[94] Sonino N, Zielezny M, Fava GA, Fallo F, Boscaro M. Risk factors and long-term outcome in pituitary-dependent Cushing's disease. *J Clin Endocrinol Metab* 1996,81:2647-2652.

[95] De Tommasi C, Vance ML, Okonkwo DO, Diallo A, Laws ER Jr. Surgical management of adrenocorticotropic hormone-secreting macroadenomas: outcome and challenges in patients with Cushing's disease or Nelson's syndrome. *J Neurosurg* 2005;103:825-830.

[96] Blevins LS Jr, Christy JH, Khajavi M, Tindall GT. Outcomes of therapy for Cushing's disease due to adrenocorticotropin-secreting pituitary macroadenomas. *J Clin Endocrinol Metab* 1998;83:63-67.

[97] Trainer PJ, Lawrie HS, Verhelst J, Howlett TA, Lowe DG, Grossman AB, et al. Transsphenoidal resection in Cushing's disease: undetectable serum cortisol as the definition of successful treatment. *Clin Endocrinol* (Oxf) 1993;38:73-78.

[98] Pouratian N, Prevedello DM, Jagannathan J, Lopes MB, Vance ML, Laws ER Jr. Outcomes and management of patients with Cushing's disease without pathological confirmation of tumor resection after transsphenoidal surgery. *J Clin Endocrinol Metab* 2007;92:3383-3288.

[99] Hammer GD, Tyrrell JB, Lamborn KR, Applebury CB, Hannegan ET, Bell S, et al. Transsphenoidal microsurgery for Cushing's disease: initial outcome and long-term results. *J Clin Endocrinol Metab* 2004;89:6348-6357.

[100] Mampalam TJ, Tyrrell JB, Wilson CB. Transsphenoidal microsurgery for Cushing disease. A report of 216 cases. *Ann Intern Med* 1988;109:487-493.

[101] Robert F, Hardy J. Cushing's disease: a correlation of radiological, surgical and pathological findings with therapeutic results. *Pathol Res* Pract 1991;187:617-621.

[102] Bochicchio D, Losa M, Buchfelder M. Factors influencing the immediate and late outcome of Cushing's disease treated by transsphenoidal surgery: a retrospective study by the European Cushing's Disease Survey Group. *J Clin Endocrinol Metab* 1995;80:3114-3120.

[103] Esposito F, Dusick JR, Cohan P, Moftakhar P, McArthur D, Wang C, et al. Clinical review: early morning cortisol levels as a predictor of remission after transsphenoidal surgery for Cushing's disease. *J Clin Endocrinol Metab* 2006;91:7-13.

[104] Pereira AM, van Aken MO, van Dulken H, Schutte PJ, Biermasz NR, Smit JW, et al. Long-term predictive value of postsurgical cortisol concentrations for cure and risk of recurrence in Cushing's disease. *J Clin Endocrinol Metab* 2003;88:5858-5864.

[105] Yap LB, Turner HE, Adams CB, Wass JA. Undetectable postoperative cortisol does not always predict long-term remission in Cushing's disease: a single centre audit. *Clin Endocrinol* (Oxf) 2002;56:25-31.

[106] Atkinson AB, Kennedy A, Wiggam MI, McCance DR, Sheridan B. Long-term remission rates after pituitary surgery for Cushing's disease: the need for long-term surveillance. *Clin Endocrinol* (Oxf) 2005;63:549-559.

[107] Rees DA, Hanna FW, Davies JS, Mills RG, Vafidis J, Scanlon MF. Long-term follow-up results of transsphenoidal surgery for Cushing's disease in a single centre using strict criteria for remission. *Clin Endocrinol* (Oxf) 2002;56:541-551.

[108] Benveniste RJ, King WA, Walsh J, Lee JS, Delman BN, Post KD. Repeated transsphenoidal surgery to treat recurrent or residual pituitary adenoma. *J Neurosurg* 2005;102:1004–1012.

[109] Friedman RB, Oldfield EH, Nieman LK, Chrousos GP, Doppman JL, Cutler GB Jr, et al. Repeat transsphenoidal surgery for Cushing's disease. *J Neurosurg* 1989;71:520-527.

[110] Hofmann BM, Hlavac M, Kreutzer J, Grabenbauer G, Fahlbusch R. Surgical treatment of recurrent Cushing's disease. *Neurosurgery* 2006;58:1108-1118.

[111] Gumbs AA, Gagner M. Laparoscopic adrenalectomy. *Best Pract Res Clin Endocrinol Metab* 2006;0:483-499.

[112] Chow JT, Thompson GB, Grant CS, Farley DR, Richards ML, Young WF Jr. Bilateral laparoscopic adrenalectomy for corticotrophin-dependent Cushing's syndrome: a review of the Mayo Clinic experience. *Clin Endocrinol* (Oxf) 2008;68:513-519.

[113] Thompson SK, Hayman AV, Ludlam WH, Deveney CW, Loriaux DL, Sheppard BC. Improved quality of life after bilateral laparoscopic adrenalectomy for Cushing's disease: a 10-year experience. *Ann Surg* 2007;245:790-794.

[114] Assie G, Bahurel H, Bertherat J, Kujas M, Legmann P, Bertagna X. The Nelson's syndrome revisited. *Pituitary* 2004;7:209-215.

[115] Assie G, Bahurel H, Coste J, Silvera S, Kujas M, Dugue MA, et al. Corticotroph tumor progression after adrenalectomy in Cushing's disease: a reappraisal of Nelson's syndrome. *J Clin Endocrinol Metab* 2007;92:172-179.

[116] Castinetti F, Nagai M, Morange I, Dufour H, Caron P, Chanson P, et al. Long-term results of stereotactic radiosurgery in secretory pituitary adenomas. *J Clin Endocrinol Metab* 2009;94:3400-3407.

[117] Estrada J, Boronat M, Mielgo M, Magallon R, Millan I, Diez S, et al. The long-term outcome of pituitary irradiation after unsuccessful transsphenoidal surgery in Cushing's disease. *N Engl J Med* 1997;336:172-177.

[118] Starke RM, Williams BJ, Vance ML, Sheehan JP. Radiation therapy and stereotactic radiosurgery for the treatment of Cushing's disease: an evidence-based review. *Curr Opin Endocrinol Diabetes Obes* 2010;17:356-364.

[119] Brada M, Ford D, Ashley S, Bliss JM, Crowley S, Mason M, et al. Risk of second brain tumour after conservative surgery and radiotherapy for pituitary adenoma. *BMJ* 1992;304:1343-1346.

[120] Fernandez A, Brada M, Zabuliene L, Karavitaki N, Wass JA. Radiation-induced hypopituitarism. *Endocr Relat Cancer* 2009;16:733-772.

[121] Minniti G, Traish D, Ashley S, Gonsalves A, Brada M. Risk of second brain tumor after conservative surgery and radiotherapy for pituitary adenoma: update after an additional 10 years. *J Clin Endocrinol Metab* 2005;90:800-804.

[122] Feelders RA, Hofland LJ. Medical treatment for Cushing's disease. *J Clin Endocrinol Metab* 2013;98:425-438.

[123] de Bruin C, Pereira AM, Feelders RA, Romijn JA, Roelfsema F, Sprij-Mooij DM, et al. Coexpression of dopamine and somatostatin receptor subtypes in corticotroph adenomas. *J Clin Endocrinol Metab* 2009;94:1118-1124.

[124] Tateno T, Kato M, Tani Y, Oyama K, Yamada S, Hirata Y. Differential expression of somatostatin and dopamine receptor subtype genes in adrenocorticotropin (ACTH)-secreting pituitary tumors and silent corticotroph adenomas. *Endocr J* 2009;56:579-584.

[125] Saveanu A, Jaquet P. Somatostatin-dopamine ligands in the treatment of pituitary adenomas. *Rev Endocr Metab Disord* 2009;10:83-90.

[126] de Bruin C, Feelders RA, Waaijers AM, van Koetsveld PM, Sprij-Mooij DM, Lamberts SW, et al. Differential regulation of human dopamine D2 and somatostatin receptor subtype expression by glucocorticoids in vitro. *J Mol Endocrinol* 2009;42:47-56.

[127] Colao A, Petersenn S, Newell-Price J, Findling JW, Gu F, Maldonado M, et al, Pasireotide B2305 Study Group. A 12-month phase 3 study of pasireotide in Cushing's disease. *N Engl J Med* 2012;366:914-924.

[128] Pivonello R, Petersenn S, Newell-Price J, Findling JW, Gu F, Maldonado M, et al. Pasireotide treatment significantly improves clinical signs and symptoms in patients with Cushing's disease: results from a phase III study. *Clin Endocrinol*(Oxf) 2014;81:408-17.

[129] Breitschaft A, Hu K, Hermosillo Reséndiz K, Darstein C, Golor G. Management of hyperglycemia associated with pasireotide (SOM230): healthy volunteer study. *Diabetes Res Clin Pract* 2014;103:458-65.

[130] Pivonello R, Ferone D, de Herder WW, Kros JM, De Caro ML, Arvigo M, et al. Dopamine receptor expression and function in corticotroph pituitary tumors. *J Clin Endocrinol Metab* 2004;89:2452-2462.

[131] Stefaneanu L, Kovacs K, Horvath E, Buchfelder M, Fahlbusch R, Lancranjan L. Dopamine D2 receptor gene expression in human adenohypophysial adenomas. *Endocrine* 2001;14:329-336.

[132] Vilar L, Naves LA, Azevedo MF, Arruda MJ, Arahata CM, Moura E, et al. (2010) Effectiveness of cabergoline in monotherapy and combined with ketoconazole in the management of Cushing's disease. *Pituitary* 2010;13:123-129.

[133] Lila AR, Gopal RA, Acharya SV, George J, Sarathi V, Bandgar T, et al. Efficacy of cabergoline in uncured (persistent or recurrent) Cushing disease after pituitary surgical treatment with or without radiotherapy. *Endocr Pract* 2010;16:968-976.

[134] Godbout A, Manavela M, Danilowicz K, Beauregard H, Bruno OD, Lacroix A.(2010) Cabergoline monotherapy in the long-term treatment of Cushing's disease. *Eur J Endocrinol* 2010;163:709-716.

[135] Pivonello R, De Martino MC, Cappabianca P, De Leo M, Faggiano A, Lombardi G, et al. The medical treatment of Cushing's disease: effectiveness of chronic treatment with

the dopamine agonist cabergoline in patients unsuccessfully treated by surgery. *J Clin Endocrinol Metab* 2009;94:223-230.

[136] Zanettini R, Antonini A, Gatto G, Gentile R, Tesei S, Pezzoli G. Valvular heart disease and the use of dopamine agonists for Parkinson's disease. *N Engl J Med* 2007,356:39-46.

[137] Pecori Giraldi F, Ambrogio AG, Andrioli M, Sanguin F, Karamouzis I, Corsello SM et al. Potential role for retinoic acid in patients with Cushing's disease. *J Clin Endocrinol* 2012;97:3577-3583.

[138] Heaney AP, Fernando M, Yong WH, Melmed S. Functional PPAR-gamma receptor is a novel therapeutic target for ACTH-secreting pituitary adenomas. *Nat Med* 2002; 8:1281-1287.

[139] Heaney AP, Fernando M, Melmed S. PPAR-gamma receptor ligands: novel therapy for pituitary adenomas. *J Clin Invest* 2003;111:1381-1388.

[140] Ambrosi B, Dall'Asta C, Cannavo S, Libe R, Vigo T, Epaminonda P, et al. Effects of chronic administration of PPAR-gamma ligand rosiglitazone in Cushing's disease. *Eur J Endocrinol* 2004;151:173-178.

[141] Suri D, Weiss RE. Effect of pioglitazone on adrenocorticotropic hormone and cortisol secretion in Cushing's disease. *J Clin Endocrinol Metab* 2005;90:1340-1346.

[142] Pecori Giraldi F, Scaroni C, Arvat E, Martin M, Giordano R, Albiger N, et al. Effect of protracted treatment with rosiglitazone, a PPAR-gamma agonist, in patients with Cushing's disease. *Clin Endocrinol* (Oxf) 2006;64:219-224.

[143] Engelhardt D, Weber MM, Miksch T, Abedinpour F, Jaspers C. The influence of ketoconazole on human adrenal steroidogenesis: incubation studies with tissue slices. *Clin Endocrinol* (Oxf) 1991;35:163-168.

[144] Sonino N. The use of ketoconazole as an inhibitor of steroid production. *N Engl J Med* 1987;317:812-818.

[145] Castinetti F, Morange I, Jaquet P, Conte-Devolx B, Brue T. Ketoconazole revisited: a preoperative or postoperative treatment in Cushing's disease. *Eur J Endocrinol* 2008;158:91-99.

[146] Ogawa R, Echizen H. Drug-drug interaction profiles of proton pump inhibitors. *Clin Pharmacokinet* 2010;49:509-533.

[147] Feelders RA, Hofland LJ, de Herder WW. Medical treatment of Cushing's syndrome: adrenal-blocking drugs and ketaconazole. *Neuroendocrinology* 2010;92(Suppl 1):111-115.

[148] Verhelst JA, Trainer PJ, Howlett TA, Perry L, Rees LH, Grossman AB, et al. Short and long-term responses to metyrapone in the medical management of 91 patients with Cushing's syndrome. *Clin Endocrinol* (Oxf) 1991;35:169-178.

[149] Hahner S, Fassnacht M. Mitotane for adrenocortical carcinoma treatment. *Curr Opin Investig Drugs* 2005;6:386-394.

[150] Kroiss M, Quinkler M, Lutz WK, Allolio B, Fassnacht M. Drug interactions with mitotane by induction of CYP3A4 metabolism in the clinical management of adrenocortical carcinoma. *Clin Endocrinol* (Oxf) 2011;75:585-591.

[151] Baudry C, Coste J, Bou Khalil R, Silvera S, Guignat L, Guibourdenche J, et al. Efficiency and tolerance of mitotane in Cushing's disease in 76 patients from a single center. *Eur J Endocrinol* 2012;167:473-481.

[152] Miller JW, Crapo L. The medical treatment of Cushing's syndrome. *Endocr Rev* 1993;14:443-458.

[153] Nader N, Raverot G, Emptoz-Bonneton A, Dechaud H, Bonnay M, Baudin E, et al. Mitotane has an estrogenic effect on sex hormone-binding globulin and corticosteroid-binding globulin in humans. *J Clin Endocrinol Metab* 2006;91:2165-2170.

[154] Alexandraki KI, Kaltsas GA, le Roux CW, Fassnacht M, Ajodha S, Christ-Crain M, et al. Assessment of serum-free cortisol levels in patients with adrenocortical carcinoma treated with mitotane: a pilot study. *Clin Endocrinol* (Oxf) 2010;72:305-311.

[155] Preda VA, Sen J, Karavitaki N, Grossman AB. Etomidate in the management of hypercortisolaemia in Cushing's syndrome: a review. *Eur J Endocrinol* 2012;167:137-143.

[156] Calhoun DA, White WB, Krum H, Guo W, Bermann G, Trapani A, et al. Effects of a novel aldosterone synthase inhibitor for treatment of primary hypertension: results of a randomized, double-blind, placebo- and active-controlled phase 2 trial. *Circulation* 2011;124:1945-1955.

[157] Amar L, Azizi M, Menard J, Peyrard S, Watson C, Plouin PF. Aldosterone synthase inhibition with LCI699: a proof-of-concept study in patients with primary aldosteronism. *Hypertension* 2010;56:831-838.

[158] Castinetti F, Brue T, Conte-Devolx B. The use of the glucocorticoid receptor antagonist mifepristone in Cushing's syndrome. *Curr Opin Endocrinol Diabetes Obes* 2012;19:295-299.

[159] Johanssen S, Allolio B. Mifepristone (RU 486) in Cushing's syndrome. *Eur J Endocrinol* 2007;157:561-569.

[160] Feelders RA, de Bruin C, Pereira AM, Romijn JA, Netea-Maier RT, Hermus AR, et al. Pasireotide alone or with cabergoline and ketoconazole in Cushing's disease. *N Engl J Med* 2010;362:1846-1848.

[161] de Bruin C, Feelders RA, Lamberts SW, Hofland LJ. Somatostatin and dopamine receptors as targets of medical treatment of Cushing's syndrome. *Rev Endocr Metab Disord* 2009;10:91-102.

[162] Melmed S, Casanueva FF, Hoffman AR, Kleinberg DL, Montori VM, Schlechte JA, et al. Diagnosis and treatment of hyperprolactinemia: An Endocrine Society Clinical Practice Guideline. *J Clin Endocrinol Metab* 2011;96:273-288.

[163] Molitch ME, Elton RL, Blackwell RE, Caldwell B, Chang RJ, Jaffe R, et al. Bromocriptine as primary therapy for prolactin-secreting macroadenomas: results of a prospective multicenter study. *J Clin Endocrinol Metab* 1985;60:698-705.

[164] Verhelst J, Abs R, Maiter D, van den Bruel A, Vandeweghe M, Velkeniers B, et al. Cabergoline in the treatment of hyperprolactinemia: a study in 455 patients. *J Clin Endocrinol Metab* 1999;84:2518-2522.

[165] Di Sarno A, Landi ML, Cappabianca P, Di Salle F, Rossi FW, Pivonello R, et al. Resistance to cabergoline as compared with bromocriptine in hyperprolactinemia: prevalence, clinical definition, and therapeutic strategy. *J Clin Endocrinol Metab* 2001;86:5256-5261.

[166] Ono M, Miki N, Kawamata T, Makino R, Amano K, Seki T, et al. Prospective study of high-dose cabergoline treatment of prolactinomas in 150 patients. *J Clin Endocrinol Metab* 2008;93:4721-4727.

[167] Webster J, Piscitelli G, Polli A, Ferrari CI, Ismail I, Scanlon MF. A comparison of cabergoline and bromocriptine in the treatment of hyperprolactinemic amenorrhea. Cabergoline Comparative Study Group. *N Engl J Med* 1994;331:904-909.

[168] Corenblum B, Donovan L. The safety of physiological estrogen plus progestin replacement therapy and with oral contraceptive therapy in women with pathological hyperprolactinemia. *Fertil Steril* 1993;59:671-673.

[169] Biswas M, Smith J, Jadon D, McEwan P, Rees DA, Evans LM, et al. Long-term remission following withdrawal of dopamine agonist therapy in subjects with microprolactinomas. *Clin Endocrinol* (Oxf) 2005;63:26-31.

[170] Kharlip J, Salvatori R, Yenokyan G, Wand GS. Recurrence of hyperprolactinemia after withdrawal of long-term cabergoline therapy. *J Clin Endocrinol Metab* 2009;94:2428-2436.

[171] Colao A, Di Sarno A, Cappabianca P, Di Somma C, Pivonello R, Lombardi G. Withdrawal of long-term cabergoline therapy for tumoral and nontumoral hyperprolactinemia. *N Engl J Med* 2003;349:2023-2033.

[172] Gillam MP, Molitch ME, Colao A. 2006 Advances in the treatment of prolactinomas. *Endocr Rev* 2006;27:485-534.

[173] Kukstas LA, Domec C, Bascles L, Bonnet J, Verrier D, Israel JM, et al. Different expression of the two dopaminergic D2 receptors, D2415 and D2444, in two types of lactotroph each characterized by their response to dopamine, and modification of expression by sex steroids. *Endocrinology* 1992;129:1101-1103.

[174] Pellegrini I, Rasolonjanahary R, Gunz G, Bertrand P, Delivet S, Jedynak CP, et al. Resistance to bromocriptine in prolactinomas. *J Clin Endocrinol Metab* 1989;69:500-509.

[175] Kaltsas GA, Nomikos P, Kontogeorgos G, Buchfelder M, Grossman AB. Clinical review: diagnosis and management of pituitary carcinomas. *J Clin Endocrinol Metab* 2005;90:3089-3099.

[176] Kars M, Roelfsema F, Romijn JA, Pereira AM. Malignant prolactinoma: case report and review of the literature. *Eur J Endocrinol* 2006;155:523-534.

[177] Lim S, Shahinian H, Maya MM, Yong W, Heaney AP. Temozolomide: a novel treatment for pituitary carcinoma. *Lancet Oncol* 2006;7:518-520.

[178] McCormack AI, McDonald KL, Gill AJ, Clark SJ, Burt MG, Campbell KA, et al. 2009 Low O6-methylguanine-DNA methyltransferase (MGMT) expression and response to temozolomide in aggressive pituitary tumours. *Clin Endocrinol* (Oxf) 2009;71:226-233.

[179] Hagen C, Schroeder HD, Hansen S, Hagen C, Andersen M. Temozolomide treatment of a pituitary carcinoma and two pituitary macroadenomas resistant to conventional therapy. *Eur J Endocrinol* 2009;161:631-637.

[180] Kovacs K, Horvath E, Syro LV, Uribe H, Penagos LC, Ortiz LD, et al. Temozolomide therapy in a man with an aggressive prolactin-secreting pituitary neoplasm: morphological findings. *Hum Pathol* 2007;38:185-189.

[181] Gillam MP, Molitch ME, Lombardi G, Colao A. Advances in the treatment of prolactinomas. *Endocr Rev* 2006;27:485-534.

[182] Gonzalez JG, Elizondo G, Saldivar D, Nanez H, Todd LE, Villarreal JZ. Pituitary gland growth during normal pregnancy: an in vivo study using magnetic resonance imaging. *Am J Med* 1988;85:217–220.

[183] Rigg LA, Lein A, Yen SS. Pattern of increase in circulating prolactin levels during human gestation. *Am J Obstet Gynecol* 1977;129:454-456.

[184] Molitch ME. Pituitary disorders during pregnancy. Endocrinol Metab *Clin North Am* 2006;35:99-116.

[185] Milker-Zabel S, Debus J, Thilmann C, Schlegel W, Wannenmacher M. Fractionated stereotactically guided radiotherapy and radiosurgery in the treatment of functional and nonfunctional adenomas of the pituitary gland. *Int J Radiat Oncol Biol Phys* 2001;50:1279-1286.

[186] Black PM, Hsu DW, Klibanski A, Kliman B, Jameson JL, Ridgway EC, et al. Hormone production in clinically nonfunctioning pituitary adenomas. *J Neurosurg* 1987;66:244–250.

[187] Ebersold MJ, Quast LM, Laws ER, Scheithauer B, Randall RV. Long-term results in transsphenoidal removal of nonfunctioning pituitary adenomas. *J Neurosurg* 1986;64:713-719.

[188] Scheithauer BW, Kovacs KT, Laws ER Jr., Randall RV. Pathology of invasive pituitary tumors with special reference to functional classification. *J Neurosurg* 1986;65:733-744.

[189] Freda PU, Beckers AM, Katznelson L, Molitz ME, Montori VM, Post KD, et al. Pituitary incidentaloma: An endocrine society clinical practice guideline. *J Clin Endocrinol Metab* 2011;96:894-904.

[190] Reddy R, Cudlip S, Byrne JV, Karavitaki N, Wass JAH. Can we ever stop imaging in surgically treated and radiotherapy naïve patients with non-functioning pituitary adenoma? *Eur J Endocrinol* 2011;165:739-744.

[191] Turner HE, Stratton IM, Byrne JV, Adams CB, Wass JA. Audit of selected patients with nonfunctioning pituitary adenomas treated without irradiation - a follow-up study. *Clin Endocrinol* (Oxf) 1999;51:281-284.

[192] Ferrante E, Ferraroni M, Castrignano T, Menicatti L, Anagni M, Reimondo G, et al. 2006 Non-functioning pituitary adenoma database: a useful resource to improve the clinical management of pituitary tumours. *Eur J Endocrinol* 2006;155:823-829.

[193] Colao A, Di Somma C, Pivonello R, Faggiano A, Lombardi G, Savastano S. Medical therapy for clinically non-functioning pituitary adenomas. *Endocr Relat Cancer* 2008;15:905-915.

[194] Horiguchi K, Yamada M, Umezawa R, Satoh T, Hashimoto K, Tosaka M, et al. Somatostatin receptor subtype mRNA in TSH-secreting pituitary adenomas: A case showing a dramatic reduction in tumor size during short octreotide treatment. *Endocr J* 2007;54:371-378.

[195] Beck-Peccoz P, Persani L. Medical management of thyrotropin-secreting pituitary adenomas. *Pituitary* 2002;5:83-88.

[196] Smallridge RC. Thyrotropin-secreting pituitary tumors. Endorinol Metab *Clin North Am* 1987;16:765-792.

[197] Greenman Y, Melmed S. Thyrotropin-secreting pituitary tumors. In Melmed S (editor): The pituitary. Blackwell Sci Inc, Boston, 1995, pp 546-558.

[198] Young WF Jr, Scheithauer BW, Kovacs KT, Hovarth E, Davis DH, Randall RV. Gonadotroph adenoma of the pituitary: a clinicopathologic analysis of 100 cases. *Mayo Clin Proc* 1996;71:649-656.

[199] Dekkers OM, Rereira AM, Romijn JA. Treatment and follow-up of clinically nonfunctioning pituitary adenomas. *J Clin Endocrinol Metab* 2008;93:3717-3726.

[200] Snyder PJ. Gonadotroph and other clinically nonfunctioning pituitary adenomas. *Cancer Treat Res* 1997;89:57-72.

[201] Ceccato F, Occhi G, Regazzo D, Randi ML, Cecchin D, Gardiman MP, et al. Gonadotropin secreting pituitary adenoma associated with erythrocytosis: case report and literature review. *Hormones* 2014;13:131-139.

[202] Karapanou O, Tzanela M, Tamouridis N, Tsagarakis S. Gonadotroph pituitary macroadenoma inducing ovarian hyperstimulation syndrome: successful response to octreotide therapy. *Hormones* 2012;;11:199-202.

[203] Saveanu A, Morange-Ramos I, Gunz G, Dufour H, Enjalbert A, Jaquet P. A luteinizing hormone-, alpha-subunit- and prolactin secreting pituitary adenoma responsive to somatostatin analogs: in vivo and in vitro studies. *Eur J Endocrinol* 2001;145:35-41.

[204] Kanner AA, Corn BW, Greenman Y. Radiotherapy of nonfunctioning and gonadotroph adenomas. *Pituitary* 2009;12:15-22.

In: Pituitary Adenoma
Editor: Dimitrios N. Kanakis

ISBN: 978-1-63484-985-2

Chapter 11

CURRENT UPDATE OF SURGICAL MANAGEMENT FOR PITUITARY ADENOMAS

Se-Youn Jang[1], MD,
and Choong-Hyun Kim[2,*], MD, PhD

[1]Department of Neurosurgery, Seoul Medical Center, Seoul, Korea
[2]Department of Neurosurgery, Guri Hospital, Hanyang University, Korea

ABSTRACT

The surgical therapeutic goal of pituitary adenoma is 1) reversing endocrinopathy and restoring normal pituitary function, 2) eliminating mass effect and restoring normal neurological function, 3) eliminating or minimizing the possibility of tumor recurrence 4) obtaining a definitive pathological diagnosis. Surgical approaches to the pituitary adenoma can be broadly divided into three groups: transsphenoidal approach (TSA), conventional craniotomy, and alternative skull base approaches. The choice of surgical approach depends on several factors. The most important of these include the size of the pituitary fossa and its degree of mineralization, the size and pneumatization of the sphenoid sinus, the position and tortuosity of the carotid arteries, the presence and direction of possible intracranial tumor extensions, the presence of any uncertainty concerning the pathology of the lesion, and whether prior therapy has been administered.

The surgical technique used to approach the pituitary adenoma has changed over the years. The microscopic TSA to the pituitary gland has undergone various modifications, since the time it was firstly introduced by Hardy. It is one of the most effective and safest approach of major neurosurgical procedures with excellent outcomes and low complication rates. Therefore, the transsphenoidal microsurgery is the most common approach for more than 95% of pituitary tumors. TSA has been refined by introduction of the endoscopic procedure for the pituitary adenoma. Although endoscope was used as an adjunct to microscopic transsphenoidal surgery, purely endoscopic transsphenoidal technique was introduced in the 1990s, and this has recently become popular. This current update will review recent advances in surgical technique for pituitary adenoma.

* Corresponding author: Choong Hyun Kim, MD, PhD, Department of Neurosurgery, Hanyang University Guri Hospital, Hanyang University College of Medicine, 249-1 Gyomun-dong Guri, Gyung-Gi Do 471-701 Korea, Tel: +82-31-560-2322, Fax: +82-31-560-2327, E-mail: kch5142@hanyang.ac.kr.

Keywords: pituitary, adenoma, endoscope, surgery, management, transsphenoidal

1. Introduction

Although the transsphenoidal approach (TSA) was originally described almost 100 years ago, this procedure remains the optimal technique for removal of pituitary and other sellar tumors. A Viennese otolaryngologist, Victor Schloffer, initially described the lateral trans-facial approach to the sphenoid bone in 1907 [1]. This was modified by Halstead and then Cushing, who adopted the sub-labial approach in 1910 [2]. The endonasal approach was described by Otto Hirsch, based on the intranasal sphenoidotomy [3]. Technical advances, including intraoperative lateral fluoroscopy, were introduced by Guiot et al. and with the microsurgical removal of the first microadenoma for Cushing's disease by Jules Hardy, reported in 1962 [4, 5].

2. Preoperative Endocrine Evaluation

For patients with pituitary tumor, endocrine evaluation should include measurement of the levels of serum prolactin, growth hormone, cortisol, T3, T4, follicle-stimulating hormone (FSH) and luteinizing hormone (LH). In approximately 71% of these adenomas, preoperative partial hypophyseal insufficiency has been demonstrated [6, 7, 8]. Moderate hyperprolactinemia (less than 200 ng/mL) is usual in 50%-65% of patients. Negative immunohistochemical staining for pituitary tumor in these cases argues strongly for hypothalamohypophyseal disconnection [6, 7, 9, 10]. Although most non-functioning pituitary adenomas are shown by immunohistochemical staining to be gonadotropic adenomas, they are commonly considered silent, with levels of plasma gonadotropins or their subunits that are usually low.

Increased basal FSH seems to be more common, especially in men [11, 12]. Increased basal LH is rare and is often combined with an excess of α-subunit [10, 13]. Overproduction of α-subunit is common, but overproduction of basal LH β-subunit is rare. In a previous study with 95 gonadotropic adenomas, immunohistochemical staining was positive to FSH β-subunit in one third, whereas two third of the patients was positive for FSH β-subunit and LH or FSH β-subunit and α-subunit [13, 14].

3. Surgical Technique: Transsphenoidal Approach

3.1. Anesthesia

The endotracheal tube is mobilized to the left side of the mouth, which is the most suitable location of the head for a right-handed surgeon, after induction of standard endotracheal intubation of anesthesia to the patient. An anesthetic technique is accompanied by normotension, normocapnia, and normovolemia. An arterial line is inserted to help monitor the systemic blood pressure, which can become elevated as a result of surgical stimulation, especially during the step of positioning and opening the transsphenoidal retractors. Unless otherwise specified, central venous pressure (CVP) monitoring is not typically used.

3.2. Positioning

The Mayfield headrest with a horseshoe is positioned to the patient's skull for the operative procedure. Fixation of the head may be necessary when certain forms of semi-recumbent guidance are used. The patient's right shoulder is positioned in the top right upper corner of the operating table. The headrest frame is positioned to the far left. The patient's head is slightly rotated toward the surgeon's side and flexed gently, so as to be face to face with the surgeon. The patient's head is oriented at a right angle to the walls of the room, to facilitate lateral intraoperative device of fluoroscopy. The left lower quadrant of the abdomen is draped for harvesting the fat graft. Before and immediately after induction of anesthesia, patients are given oxymetazoline intranasally. After positioning has been completed, the nasal entry is washed with Betadine solution followed by packing with Afrin-soaked pledgets.

3.3. Exposure

There are several options to access the pituitary fossa via transsphenoidal route. Three main typical approaches are the following: the transnasal transseptal TSA, the endonasal TSA, and the recently used endoscopic TSA.

4. Transseptal Transsphenoidal Approach

Although the cartilaginous portion of the nasal septum is approached through the right nostril, submucosal dissection is carried out under the left side of the septum. The mucosa in the anterior part of the septum is tightly adherent. Because of this, the initial submucosal dissection is performed very slowly and very carefully until the shining white cartilage septum is well visualized. This operative field should be avascular and the surgical plane could be easily dissected. Until the bony septum is reached, the mucosal resection is carried out posteriorly, with enlargement of the submucosal window, along the superoinferior plane. In addition, until the left side of the anterior surface of the sphenoid bone is visible, the submucosal dissection on the left side of the septum is carried out posteriorly.

The direction of the nasal speculum during dissection must have at least a 20 angle from the floor of the maxilla. The bony septum at the level of anterior surface of the sphenoid bone is often soft and thin. In cases that the bony septum is too difficult to remove, this implies either that the speculum is too close to the bony spine of the maxilla, which means that the direction of the speculum is too low, or that the latter is against the perpendicular plate of the ethmoid, which means that its direction is too high. The 130-150 mm deepest nasal speculum is sufficient to reach the front of the sphenoid sinus. If the end of the speculum is so deep inside the nose, reaching the anterior site of the sphenoid bone, then it is either too low along the roof of the nasopharynx or it is too high and pointing toward the ethmoid air cells and anterior frontal fossa. When the location of the front surface of the sphenoid bone is identified, the speculum is further opened and rotated to crush the thin portion of the septum by the left arm of the nasal speculum which is followed by introducing it in the submucosal plane on the right side of the patient's nose. The transsphenoidal suction is used to further dissect this submucosal plane superiorly and inferiorly on both sides of the septum. An indwelling transsphenoidal retractor is applied in subsequent place. This procedure can cause intraoperative hypertension, therefore the surgeon should notify the anesthesiologist for such a possibility. The application of the self-retaining transsphenoidal retractor results in some submucosal oozing, which can easily be controlled by applying cotton balls.

Moreover, submucosal resection aids in reducing bleeding and decreases the risk of postoperative mucocele formation. The front face of the sphenoid sinus has a characteristic appearance, looking like the keel of a boat. The anterior face of the sphenoid bone is then removed by identifying the sphenoid ostium that central ridge of sphenoid by Kerrison rongeurs. At this stage the dimensions and features of the sella are evaluated and the lateral walls of the anterior face of the sphenoid are further removed until both lateral aspects of the sella are well visualized, especially the infrasellar prominences of the internal carotid arteries.

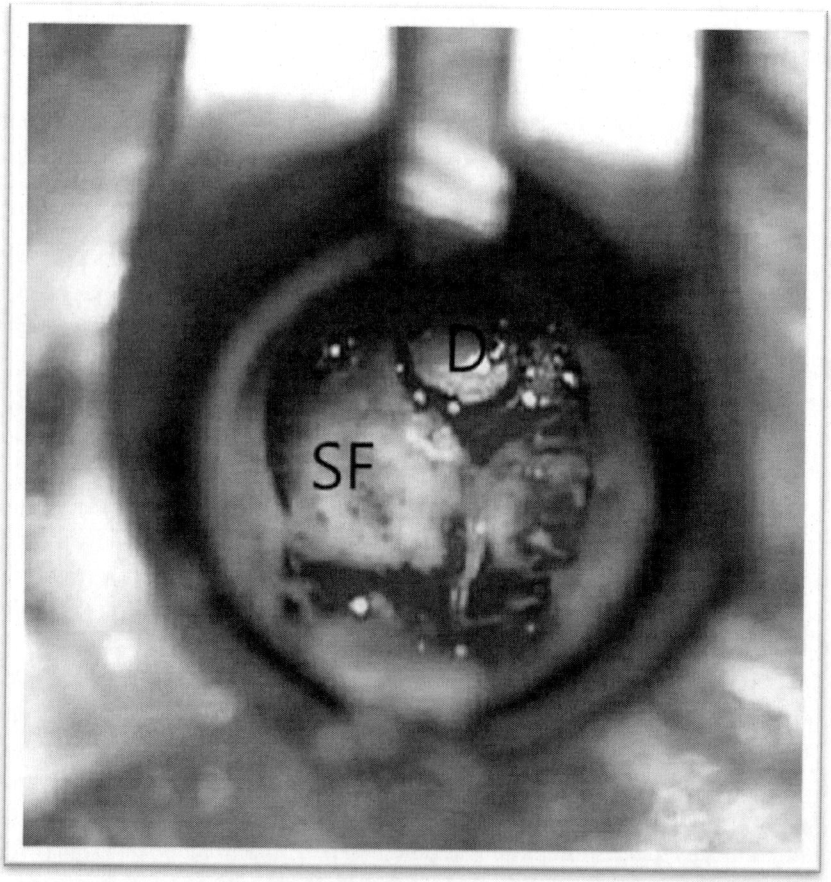

Figure 1. An intraoperative photograph showing opening of the sellar floor in a patient with a pituitary microadenoma (SF: sellar floor, D: dura).

In the most cases of pituitary adenomas, the sellar floor is thin enough to be easily cracked by gently pressing against it with a curette or a dissector easily. Then, it is removed by using Kerrison rongeurs (Figure 1).

In some tumors, the sellar floor is either eroded or it is extraordinarily thin, and it can be thus fractured with a blunt hook. The removal of the bone is done without extension to the frontal skull base, so as to prevent any possible bleeding from the anterior intercavernous sinus.

However, if bleeding occurs, gentle pressure with Avitene® (C. R. Bard, Inc., Murray Hill, NJ) is the fastest way to stop it. The dura is then opened for tumor removal, after hemostasis has been established. It is very important to cut the dura without the insertion of the knife deep into the sellar space. In this stage, the surgeons should be particularly careful to avoid major vessel injury, because in some cases the carotid artery could be displaced both medially and anteriorly, and it can thus be easily injured while opening the dura. The exposed sellar floor is gradually expanded as the tumor resection progresses (Figure 2).

5. Endonasal Transsphenoidal Approach

The anterior portion of the septum is bypassed and the sphenoid sinus is directly approached through its anterior wall, when the endonasal approach is chosen.

The landmarks regarding the location of the sphenoid sinus level are the different anatomical structures of the nasal cavity. The sphenoid ostium is usually located at the level of the middle turbinate. In addition, it can be traced by following the roof of the nasopharynx as it curves forward and upward. The meeting point of this course with the middle turbinate, leads to the floor of the pituitary fossa.

The mucosa is cut on the side of the nostril through which the approach is carried, and then the thin bony septum is mobilized with gentle pressure using the blade of the nasal speculum. Subsequently, the septum is placed between the two blades of the speculum, blades are arranged in the submucosal plane.

Further dissection with the tip of a suction instrument is made, until adequate exposure of the anterior surface of the sphenoid bone is achieved, similar to what is finally visualized using the transseptal TSA.

The endonasal transsphenoidal approach is similar to what was described above, when the transsphenoidal transseptal approach after transsphenoidal self-retaining retractor is applied. The advantage achieved by the use of the endonasal approach is best appreciated in pituitary macroadenomas when the suprasellar component of the tumor and the diaphragm sella do not fall down into the surgical field.

6. Endoscopic Endonasal Approach

6.1. Introduction

Compared with other methods, the main advantage of the endoscopic surgery can be improved visualization.

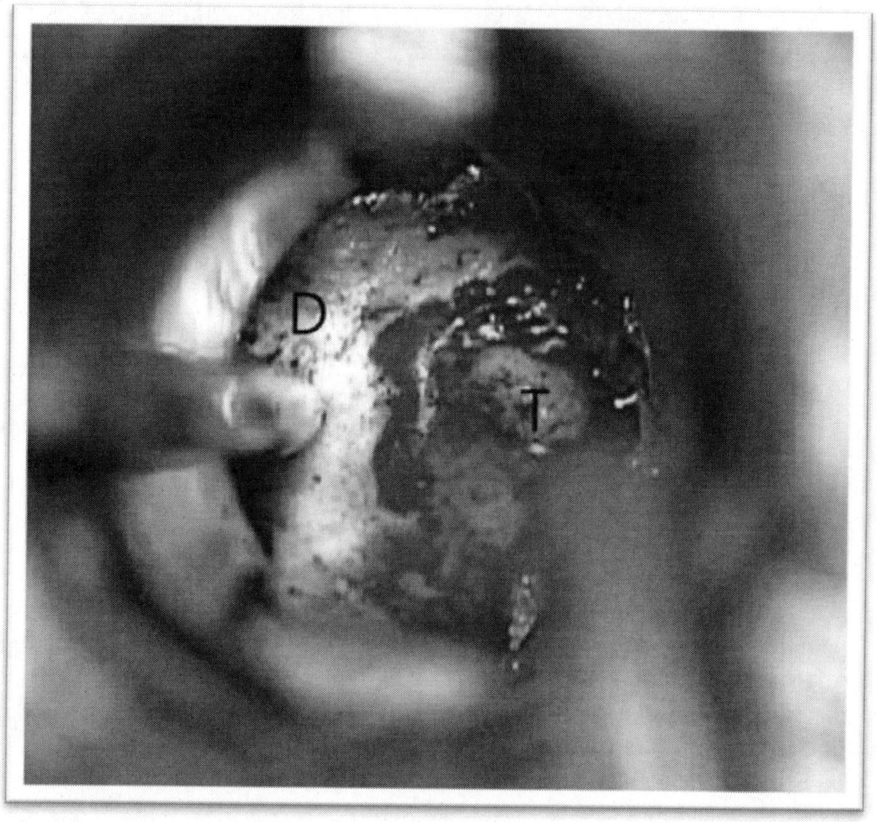

Figure 2. Dura is incised and tumor is resected carefully by the use of a ring curette (D: dura, T: tumor).

The latter method results in increased approach to inaccessible areas, and it is therefore possible to facilitate the avoidance of complications, resulting from incomplete tumor resection. Another potential advantage of endoscopic surgery is improving cosmesis and reduction in morbidity from tissue trauma, injury of blood vessels and nerves. The reduced morbidity results in rapid recovery, shorter hospital stay, and decreased cost of medical care.

6.2. Patient Selection

There are some absolute contraindications of the endoscopic surgery for the surgical management of the pathological processes concerning the skull base. It is recommended to use a different approach for operation on the distal or deep to carotid neurovascular structure. In other words, the endoscopic tumor removal is not normally suitable for endoscopic resection if tumors are located on the lateral side of optic nerve. However, the endoscopic surgery is occasionally available in case that the important anatomical structures are displaced by tumor. Therefore, the endoscopic surgery is suitable for lesions that are accessible to the tumor with minimal manipulation of normal structure. When the ablation or reconstruction of major vessels is necessary, endoscopic surgery is not indicated. If the tumor involves superficial tissues, a microscopic open surgery may be more practical. Tumor volume has not been a limiting factor in appropriately selected cases.

6.3. Operating Room Setup

The surgeons are placed on the right side of the patient opposite to the anesthesia team. The nurse is positioned towards the foot of the bed. This arrangement provides access to the nasal area by the surgeon, without the latter having to be interrupted during the surgery. Additional monitors for image guidance are placed beside the patient's head. Electrical cords and suction tubes are connected away from the surgical field toward the head and foot of the bed to minimize interference with surgical instruments. Furthermore, a three Mayfield pin fixation system reduces the intraoperative movement of the head, especially during drilling and neurovascular dissection. The head is fixed following endotracheal intubation with the neck in slight extension turned to the right by 10-15, and with the patient as close as possible to the right-hand side of the surgical bed. If the lesion extends anterior to the cribriform plate or if a frontal sinusotomy is necessary, extension of the neck provides a better angle for the visualization of the lesion. The proposal of this positioning can help the surgeon to adjust him- or herself in a manner that avoids distortion and fatigue of the surgeon's back, neck, and hands. Similarly, in order to avoid excessive burden on the surgeon's neck, the monitors of the operative field should be placed on the eye level of the surgeon.

Neurophysiological monitoring of cortical function (somatosensory evoked potentials) with/without brainstem function (brainstem evoked responses) is regularly carried out in all cases with exposure of the dura or dissection near the carotid arteries. Neurophysiological monitoring can identify the change in cerebral blood flow which can alert the anesthesiologist to adjust blood loss or changes of blood pressure. The cranial nerve monitoring by electromyography may be performed adequately. In a next step, a nasal decongestant, for example oxymetazoline 0.5%, will be topically applied to the nasal mucosa by using cottonoids. The skin of external nose, nasal vestibule, and fat graft donor site are prepared with a sterilized povidone solution. In addition, the patient is given a fourth-generation cephalosporin for perioperative antibiotic prophylaxis.

6.4. Operative Procedure

The endoscope is introduced at the 12 o'clock position of the nostril (usually the right) and the nasal vestibule is retracted upward. In this way the available space in the nostrils is increased and another device instrument can also be introduced. A suction tip is introduced at the 6 o'clock position on the same side. The dissector can be introduced through the left nasal cavity. The continuous suction-irrigation performed by an assistant, in order the lens of the scope to remain clean, ensures that the surgeon can keep the visualization without removing the scope for frequent cleaning. Removal of one or both middle nasal turbinates is initially performed, for widening of the nasal corridor, and then out-fracturing of the inferior turbinates is followed so as to provide room for the endoscope. These steps will provide a wider access to the posterior nasal cavity including the sphenoethmoid recess and the posterior choanae. Injection of vasoconstrictors is optional and is carried out according to the preferences of surgeon. The sphenoidotomy is initiated by identifying and expanding the natural ostium of the sphenoid sinus or by entering the sphenoid sinus at the junction of the nasal septum and the rostrum of the sphenoid sinus (Figure 3). Instruments are used to incise and disarticulate the posterior septum from the rostrum of the sphenoid bone. Removal of the bony rostrum is completed using Kerrison rongeurs and a high-speed drill. Wide bilateral sphenoidotomies are carried out by extending laterally to the level of the medial pterygoid plates and lateral wall of the sphenoid sinus, superiorly to the level of the planum sphenoidale and inferiorly to the floor of the sphenoid sinus. The resection of rear edge on the nasal septum is performed with a backbiting forceps. The removal of the posterior septum facilitates bilateral instrumentation without displacement of the septum into the path of the endoscope, and improves the lateral angulation and range of motion of all used instruments (Figure 4). As a conclusion, wide bilateral sphenoidotomies and a posterior septectomy provide both access and visualization of the related anatomical structures.

7. Intradural Endoneurosurgical Dissection

Endoneurosurgical tumor removal belongs to the same dissection principles of open approaches, since the surgeon also with this procedure can avoid blind dissection of tumors from blood vessels and nerves.

In any case, the tumor can be easily extracted by pulling without looking at the underlying structure. If it is not possible to carry out the above method, the resection of the tumor should be abandoned. In particular, this approach includes the steps described in the following lines. A small diameter suction tip is used in the left hand to maintain gentle traction while a dissecting or debulking instrument is used in the right hand. For the debulking of soft lesions, such as pituitary tumors, a 6-8 Fr. suction tip is suitable. A gentle suction allows distal angulation to improve the range of access, and provide more space for the tip of the endoscope.

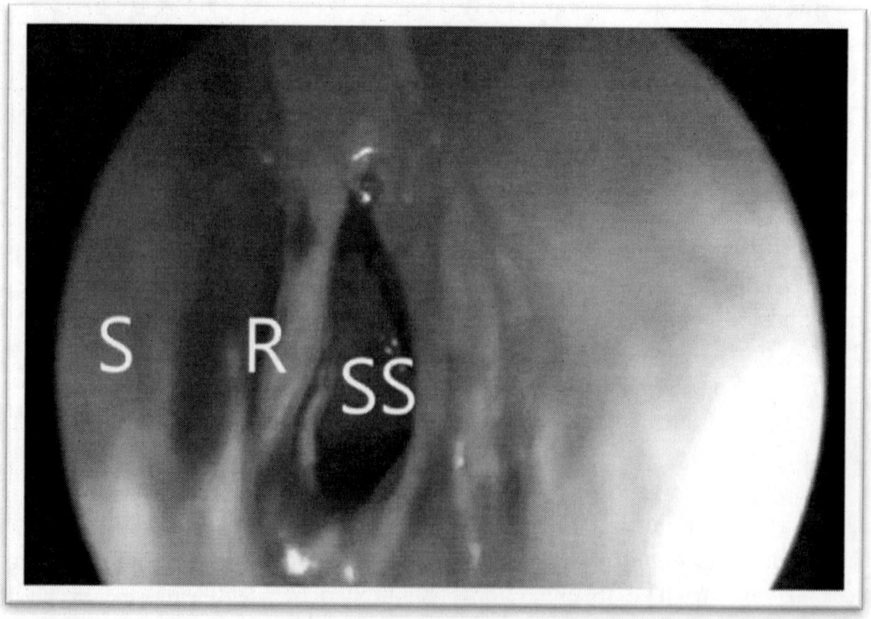

Figure 3. Endonasal endoscopic view demonstrating sphenoid ostium and inner aspect of sphenoid sinus (SS: sphenoid sinus, R: rostrum of the sphenoid bone, S: posterior septum).

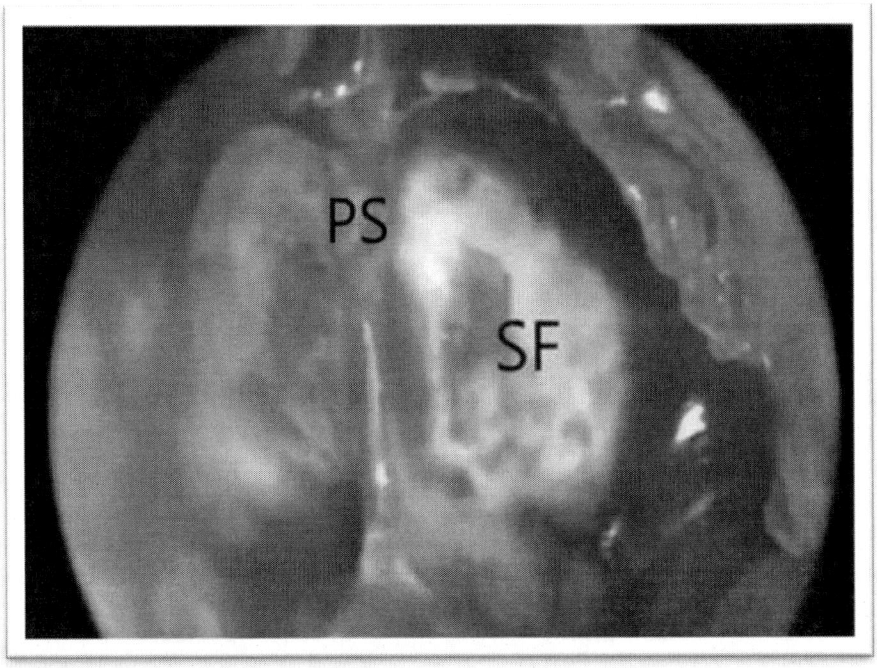

Figure 4. Endoscopic view revealing the outer side of sellar floor and structures in the sphenoid sinus (SF: sellar floor, PS: posterior sphenoid wall mucosa).

Internal debulking is continued until the tumor capsule can be freely mobilized by smooth traction applied with a 4-6 Fr. suction tip. Sharp dissection is used to divide intratumoral bands and enable the extracapsular dissection. The extracapsular dissection should be performed as rapidly as possible or alternatively by a fine blunt endoscopic dissector. The critical neurovascular structures are identified and protected using small cotton ball.

The tumor capsule is coagulated using the appropriately shaped endoscopic bipolar cautery. Continuous irrigation is important in order to avoid thermal damage to critical neurovascular structures from the heat produced by the cauterization.

8. Hemostatic Techniques

Preoperative strategies include devascularization of the tumor by angiographic embolization of the vascular supply when possible. However, the most tumors receive blood supply from the intracranial circulation, and embolization is either not available or is too dangerous to perform. The first step is to devascularize the tumor as part of the approach or sequentially during the resection. Bulky intranasal tumors are first partially resected to expose the dural base. The endoscopic bipolar electrocautery is used in the initial stage of hemostasis. Then, circumferential dissection around the margin of the tumor should be performed, and cauterize the feeding arterial vessels. Afterwards, the hypertrophied bone of the anterior cranial base is removed by the drilling, and the dura is cauterized for effective devascularization of the tumor. Intracapsular tumor dissection is often performed in a relatively bloodless field.

9. Sphenoidal Surgery

The purpose of this exposure is to make the sphenoid sinus cavity into a large single rectangular cavity with walls that are completely flat, devoid of septation that would interfere with the visualization of neurovascular landmarks or with the manipulation of the endoscope or dissecting instruments. It enables the surgeon to have the unobstructed maneuverability of endoscope and prevents simultaneously the lens of endoscope to become dirty by the blood, which is essential in case of bleeding on operative field. Utilizing the available space fully is made with widening of the sphenoidotomy toward the lateral recesses, lateral to the vertical carotid canal, and superiorly to expose the posterior cells of the ethmoid sinus, the planum-tuberculum junction and optic-carotid recesses. The sphenoid sinus mucosa is removed, and venous bleeding should be controlled either by irrigation of warm saline solution or by topical application of bone wax. Thereafter, the key anatomical landmarks have to be identified. The key landmarks are the outer and inner optic-carotid recesses, the parasellar and paraclival carotid canal, the sellar and clival recesses, and the strut over the superior intercavernous sinus. The intracranial entrance at the level of the medial opticocarotid recess allows simultaneous access to the carotid canal, optic canal, pituitary fossa, and medial part of the cavernous sinus. When removing the bone adjacent to the carotid canal, it is important to weaken the bone with a blunt elevator or with the tip of the bone forceps. Finally, the bone is removed by Kerrison rongeur with the 1-mm angled tip.

10. Intrasellar Dissection

The debulking of the tumor is used by the two suctions technique, or by ultrasonic aspirator in case of a firm tumor. These techniques can achieve more effective and less traumatic serration of the tumor from the normal gland, stalk, cavernous sinus contents, but also controlled removal of the tumor. In many cases, extracapsular dissection is actually available, as a result of the improved visualization provided by the endoscope. After removal of macroadenoma, the diaphragm can be lowered to allow the direct visualization. A systematic intrasellar dissection is essential to optimize visualization while protecting the normal gland. After the bipolar cauterization, the dura is opened by using a sickle knife or retractable blade in the center of the sella. The opening is extendedcaudally and obliquely towards "8 o'clock" and "5 o' clock" positions, to create an inferior flap of dura as the initial opening. The superior flap is left intact to act as a retractor and hold the anterior face of the tumor overlying the diaphragm. Macroadenomas often herniate through this inferior opening. The inferior part of the tumor is removed in a posterior trajectory towards the clival-dorsum junction, proceeding widely, from one cavernous sinus to the opposite one. The macroadenomas must be carefully removed because the posterior dorsum of the sella turcica may be eroded, thus leaving the dura of the basilar cistern at risk for transgression, which can result in injury to the basilar artery. The pituitary stalk is most commonly located in this position. We should carefully examine the angle between the optic nerve and carotid artery, and the inside of the medial optic-carotid recesses. These are two common sites for remnant tumor. The other common site is under the anterior lip of dura, at the level of the anterior intercavernous sinus, directly just below the sella-tuberculum junction. In order to optimize visualization of this latter segment, it is necessary to remove the bone and underlying tumor along the anterior aspect overlying the diaphragm. The descending of diaphragm will allow opening up the superior angle. Final inspection of the sella turcica is undertaken in a clockwise fashion starting downward at the "6 o'clock" position and performed using angled endoscopes as required. At this stage, the diaphragm must descend concentrically. If the diaphragm fails to fall down concentrically, it is required to hold the tumor in the suprasellar space for complete resection.

If the main purpose of surgery is optic nerve decompression, tumor removal is deemed adequate only when pulsations are visible in the diaphragm. In case that the diaphragm does not descend concentrically, additional removal of the diaphragm may be considered electively. Finally, the residual tumor in the suprasellar cistern can be removed easily under direct visualization, until the optic nerves are fully visible.

11. Reconstruction

The basic principle of reconstruction is to maintain the separation of the sinonasal tract and intracranial cavity. The aim of sellar repair is to create a protective barrier, reducing the dead space, and preventing the descent of the chiasm into the sellar cavity. To guarantee these results, different materials have been used. The best choice is to use autografts. On top of fascial graft, an abdominal fat graft has been used as a bolster and subsequently a biological dressing is applied. A fibrin sealant is also applied to secure the fat graft (Figure 5). Moreover, sponge packings are placed intranasally to support the fat graft.

12. Advantages and Disadvantages of the Procedure

The advantages of endoscopic surgery compared to microscopic surgery are that the former is able to provide the visualization through a narrow corridor and to reserve the angled portion, so as to ensure visibility.

However, the disadvantage of endoscopic surgery is that the progression of the operation may be difficult when the lens become turbid by blood and massive bleeding occurs. Besides, the surgeon cannot use both hands because of holding the endoscope by another hand. Since the visual field of the endoscope moves according to the hand movement in the unfamiliar stage of endoscopic surgery, it is possible to shake images and move to undesired directions. Moreover, the endoscopic surgery may cause undesired intraoperative complications because the endoscope cannot give a three-dimensional image and perspective. It is also difficult to reconstruct the sellar floor because of inevitable difficulty to collect the large bony fragment by endoscope. Transseptal TSA has the advantage of access to the sellar floor without damages of the surrounding structures close to the midline, but the deformity of nose or septal perforation is likely to occur.

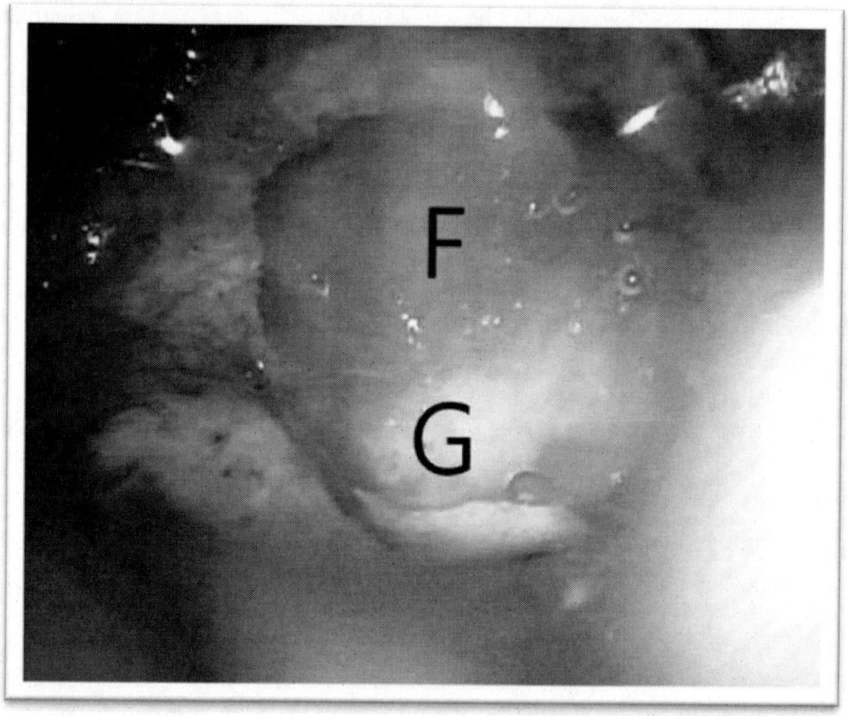

Figure 5. Intraoperative view showing reconstruction of sellar floor with fat graft and fibrin glue (F: fat graft, G: fibrin glue).

The transnasal TSA has all the advantages of the transseptal TSA and endoscopic surgery. In the transnasal TSA, exposure of the sellar floor is faster, and easy to take nasal reconstruction compared to conventional approaches. Furthermore, cosmetic results are excellent because the incision does not occur in the nasal septum. In most cases, nasal septum following pituitary surgery is replaced in the midline with packing of each nostril. However, this procedure may be potential to hurt the nasal mucosa if the nostril is too narrow. The major advantage of the endoscopic approach is that nasal complications are quite few compared to other approaches.

13. Postoperative Management

Perioperative prophylactic antibiotics are administered until the packing is removed. To prevent adhesions between the nasal septum and turbinates, silastic splints which are placed at the time of surgery are usually removed in postoperative 5-21 days. If a septal mucosal flap is used, the splints are maintained for 2-3 weeks to promote healing of the donor site. Patients are instructed to use a saline nasal spray for nasal hygiene, and should not do any activity that may raise the intracranial pressure or may stress the graft, such as nose blowing, physical exertion, or bending over. They are followed-up for 2-4 weeks initially to debride nasal crusting until healing is complete. Any clear rhinorrhea should be evaluated with endoscopic examination and testing of the fluid for β2-transferrin. Complete healing of fat grafts can be prolonged for several months while the non-viable part of the fat graft separates from the vascularized portion. If necessary, after the risk of leakage of CSF has elapsed, saline irrigation for nasal hygiene can be established.

14. Complications of Surgery

TSA is well known as one of the safe procedures in neurosurgical field. In several retrospective studies, operative mortality and major morbidity rates are 0.5% and 2.2%, respectively [15]. Endoscopic series have reported the rates of complications that vary from 10% to 26.9% [16, 17, 18, 19]. The most common complications are permanent diabetes insipidus, newly developed pituitary insufficiency, and postoperative cerebrospinal fluid (CSF) leakage. The rate of CSF leakage following endoscopic endonasal surgery for pituitary adenomas varies from 1.2% to 14% [16, 20, 21]. There is also a great risk, such as CSF leakage in patients with pituitary macroadenomas, especially if there is significant extrasellar extension. CSF leakage is almost controlled within 3 days of lumbar drainage. Diabetes insipidus is reported as the frequent complication following pituitary surgery, with incidence of transient diabetes insipidus of 2.5% to 20% and permanent diabetes insipidus in 1% to 14.8% in endoscopic series [17, 19, 22]. Major causes of operative death are intracranial hemorrhage, hypothalamic damage, or meningitis related to the development of CSF fistulas.

References

[1] Schloffer H. Erfolgreiche Operation eines hypophysentumors auf nasalem Wege. *Wien Klin Wochenschr* 1907;20:621-624.

[2] Cushing H. The weir mitchell lecture: Surgical experiences with pituitary disorders. *JAMA* 1914;LXIII:1515-1525.

[3] Hirsch O. Endonasal method of removal of hypophyseal tumors with report of two successful cases. *JAMA* 1910;55:772-774.

[4] Bigos ST, Robert F, Pelletier G, Hardy J. Cure of Cushing's disease by transsphenoidal removal of a microadenoma from a pituitary gland despite a radiographically normal sella turcica. *J Clin Endocrinol Metab 45* 1977;45:1251-1260.

[5] Bouche J, Guiot G..[Unrecognized sphenoidal empyema. Approach by means of low transseptal route] *Ann Otolaryngol* 1962;79:876-878.

[6] Comtois R, Beauregard H, Somma M, Serri O, Aris-Jilwan N, Hardy J. The clinical and endocrine outcome to trans-sphenoidal microsurgery of nonsecreting pituitary adenomas. *Cancer* 1991;68 :860-866.

[7] Greenman Y, Tordjman K, Kisch E, Razon N, Ouaknine G, Stern N. Relative sparing of anterior pituitary function in patients with growth hormone-secreting macroadenomas: Comparison with nonfunctioning macroadenomas. *J Clin Endocrinol Metab* 1995;80:1577-1583.

[8] Marazuela M, Astigarraga B, Vicente A, Estrada J, Cuerda C, Garcia-Uria J, et al. Recovery of visual and endocrine function following transsphenoidal surgery of large nonfunctioning pituitary adenomas. *J Endocrinol Invest* 1994;17: 703-707.

[9] Arafah BM. Reversible hypopituitarism in patients with large nonfunctioning pituitary adenomas. *J Clin Endocrinol Metab* 1986;62:1173-1179.

[10] Boute D, Dewailly D, Fossati P..[Gonadotropic adenoma] *Ann Med Interne* (Paris) 1990;141:42-52.

[11] Chanson P, Pantel J, Young J, Couzinet B, Bidart JM, Schaison G. Free luteinizing-hormone beta-subunit in normal subjects and patients with pituitary adenomas. *J Clin Endocrinol Metab* 1997;82:1397-1402.

[12] Kwekkeboom DJ, de Jong FH, Lamberts SW. Gonadotropin release by clinically nonfunctioning and gonadotroph pituitary adenomas in vivo and in vitro: Relation to sex and effects of thyrotropin-releasing hormone, gonadotropin-releasing hormone, and bromocriptine. *J Clin Endocrinol M*etab 1989;68:1128-1135.

[13] Daneshdoost L, Gennarelli TA, Bashey HM, Savino PJ, Sergott RC, Bosley TM, et al.: Identification of gonadotroph adenomas in men with clinically nonfunctioning adenomas by the luteinizing hormone beta subunit response to thyrotropin-releasing hormone. *J Clin Endocrinol Metab* 1993;77:1352-1355.

[14] Snyder PJ: Gonadotroph cell adenomas of the pituitary. *Endocr Rev* 1985;6:552-563.

[15] Zervas N: Surgical results for pituitary adenomas: Results of an international survey. In Black P, Zervas N, Ridgeway E, et al. (editors): Secretory tumors of the pituitary gland: Raven, New York 1984, pp 377-385.

[16] Berker M, Hazer DB, Yucel T, Gurlek A, Cila A, Aldur M, et al. Complications of endoscopic surgery of the pituitary adenomas: Analysis of 570 patients and review of the literature. *Pituitary* 2012;15:288-300.

[17] Gondim JA, Almeida JP, Albuquerque LA, Schops M, Gomes E, Ferraz T, et al.: Endoscopic endonasal approach for pituitary adenoma: Surgical complications in 301 patients. *Pituitary* 2011;14:174-183.

[18] Hofstetter CP, Shin BJ, Mubita L, Huang C, Anand VK, Boockvar JA, et al. Endoscopic endonasal transsphenoidal surgery for functional pituitary adenomas. *Neurosurg Focus* 2011;30: E10.

[19] Tabaee A, Anand VK, Barron Y, Hiltzik DH, Brown SM, Kacker A, et al.: Endoscopic pituitary surgery: A systematic review and meta-analysis. *J Neurosurg* 2009;111:545-554.

[20] Cappabianca P, Cavallo LM, Colao A, de Divitiis E: Surgical complications associated with the endoscopic endonasal transsphenoidal approach for pituitary adenomas. *J Neurosurg* 2002;97: 293-298.

[21] Loyo-Varela M, Herrada-Pineda T, Revilla-Pacheco F, Manrique-Guzman S. Pituitary tumor surgery: Review of 3004 cases. *World Neurosurg* 2013;79:331-336.

[22] Jho HD: Endoscopic transsphenoidal surgery. *J Neurooncol* 2001;54:187-195.

In: Pituitary Adenoma
Editor: Dimitrios N. Kanakis
ISBN: 978-1-63484-985-2

Chapter 12

VASCULAR ANATOMY OF THE SELLAR REGION AND COMPLICATIONS DURING ENDOSCOPIC ENDONASAL TRANSSPHENOIDAL SURGERY FOR PITUITARY ADENOMAS

Yasuhiko Hayashi**, *MD, PhD
Department of Neurosurgery, Graduate School of Medical Science,
Kanazawa University, Kanazawa, Japan

ABSTRACT

In general, transsphenoidal surgery has been considered to have a low rate of complication and mortality. Among the postoperative complications associated with transsphenoidal surgery (TSS), such as cerebrospinal fluid leakage, hypopituitarism, diabetes insipidus, vascular injury, meningitis, cranial nerve neuropathy, and nasal bleeding, vascular injury is unusual, but most possibly fatal complication. Therefore, the pituitary neurosurgeons need to have the knowledge about the possible incidence during the intra- and post-operative phase. Vascular injuries during the TSS described in the literature include fatal hemorrhage from internal carotid artery (ICA), ICA occlusion, pseudoaneurysm formation, carotid cavernous fistula, subarachnoid hemorrhage, vasospasm, and distal embolism with cerebral infarction. It is important to understand the patient's vascular anatomy at the sella and its surrounding structures, during the preoperative examination of the TSS, to avoid the vascular complications. Although recent advancement of the operative techniques and instruments of transsphenoidal approach enable the neurosurgeons to dissect arteries derived from the ICA and external carotid artery (ECA) during the surgery, it remains a difficult problem to preserve intact vessels even for the expert pituitary neurosurgeons. In particular, the introduction of endoscope into the TSS dramatically improved intraoperative visualization and diminished traumatization. Subsequently, the operative indication for performing TSS gradually developed to include the suprasellar, parasellar, clival, and cervicomedullary junction (extended transsphenoidal surgery). However, since the indications for the use of

* Corresponding author: Yasuhiko Hayashi, MD, PhD, 13-1 Takara-machi, Kanazawa, Ishikawa, 920-8641, Japan, Tel: +81-076-265-2384, Fax: +81-076-234-4262, E-mail: yahayashi@med.kanazawa-u.ac.jp.

TSS have grown, this fact can lead to increasing chances of intraoperative vascular injuries, and till now has not been reached a definite conclusion, whether TSS has a significant difference in the complication rate between endoscope and microscope techniques. Another advancement of preoperative neuroradiological investigation to detect such arteries derived from the ICA and the ECA is also useful for their precise localization and avoidance of fatal complications. Especially, the role of digital subtraction angiography in the operating room is significant, because, once the arterial injury during TSS happens, the emergent detection of affected vessel(s) and the management of the trauma is required. In addition, the development of endovascular surgery both in the techniques and the instruments remarkably changed the principles of treatment for intraoperative vascular injury during the TSS. Especially, in cases of ICA injury, the endovascular treatment with parent artery occlusion can be performed with acceptable morbidity and mortality rates. This technique can be also applied to the pseudoaneurysm, which arises from the injury site of the ICA at the postoperative delayed period, and causes fatal and massive epistaxis. However, vascular injury during endoscopic endonasal TSS is not well studied or reported, despite it is still a feared complication. The anatomic substrate for such complication in each stage of the TSS (naso-sphenoidal, spheno-planum, dural, intrasellar, and suprasellar phase) is discussed with respect to operative and neuroradiological aspects, identification of risk factors, management strategies for avoidance of such serious vascular complications, and their outcomes.

Keywords: transsphenoidal surgery, pituitary, vascular, complication, endoscope

1. Introduction

Pituitary adenomas constitute approximately 10-22.5% of all primary intracranial tumors, and surgical removal is the first optional management except for prolactinoma [1-4]. The transsphenoidal surgery (TSS) for removal of pituitary tumors has been originally applied due to its effectiveness and safety, with serious morbidity and mortality rates typically less than 1% [5, 6]. Recent advancement in operative and neuroradiological technologies has had a major impact on the treatment strategies for pituitary tumors, and TSS has become increasingly popular all over the world. In particular, the introduction of endoscope into the TSS has made a great progress not only on the resection rate of the tumor but also on the preservation of normal endocrinological function and the remission rate for the functioning adenoma [1, 7-9]. Moreover, the indication for the use of TSS has grown for the suprasellar, parasellar, clival, and craniocervical junction, since it has been regarded as extended TSS, and many surgeons reported its effectiveness in the management of craniopharyngioma, clival chordoma, and pituitary adenoma with invasion into the cavernous sinus [10-12].

Historically, the TSS was originally introduced by Schloffer and Cushing during the first decade of the 20th Century [13-15]. The adaptation of the transsphenoidal route as a surgical corridor is based on the concept that this surgery is significantly less dangerous for the patients with pituitary tumors compared to the craniotomy, which was considered to be extraordinary difficult on the contrary, because the instrumentation, lightning, cautery, anesthesia, and medication were not available in those days [13, 14]. This revolutionary introduction was followed by the addition of the radiofluoroscopy by Guiot, as well as the operating microscope and specialized instruments by Hardy 60 years later [16, 17]. Therefore, concerning TSS, safety should be secured both through the operation by the surgical techniques and the anatomical knowledge of the pituitary region. However, many authors have reported various complications associated with the TSS including cerebrospinal fluid leakage, hypopituitarism, diabetes insipidus, meningitis, cranial nerve neuropathy, nasal bleeding, and vascular injury [1-7, 16, 18].

Despite the advancement of TSS, one of the most serious problems during this approach is vascular complications, in which injury to the cavernous ICA most commonly occurs at the sellar dural incision, and has been reported tooccur in 0-3.8% of cases [5, 18-22]. Even expert pituitary neurosurgeons experienced a 0.6-0.8% incidence of vascular injuries [23-25]. Therefore, all neurosurgeons trying to perform TSS should try to avoid the ICA injury and prepare to manage its risk with the appropriate preoperative evaluation, such as digital subtraction angiography (DSA) or 3-dimensional computed tomographic angiography (3D-CTA), fusion images with magnetic resonance imaging (MRI) and 3D-CTA, and computer graphics. The overall incidence of ICA injury was reported to be 1.1%, and the rate of ICA injury was inversely proportional to the surgeon's transsphenoidal experience, being 1.4% for the least experienced surgeons, 0.6% for those with intermediate experience, and 0.4% for the most experienced [19].

Anatomical studies of the sphenoid sinus and sellar region are relevant, because they can improve spatial orientation to the landmarks. Injury to ICA is the most feared complication leading to the catastrophic clinical deterioration of the patients [3, 11, 26, 27]. Historically, emergency surgical ligation of the ICA, to cease massive bleeding during pituitary surgery, has been required. However, this treatment was associated with an unacceptable high incidence of major clinical neurological deficit [20, 21]. Therefore, the development of endovascular treatment, combined with bypass surgery can provide dramatic changes on the aspect of control of the bleeding, embolization of carotid cavernous fistula and pseudoaneurysm, and cerebral revascularization to maintain good clinical outcomes [28-31]. In addition, the cavernous sinuses on both sides, which exist on the boundaries of the sella turcica, are vulnerable to injury during the TSS [21, 32]. The vascular complications should be discussed in each stage of the TSS (naso-sphenoidal, spheno-planum, dural, intrasellar, and suprasellar phase) with respect to the operative and neuroradiological aspects, identification of risk factors, management strategies for the avoidance of such serious vascular complications, and their outcomes.

2. Vascular Anatomy of the Transsphenoidal Surgery

The process of the TSS was divided into five phases including naso-sphenoidal, sphenoid-planum, dural, intrasellar, and suprasellar. Vascular anatomic aspects of each stage are described.

2.1. Naso-Sphenoid Phase

Vascular injury can be frequently encountered on removal of the base of middle turbinate. The sphenopalatine arteries, branches of the internal maxillary artery, emerge through the sphenopalatine foramen (the height of lower margin of superior turbinate), run under the nasal mucosa, and supply the nasal structures, including nasal septum (anterior ~ posterior part: posterior septal nasal artery, inferior part: descending palatine artery) and middle turbinate (posterior lateral nasal artery). Posterior septal nasal artery, distributing nasal septum, has anastomoses with the posterior ethmoidal artery (PEA) [26]. Endoscopic observation sometimes reveals the pulsation of the artery. All the above mentioned arteries are important and should be kept in mind not to be injured. Careful attention should be paid at the procedure for dissection of mucosa at the nasal septum from the anterior wall of the sphenoid sinus. The sphenopalatine artery can be caught at the sphenopalatine foramen, through which the artery emerges, so as not to cause massive bleeding when removal of the anterior wall of the sphenoid sinus is widely required (Figure 1A) [34]. Law reported that the bleeding from the sphenopalatine artery could occur from the bone directly, from the venous diploic space or from the blood supply to stout bony structure, particularly in patients with acromegaly [20]. If the bleeding from the sphenopalatine artery is difficult to control, endovascular management, coil embolization of the maxillary artery, can be indicated. Although the midline approach would not disturb the main trunks of the sphenopalatine arteries, hemostasis of the posterior attachment of the middle turbinate, containing a branch of the sphenopalatine artery, is achieved with a suction electrocautery [34]. However, when nasoseptal pedicled flap, which is used for reconstruction of the skull base, should be made intraoperatively from the nasal septal mucosa, it is important to keep the sphenopalatine artery intact within the nasoseptal flap, whose base is required to be narrow in order to be adhered to the skull base. Therefore, the sphenopalatine artery should be stored within the narrow base of the pedicled flap [35].

Maxillary artery is the largest terminal branch of the ECA. It arises at the level of the neck of the condylar process and passes medial to it. Then, it ascends to the posterior part of the pterygopalatine fossa, and sphenopalatine artery is divided from it and run into the sphenopalatine foramen (Figure 1B). When exploring tumors, extending into the pterygoid fossa such as pituitary adenoma, adenocystic carcinoma and neurinoma, the course of the maxillary artery, which is buried in the adipose tissue at the pterygoid fossa, needs to be recognized in order to avoid an injury. Therefore, preoperative evaluation of the maxillary artery, such as 3D-CTA, is important.

2.2. Spheno-Planum Phase

Vascular injury can be frequently encountered on removal of the planum sphenoidale and the posterior base of superior turbinate, especially in the case of extended TSS for the suprasellar lesion, an unusual TSS targeting for the pituitary adenoma. PEA, which has a smaller diameter than the anterior ethmoidal artery, diverges from the ophthalmic artery and passes between the medial rectal muscle and the superior oblique muscle. Afterwards, it runs through a thin, bony channel at the medial wall of the orbit along the ethmoidal roof, seen after submucosal dissection in the posterior ethmoidal sinus [12, 33].

Although the distribution of PEA has been reported to be variable, mainly it perfuses into the superior turbinate, the posterior ethmoid sinus, the posterior part of the lamina cribrosa, and the planum sphenoidale [33]. Neurosurgeons can find the unexpected hemorrhage from PEA, if the dissection around the superior turbinate and the posterior ethmoidal sinus is carried out [11]. Although the injury of PEA is considered as an extremely rare complication during TSS, the pituitary neurosurgeon should always have in mind the possibility of PEA injury.

In order to expose suprasellar lesions in the extended TSS approach, the superior and/or supreme turbinates should be removed along their base, taking care not to damage the turbinate lamina. During such maneuvers, it is important to avoid damaging the PEA, which frequently arises from the first segment of the ophthalmic artery and passes medially from the dura of the planum sphenoidale, to the posterior lamina cribrosa and then to the posterior ethmoidal cells [12]. Cavallo et al. reported that wide sphenoidectomy and bilateral posterior ethmoidectomy, to obtain a wider view of the planum sphenoidale, enable surgeons to clearly identify both PEAs, which are considered as "dangerous" landmarks and represent the anterior limit when opening the planum sphenoidale [10, 36]. Because the PEA branches the proximal portion of the ophthalmic artery with high blood pressure, injury of the PEA can cause massive and severe bleeding that should be avoided as much as possible.

As the PEA is a large branch stemming from the ophthalmic artery, it can be detected at the planum sphenoidale or posterior ethmoidal sinus on preoperative examinations, such as CTA. If this is the case performing the extended TSS, more attention should be paid in order to avoid unexpected severe arterial bleeding during submucosal dissection of the superior and lateral nasal cavity.

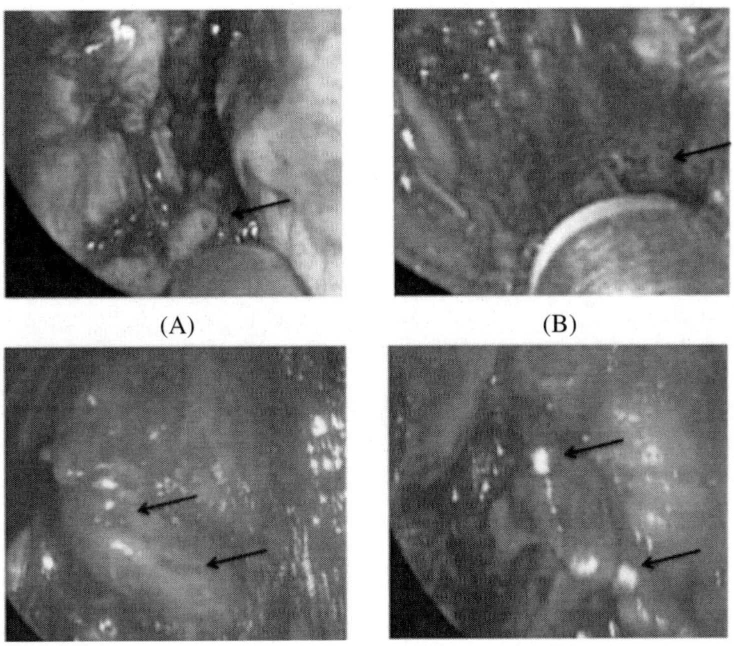

(A) (B) (C) (D)

Figure 1. A. Intraoperative endoscopic view shows the bleeding from the branch of sphenopalatine artery (posterior lateral nasal artery, A, arrow) B. is successfully coagulated with single-shaft bipolar coagulator (B, arrow) C. Intraoperative endoscopic view shows the maxillary artery (arrows) running in the pterygopalatine fossa after removal of the posterior wall of the maxillary sinus D.Hemoclips (arrows) were applied to resect the maxillary artery in the pterygopalatine fossa.

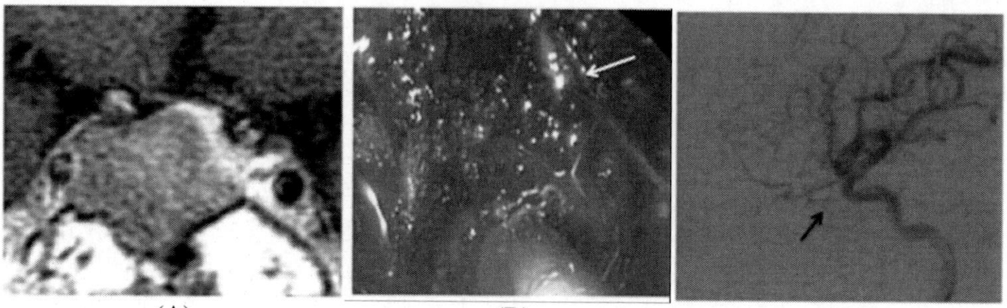

(A) (B) (C)

Figure 2. A. Magnetic resonance imaging of pituitary adenoma extending into the suprasellar region and compressing the optic nerves, with further invasion into the right cavernous sinus B. Intraoperatively, a massive hemorrhage suddenly appeared during mucosa dissection just above the sellar floor, suggesting the posterior ethmoidal artery (PEA) as the origin of the bleeding (white arrow) C. Digital subtraction angiography performed after the operation showed left PEA (arrow) to be responsible for this hemorrhage.

3. Illustrative Case

A 69-year-old man presented with a 6-month history of activity loss and visual field disturbance. MRI identified a pituitary tumor extending into the suprasellar region, compressing the optic nerves and invading the right cavernous sinus (Figure 2A). Neuro-ophthalmological investigation showed bitemporal hemianopsia, and endocrinological evaluation showed a decline of adrenocorticotrophic hormone (ACTH).

During the routine endoscopic TSS, a massive hemorrhage was suddenly encountered in the sphenoidal phase during mucosa dissection just above the sellar floor (Figure 2B). It was difficult to control this arterial bleeding, and the massive hemorrhage obstructed our endoscopic view, with the total amount of blood rising up to 2280ml. The bleeding point was found to originate from the left PEA was captured under the direct endoscopic view and was controlled with the single shaft bipolar coagulator (Karl Storz Endoscopy, Tuttlingen, Germany). Partial resection of the hard adenoma was performed, and the visual field defect and decline of ACTH level were restored. DSA performed after the operation showed left PEA, stemming from the ipsilateral ophthalmic artery, to be responsible for this hemorrhage (Figure 2C). Postoperative course was uneventful, and the residual tumor has been unchanged for four years.

3.1. Dural Phase

Vascular injury can be frequently encountered on opening of the dura mater of sellar floor, especially in the case of extended TSS for a suprasellar lesion, such as craniopharyngioma. Pituitary adenomas, further manifest with ballooning of the sellar floor, and compression of the intercavernous sinus for a long period and thus leading even to its complete occlusion.

The cavernous sinuses on either side of the sella are vascular structures filled with venous blood under venous pressure. The two cavernous sinuses frequently connect through dural channels, most commonly superior and inferior intercavernous sinus. These connecting channels can be injured during the opening of the dura mater. The dura itself consists of two layers, and between them, vascular channels commonly proliferate and are diminished by compression of macroadenoma for a long period. In particular, superior intercavernous sinus usually locates between the sellar floor and the tuberculum sellae (tuberculum recessus), and coagulation and cut off of the superior intercavernous sinus is required, to advance into the suprasellar lesion during the extended TSS (trans-tuberculum sellae approach). The size and location of the superior intercavernous sinus can also influence the bone removal of the tuberculum sellae [20]. If bleeding once occurs in the cutting of the sinus, the surgical procedure will be slow and more difficult. Therefore, the incisions are made in the dura mater anteriorly and inferiorly to the superior intercavernous sinus, and the sinus is coagulated and then divided to obtain a direct view of the suprasellar cistern without disturbance by the pituitary gland [37]. In order to coagulate this sinus, the low-profile, single shaft bipolar coagulator is very useful (Figure 3).

The capsular artery, which feeds the capsule (dura mater) of the pituitary, usually is clinically insignificant and arises from the distal and medial portion of the cavernous ICA, commonly supply the sellar dura, and can also proliferate to feed any possible pituitary lesion [20, 21]. These vessels have anastomosis with the contralateral ones at the midline, and have the potential of causing technical difficulty, when dealing with the lesion directly. Zada et al. reported the midline dural filum at the sellar floor, in half of the cases examined. This filum is identified as a strand-like dural extension or as a small vascular dural structure [38]. From our intraoperative observation, active bleeding was identified from the dural filum in many of the cases, which was thought as a result of the blood supply from the anastomosis of the capsular arteries (Figure 4).

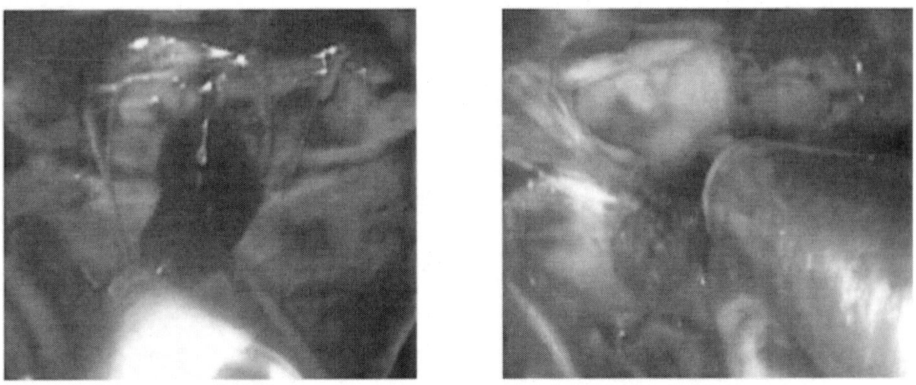

(A) (B)

Figure 3. A. Bleeding from the superior intercavernous sinus is detected when cutting with a micro-knife and B. Coagulating with the single-shaft bipolar coagulator, in order to obtain a direct view of the suprasellar cistern without disturbing the pituitary gland.

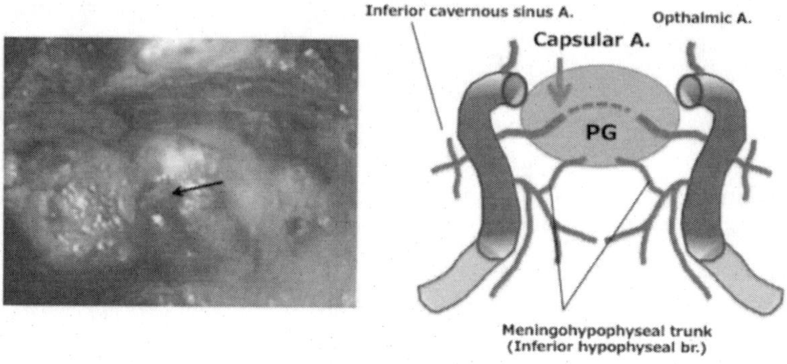

(A) (B)

Figure 4. A. Intraoperative endoscopic observation identifies the dural filum and the bleeding from it (arrow), which was thought to originate from the capsular arteries
B. A scheme of the arterial supply over the dura mater of the sella.

The carotid artery frequently produces a bony prominence into the sphenoid sinus wall, below the floor and along the anterior margin of the sella bilaterally (carotid prominence). Moreover, usually the optic canals protrude into the superolateral portion of the sinus, and the carotid prominence, a diverticulum of the sinus, often projects laterally between the optic canal and the carotid prominence. The dura mater over the medial surface of the cavernous sinus is exposed after removing the mucosa and bone at the lateral wall of the sphenoid sinus. Subsequently, the cavernous ICA is exposed after dural opening of the sella. Rhoton reported that there is an area between optic nerves and carotid arteries where bone thickness less than 0.5 mm from the mucosa of the sphenoid sinus in some of the cases, and meanwhile, no bony thickness is found between these structures in a few cases. The absence of such bony protection over the wall of the cavernous sinus may lead to a serious injury of the cranial nerves and the ICA during the TSS. The bone of the calvaria is often thinner over the carotid arteries than over the anterior margin of the pituitary gland [39]. Pituitary neurosurgeons are required to recognize these bony structures, related to the ICA, in order to avoid unnecessary ICA injury. 3D-CTA with thin slices of bone images is useful as a preoperative evaluation. In our institute, oblique-coronal image (sections perpendicular to the line from lower margin of the nostril to the top of the posterior clinoid process) as "transsphenoidal view" is taken routinely in the preoperative evaluation of the TSS (Figure 5).

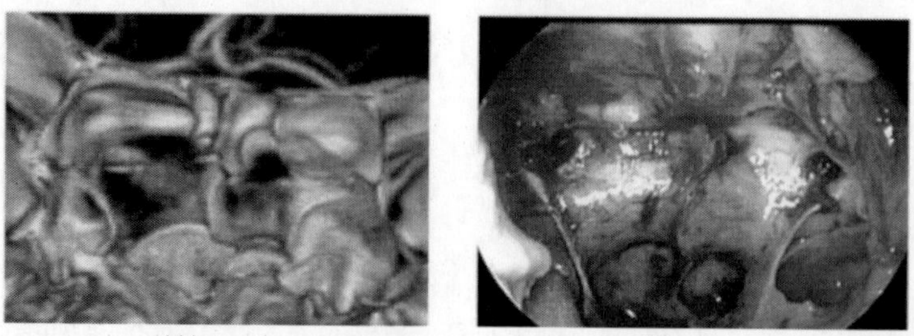

(A) (B)

Figure 5. A. 3D-CT reconstruction of oblique-coronal image (sections perpendicular to the line, from lower margin of the nostril to the top of the posterior clinoid process) as "transsphenoidal view," is obtained as a routine preoperative evaluation of the transsphenoidal surgery for the pituitary tumors B. Intraoperative endoscopic view for the sellar floor and its surroundings after wide sphenoidectomy.

During the TSS approach to the sella, complete midline orientation should be maintained all the time to avoid the injury of the ICAs. Besides, the cavernous portion of the ICA is vulnerable to damage during the exposure of the sella. In the dural phase, in most cases, the injury of ICA can be encountered with the dural opening of the sellar floor. Therefore, careful preoperative evaluation of bony structure in the sphenoid sinus as well as measurement of intercarotid distance is essential to avoid the serious ICA injury [20]. Perdoni et al. reported that the mean intercarotid distances found at the level of tuberculum sellae, sellar floor and clivus were 13.32, 18.00 and 18.90 mm respectively. The distance between ICAs at the tuberculum sellae is narrower than that at the sellar floor. The mean distance found between the ICAs at the level of the 18 mm sellar floor can be considered a “safe zone” to access the hypophysis, and other researchers reported similar value [40]. However, endoscopy is very useful in providing a panoramic view of the depth in the sphenoid sinus, including bilateral carotid prominence and opticocarotid recessus. Fujii et al. reported an interesting study, showing the various parts regarding bony thickness of the posterior wall of the sphenoid sinus. In this chapter, the thickness of the bone of the sphenoid sinus together with the intracranial ICAs was described as follows, the thickness of the bone separated the ICA and sinus is less than 0.5 mm in 88% of cases, and areas of bone defect were present in 8% of them [41]. Therefore, fine maneuvers are required and easy cautery should be avoided as much as possible. In this connection, the vidian canal can be a critical landmark for the petrous and parasellar ICA [12]. Identification of this landmark and the parasellar and paraclival carotid prominence is also critical in staying oriented to the petrous ICA [42]. The bone over these prominences can be carefully and safely removed to have the ICA in view [43].

4. Illustrative Case

A 38-year-old man presented with activity loss and visual field deficits that had been ongoing for the last two months. He had consulted previously another clinic, where a large-sized suprasellar extended tumor was detected with MRI, and was referred to our department where neurological evaluation revealed bitemporal hemianopsia, and endocrinological evaluation showed reduced levels of baseline cortisol, ACTH, and thyroid hormones. MRI showed a calcified solid mass with remarkable suprasellar extension compressing both optic nerves upward (Figure 6A). Extended endoscopic endonasal TSS was performed, and gross total removal of the tumor was achieved and subsequently visual function was remarkably improved. Pathological diagnosis of the surgical specimen was non-functioning pituitary adenoma.

Intraoperatively, during right-sided dissection of the dural phase of the TSS, arterial bleeding emerged from the right ICA, during the removal of the bone at the carotid prominence (Figure 6B). Hemostasis was immediately carried out with continuous aspiration of the hemorrhage without leading to catastrophic hemorrhage. Tumor was successfully removed via extended TSS, and the patient was discharged without any neurological deficit.

However, one month later, follow-up MRI revealed de novo flow void mass at the cavernous ICA (Figure 6C). DSA was performed to demonstrate aneurysm formation at the right cavernous ICA, and it was most suspected to be pseudoaneurysm (Figure 6D). The risk of aneurysm rupture is considered to be quite high. Therefore, in order to prevent rupture the aneurysm, endovascular embolization of parent ICA to occlude pseudoaneurysm and superficial temporal artery-middle cerebral artery anastomosis for cerebral revascularization was successfully performed. Postoperative DSA revealed disappearance of aneurysm and restoration of the blood supply from the ECA to the ICA (Figure 6E, 6F). Cerebral blood flow measurement showed no perfusion defect and MRI showed no ischemic changes on the right hemisphere. The patient left the hospital with no neurological deficit. In a later time-point, residual tumor was managed with conservative treatment.

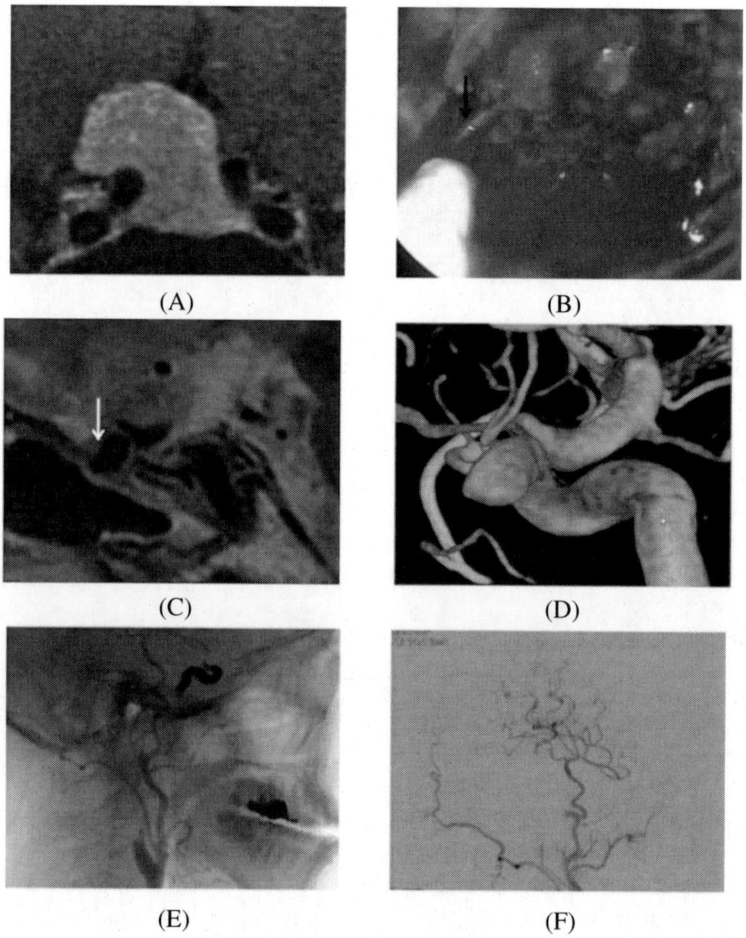

Figure 6. A. Magnetic resonance imaging (MRI) reveals the non-functioning pituitary adenoma extending into the suprasellar cistern B. During right-sided dissection of the dural phase of the transsphenoidal surgery, arterial bleeding emerged from the small branch of the right ICA (arrow) during the removal of the bone at the carotid prominence C. MRI obtained one month later revealed de novo flow void mass with anterior protrusion at the right cavernous ICA D. DSA demonstrated aneurysm formation at the right cavernous ICA, suggesting pseudoaneurysm E. Endovascular embolization of parent ICA to occlude pseudoaneurysm and superficial temporal artery-middle cerebral artery anastomosis for cerebral revascularization was successfully performed. Postoperative DSA revealed disappearance of the aneurysm and F. excellent restoration of the blood supply from the ECA to the ICA.

4.1. Intrasellar Phase

Vascular injury of ICA and its perforator can be encountered on removal of tumor invading into the cavernous sinus or incision of cavernous sinus wall. The ICA sometimes can be tortuous and protrude to the midline [32]. Therefore, ICA injury in this phase frequently leads to the fatal neurological and systemic complications, with published rates, occurring by the use of traditional open approaches ranging from 3% to 8% [44, 45], whereas for standard microscopic TSS for pituitary tumors ranging from 0.2% to 1.4% [5, 18, 20]. On the other hand, cases in which endoscopic endonasal surgery was used, a limited number of ICA injuries were reported, suggesting that these were indeed rare [37, 46, 47]. Moreover, increased use of the endoscopic endonasal approach for skull base lesions can provide wide exposure and visualization of its surroundings with remarkable advancement of the specialized instrumentation [8, 9]. It can allow improved localization and control of the ICAs. However, increased chances of dissection due to endoscopic wide visualization around the ICAs may result in a higher rate of ICA injury [26]. In some cases, the parasellar ICA protrudes inside the adenoma with remarkably tortuosity. Cautious preoperative evaluation is required to prevent fatal ICA injury and remove the tumor efficiently (Figure 7).

Because little or no separation exists between the medial portion of the ICA and the lateral surface of the pituitary gland, blunt instrument should be used for the dissection of the tumor periphery inside the sella. Perforation or laceration of the ICAs in the cavernous sinus represents a very serious problem and unfortunately is a common type of injury in the TSS [21]. In the cases of large invasive pituitary adenomas eroding the skull base, tumors may actually surround the ICAs and, occasionally, may invade the adventitial wall of the vessels, which causes injury to the integrity of the ICAs, when the tumor is removed radically. Dissection of tumors away from the ICAs or displacement of the ICAs in the cavernous sinus during an attempt to achieve hemostasis can lead to thrombosis of the ICAs, resulting in occlusion and occasionally embolization.

Important branches of the ICA, supplying the pituitary gland with blood, arise from the meningohypophyseal trunk, which arises between the carotid segment C4 and C5 and supplies the pituitary gland and the pituitary stalk [20]. This trunk can also proliferate to provide blood supply to pituitary tumors. It divides into three branches, inferior hypophyseal branch, dorsal meningeal branch, and tentorial branch. Inferior hypophyseal branch is the largest of these three, and runs medially to supply the posterior pituitary lobe, appearing as the latter's net of terminal vessels [12, 44].

Direct injury to the carotid artery frequently leads to formation of a pseudoaneurysm, like in our case described above, even if the artery appears to be intact up to the point of maintaining its flow inside the ICAs without further bleeding. According to some authors' reports, the rates of pseudoaneurysm formation after ICA injury are generally very high, and carotid cavernous fistula and thrombosis can occur either [26, 48]. Kai et al. reported a case of a patient who suffered a pseudo ICA aneurysm following TSS, and cerebral angiograms showed a pseudoaneurysm arising from the C4 portion of the left ICA. It was successfully treated with bypass surgery and ICA occlusion involving the pseudoaneurysm using coil embolization. Postoperative angiograms showed that the pseudoaneurysm was completely occluded and the bypass was fully patent. Authors addressed that massive arterial bleeding is encountered during TSS, therefore the patient should be carefully monitored to detect early the development of a pseudoaneurysm. When such an aneurysm is found to have ruptured, interventional surgery has proved effective in the management of this complication [49].

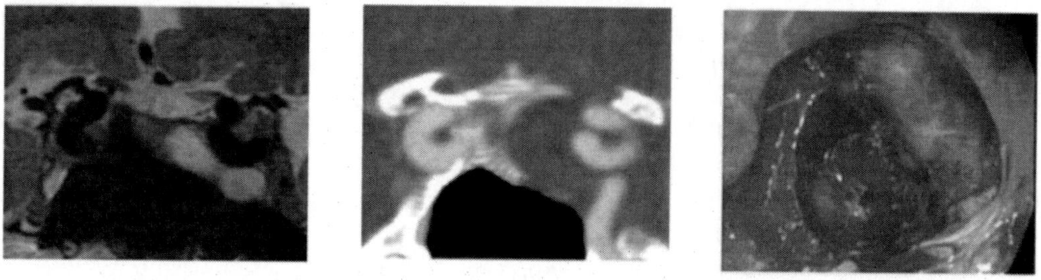

(A) (B) (C)

Figure 7. In a representative case was shown the ICA protrusion into pituitary adenoma, the latter invading into the cavernous sinus. A. Preoperative MRI revealed that the cavernous ICA was involved in the adenoma. An intratumoral cyst was identified B. Preoperative CTA revealed tortuous cavernous ICA protruding into the adenoma C. Intraoperative endoscopic view after opening of the intratumoral cyst clearly showing the tortuous ICA to be adjacent to the cyst.

The ICA can be placed into mechanical spasm by causing dissection around the ICAs or injury to them. TSS complicated by peritumoral hemorrhage is associated with a significant rate of neurological deterioration, due to delayed cerebral vasospasm, and this spasm can clearly cause arterial insufficiency and stroke [26]. Therefore, early recognition and proper management, according to guidelines used for postaneurysmal subarachnoid hemorrhage (SAH), may help to prevent deterioration of outcomes in those patients [19, 50]. Puri et al. reported three cases of developed vasospasm of the intracranial vessels after TSS, with extension of peritumoral hemorrhage into the subarachnoid space, starting as early as postoperative day 5 and continued as late as postoperative day 10. The outcomes of these three cases were not excellent, therefore, they concluded that the vasospasm after TSS associates with the significant risk of neurological morbidity [50]. The timing and distribution of cerebral vasospasm after TSS is similar to that observed in the patients after SAH due to aneurysmal rupture. Therefore, the management of the vasospasm including early vascular imaging evaluation, aggressive hyperdynamic therapy, and neurointerventional procedures should be applied to prevent upcoming ischemic complications [50-52].

4.2. Suprasellar Phase

Pituitary adenoma with remarkable suprasellar extension, in particular, in the case with significant anterior skull base extension, the extended transtuberculum sellae-transplanum sphenoidale approach is required to remove the pituitary adenoma. With this approach, the suprasellar cistern is fully exposed during and after the surgery [53, 54]. Vascular injury, at the level of supraclinoid ICAs and their branches, can be encountered on dissection between the tumor and the vessels involved or adhered to the tumors at the suprasellar, the interpeduncular, and the prepontine cisterns. Thus, ICA, superior hypophyseal artery, anterior and posterior communicating arteries, posterior cerebral artery, basilar artery and its perforators, and superior cerebellar artery, are the vessels affected during the extended endoscopic TSS (Figure 8). Therefore, during the manipulation of the vessels in the suprasellar phase, neurosurgeons should take into consideration the anatomy of the Circle of Willis and its integrity with respect to its collateral flow [48]. Concerning their branches and perforators, special attention should be paid to the injuries of the hypothalamic arteries, but also prevention of a direct hypothalamic trauma, which could cause recent memory disturbance [25]. Once the pituitary stalk can be seen in the subchiasmal spaces, the superior hypophyseal artery and the perforating branches for the inferior surface of the chiasm are apparent, and the posterior communicating artery and its perforator are also detected in the deeper parts of the operative field [10]. During the removal and dissection of the tumors at the TSS, the vascular anatomy around the suprasellar cistern turns to be very complex and is frequently distorted in the cases of large tumors. Besides, above the diaphragm sellae, a circuminfundibular venous plexus exists and can elaborate to feed pituitary lesions. As mentioned above, more expanded approach to obtain wide operative field and excellent visualization, with greater ICAs manipulations and subsequent ICAs' exposure, could increase the risk of vascular injuries [12, 27]. However, in some series, it was indicated that lateral exposure of pituitary tumors enable wider range of endoscope access than microscope and does not lead to a remarkable incidence of injuries overall of for tumors. In the cases of vascular injuries described above, massive bleedings flow into the sphenoid sinus and nasal cavity. However, in this phase, massive bleeding due to the vascular injuries "attacks" hypothalamus, intraventricle and brainstem, causing fatal neurological deteriorations. Besides, once the vascular injury occurs, it is very difficult to control the bleeding, so as to maintain visualization at the deep and narrow operative field, thus higher techniques are required to find the bleeding point [27].

Needless to say, the best strategy for managing ICA injuries during the TSS is prevention. Therefore, considerable preoperative neuroradiological assessment of the course of the ICAs at the suprasellar cistern is essential, as well as tumor and patient risk factors (e.g., ICA involvement with tumor, atherosclerosis in patients with acromegaly or Cushing disease) [27].

When exploring a suprasellar lesion below the optic chiasm such as craniopharyngioma, preservation of chiasm vascularization, fed from the superior hypophyseal artery is partially important, and extended transsphenoidal approach with endoscope offers an excellent visualization, in order to avoid any vascular injury resulting during the dissection between the tumor and the vessels [11]. An avulsion of perforator arising from the P1 portion of posterior cerebral artery during the resection of the part of suprasellar extension of pituitary adenoma may occur, and Kassam et al. used a topical hemostatic agent to control the bleeding, but as a result of this forcible tearing, the patient suffered from severe transient dysphagia [36].

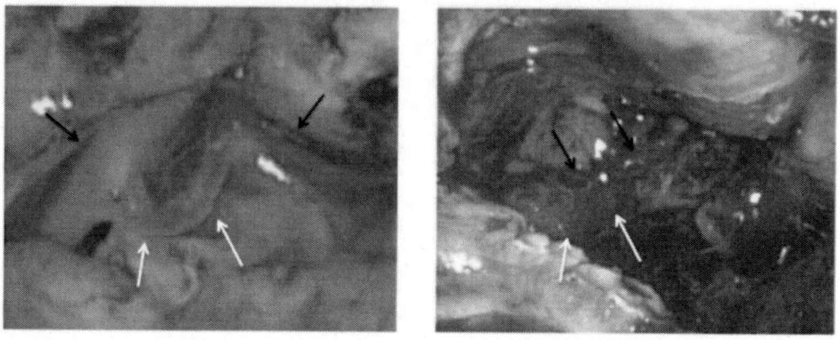

(A) (B)

Figure 8. A. Intraoperative endoscopic view clearly revealed the anterior communicating artery (white arrows) and anterior cerebral arteries (black arrows) and B. the ICA (white arrows) and the superior hypophyseal artery (black arrows) after removal of pituitary adenoma via the extended transtuberculum sellae approach.

5. Procedures and Instrumentations for the Prevention and Control of Bleeding

As mentioned above, the first problem related to this approach concerns the control and prevention of bleeding, especially in the procedures of intra- and supra-sellar phases. Because it is difficult to control massive bleeding coming from the main vessels, as many neurosurgeons addressed, it is important to make all surgical maneuvers under the direct endoscopic view [16].

In particular, in the suprasellar phase, angled 30° or 45° 4 mm rigid endoscope was used to assess the completeness of tumor removal and to help observe the tumor-neurovascular interface clearly [1, 9, 37]. Dusick et al. reported that the use of the micro-Doppler probe for carotid localization before dural opening and angled hook blades for lateral dural opening are potentially simple and effective surgical adjuncts that can help minimize the risk of ICA injury, and recommended for all TSS as routine intraoperative examination (Figure 9)[19, 22]. Kitano and Taneda reported the use of the micro-Doppler probe later during tumor resection within the cavernous sinus, in order to confirm the ICA course, as a technique that they strongly recommended [55]. In addition, the Doppler is more reliable than neuronavigation systems, because it gives real time feedback, whereas the latter are prone to varying degrees of inaccuracy even for fixed cranial-base landmark [2, 56]. Indocyanine green fluorescence shows promise as an intraoperative marker in differentiating pituitary tumors from normal gland, and virtually identifying areas of dural invasion without development of any adverse events [57]. Yano et al. clearly demonstrated intraoperative visualization of the intercavernous sinus before dural incision and the cavernous ICA in the intrasellar phase, and encouraged the improvement of the tumor resection with more safety and effectiveness [35]. Although the indocyanine green fluorescence has not yet become popular in the TSS, these results support the further development of fluorescence-guided tumor resection techniques, since these can lead to improved outcomes, from the aspect of preservation of normal gland, extent of tumor resection, and avoidance of vascular injury. Dusick et al. also addressed that the use of low-profile hook blades for dural opening can reduce the risk of the ICA and other vascular injuries because the blade angle allows the cutting force to be directed away from the intradural surface and back toward the surgeon instead [19]. Rhoton proposed that angled piston-gripped dural scissors could be used for this purpose [58].

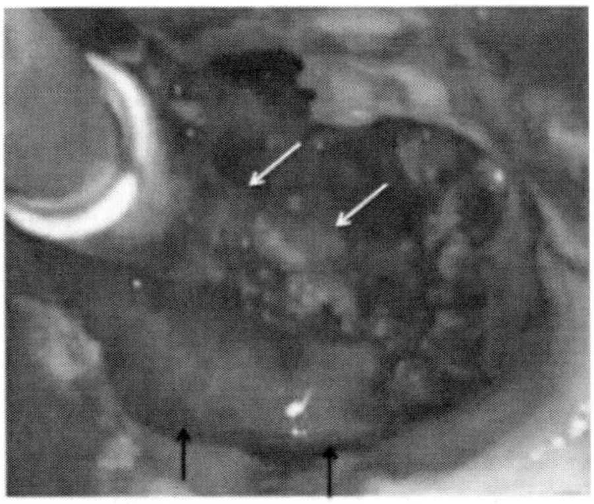

Figure 9. Micro-Doppler probe (black arrow) for localizing carotid artery (white arrow) during the removal of pituitary adenoma, to prevent the ICA injury. The procedure is recommended for every kind of transsphenoidal surgery as routine intraoperative examination.

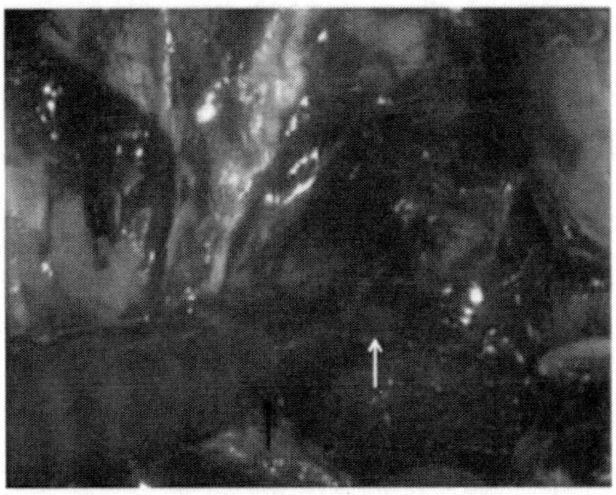

Figure 10. Low-profile bipolar coagulator for the coagulation of vessels of the tumor capsule, making possible the bipolar coagulation of arterial bleeding in narrow spaces.

Low-profile bipolar coagulator, specially designed to work through the nose, with tips up to 0.3 mm and single shaft, are now available for the coagulation of vessels of the tumor capsule, making possible the bipolar coagulation of arterial bleeding in narrow spaces (Figure 10). Vascular clips with an applicator designed for endonasal use can be useful for the bleeding control of the vascular injuries in the naso-sphenoid and sphenoid-planum phase [20]. However, these devices are not practical for the ICA injury for the fear of enlarging the hemorrhage point.

Although the bleeding due to the ICA injury during the TSS is so massive and difficult to control in the operative field, most ICA injuries originated from small puncture wounds that can be fortunately controlled in an initial phase with Gelform and cottonoids. Therefore, when the neurosurgeons encounter the ICA injury during the TSS, they must detect the accurate bleeding point of the ICA injury despite of the difficulty in controlling a massive bleeding at first moment [30]. Following the initial care, the next steps include a two-layered muslin gauze patch or collagen sponge immersed in fibrin glue or BioGlue, and then a fat graft put over the puncture point accurately. Harvested fascia with fibrin glue is strong and adhesive material, which can be applied to the puncture point for the control of the bleeding [59]. But neurosurgeons need to prepare the fascia and fat graft from abdomen or thigh in advance intraoperatively. However, overpacking the repair of injured site should be refrained, because it could result in carotid occlusion and subsequent cerebral infarction. The use of the clip to control the bleeding and preservation of the vessel patency is reported in some cases [20]. Direct suturing repair for the larger laceration of the vessel is basically not practical, because suturing technique is quite difficult and time consuming at that serious situation.

Unfortunately, if the arterial bleeding from the injured vessels is not controlled finally, trapping of the vessels with aneurysm clip is applied to the injured site or the parent artery, thus "sacrificing" the vessels. However, recent advancement of endovascular surgery has changed the methods to repair the vascular injuries [28]. As some authors have already described and vascular group of our institute performs, urgent cerebral angiography should be carried out in the operating room. After the detection of the extravasation and presentation of a pseudoaneurysm or carotid cavernous fistula, balloon is approached to the injured site and inflated to occlude the parent vessels [28, 29, 48]. After the repair of the injured site, ICAs are supposed to be involved in most of the cases, it is needed to confirm that the injured site is successfully repaired after deflation of the balloon and collateral circulation via the Circle of Willis in the case of ICA occlusion should be assessed [30]. With the appearance of pseudoaneurysm or carotid cavernous fistula, endovascular treatment, involving ICA embolization, should be immediately achieved [31, 60, 61]. In this case, since the collateral circulation is not excellent via anterior communicating artery or posterior communicating artery, the ECA-ICA bypass surgery, including superficial temporal artery-middle cerebral artery anastomosis, high flow bypass using arterial graft, should be immediately performed to prevent the subsequent ischemic complication due to the ICA embolization [49]. Even if the result of the angiography is normal after the vascular injury, it is strongly recommended to repeat DSA or 3D-CTA within five days to detect the delayed occurrence of any possible pseudoaneurysm. MRI should be also carried out and evaluated, whether cerebral infarction emerges in the case of the ICA embolization, and CT scan should be also obtained immediately after endovascular procedure, whether SAH occurred, which can lead to clinically significant cerebral vasospasm [50, 62].

References

[1] Halvorsen, H, Ramm-Pettersen, J, Josefesen, R, Ronning, P, Reinlie, S, Meling, T, et al. Surgical complications after transsphenoidal microscopic and endoscopic surgery for pituitary adenoma: a consecutive series of 506 procedures. *Acta Neurochir (Wien)*, 2014;156:441-449.

[2] Central Brain Tumor Registry of the United States: Primary Brain Tumors in the United States Statistical Report 1998-2002. Hinsdale II, CBTRUS, 2005 (http://www.cbtrus.org/reports/2005-2006/2006report. pdf).

[3] Ramakrishman, VR, Suh, JD, Lee, JY, O'Malley, BW, Grady, MS, Palmer, JN. Sphenoid sinus anatomy and suprasellar extension of pituitary tumors. *J Neurosurg*, 2013;119:669-674.

[4] Surawicz, TS, McCarthy, BJ, Kupelian, V, Jukich, PJ, Bruner, JM, Davis. FG. Descriptive epidemiology of primary brain and CNS tumors: results from the Central Brain Tumor Registry of the United States, 1990-1994. *Neuro Oncol*, 1999;1:14-25.

[5] Ciric, I, Ragin, A, Baumgartner, C, Pierce, D. Complications of transsphenoidal surgery: results of a national survey, review of the literature, and personal experience. *Neurosurgery*, 1997;40:225-236.

[6] Gondim, JA, Almeida, JP, Albuquerque, LA, Schops, M, Gomes, E, Ferraz, T, et al. Endoscopic endonasal approach for pituitary adenoma: surgical complications in 301 patients. *Pituitary*, 2011;14:174-183.

[7] Berker, M, Hazer, DB, Yücel, T, Gürlek, A, Cila, A, Aldur, M, Onerci, M. Complications of endoscopic surgery of the pituitary adenomas: analysis of 570 patients and review of the literature. *Pituitary*, 2012;15:288-300.

[8] Schwartz, TH, Stieg, PE, Anand, VK. Endoscopic transsphenoidal pituitary surgery with intraoperative magnetic resonance imaging. *Neurosurgery*, 2006;58(Suppl 1): ONS44-51.

[9] Saeki, N, Murai, H, Hasegawa, Y, Horiguchi, K, Hanazawa, T. Endoscopic endonasal transsphenoidal surgery for pituitary adenomas. *No Shinkei Geka*, 2007;35:971-985.

[10] Cavallo, LM, de Divitiis, O, Aydin, S, Messina, A, Esposito, F, Iaconetta, G, et al. Extended endoscopic endonasal transsphenoidal approach to the suprasellar area: anatomic considerations--part 1. *Neurosurgery*, 2007;61(Suppl 3):24-33.

[11] de Divitiis, E, Cavallo, LM, Cappabianca, P, Esposito, F. Extended endoscopic endonasal transsphenoidal approach for the removal of suprasellar tumors *Neurosurgery*, 2007;60:46-58.

[12] Kassam, A, Snyderman, CH, Mintz, A, Gardner, P, Carrau, RL. Expanded endonasal approach, the rostrocaudal axis. Part I. Crista galli to the sella turcica. *Neurosurg Focus*, 2005;19:E3.

[13] Cohen-Gadol, AA, Laws, ER, Spencer, DD, De Salles, AA. The evolution of Harvey Cushing's surgical approach to pituitary tumors from transsphenoidal to transfrontal. *J Neurosurg*, 2005;103:372-377.

[14] Cushing, H. Papers relating to the pituitary body, hypothalamus and parasympathetic nervous system. Charles C. Thomas. Springfield: IL, 1932.

[15] Schloffer, H. Erfolgreiche Operation eines Hypophysentumors auf nasalem Wege (In German). *Wien Klin Wochenschr*, 1907;20:621-624.

[16] Guiot, G. Transsphenoidal approach in surgical treatment of pituitary adenomas: General principals and indications in non-functioning adenomas. In Kohler PO, Ross GT (editors): Diagnosis and Treatment of pituitary tumors: Proceedings of a conference. International Congress Series. Excerpta Medica, Amsterdam, 1973, pp. 159-179.

[17] Hardy, J. Transsphenoidal hypophysectomy. *J Neurosurg*, 1971;34:582-594.

[18] Fatami, N, Dusick, JR, de Paiva Neto, MA, Kelly, DF. The endonasal microscopic approach for pituitary adenomas and other parasellar tumors: a 10-year experience. *Neurosurgery*, 2008;63(Suppl 2):244-256.

[19] Dusick, JR, Esposito, F, Malkasian, D, Kelly, DF. Avoidance of carotid artery injuries in transsphenoidal surgery with the Doppler probe and micro-hook blades. *Neurosurgery*, 2007;60(Suppl 2):322-328.

[20] Laws, ER. Jr. Vascular complications of transsphenoidal surgery. *Pituitary*, 1999;2: 163-170.

[21] Oskouian, RJ, Kelly, DF, Laws, ER. Jr. Vascular injury and transsphenoidal surgery. *Front Horm Res*, 2006;34:256-278.

[22] Yamasaki, T, Moritake, K, Hatta, J, Nagai, H. Intraoperative monitoring with pulse Doppler ultrasonography in transsphenoidal surgery: technique application. *Neurosurgery*, 1996;38:95-98.

[23] Mortini, P, Losa, M, Bazaghi, R, Boari, N, Giovanelli, M. Results of transsphenoidal surgery in a large series of patients with pituitary adenoma. *Neurosurgery*, 2005;56: 1222-1233.

[24] Oskoulan, RJ, Laws, ER. Vascular complications in transsphenoidal surgery. Presented at the annual meeting of the American Association of Neurological Surgeons, May 1-6. *J Neurosurg*, 2004;100:806.

[25] Raymond, J, Hardy, J, Czepko, R, Roy, D. Arterial injuries in transsphenoidal surgery for pituitary adenoma: the role of angiography and endovascular treatment. *AJNR Am J Neuroradiol*, 1997;18:655-665.

[26] Gadhinglajkar, SV, Sreedhar, R, Bhattacharya, RN. Carotid artery injury during transsphenoidal resection of pituitary tumor: anesthesia perspective. *J Neurosurg Anesthesiol*, 2003;15:323-326.

[27] Gardner, PA, Tormenti, MJ, Pant, H, Fernandes-Miranda, JC, Snyderman, CH, Horowitz, MB. Carotid artery injury during endoscopic endonasal skull base surgery: incidence and outcomes. *Neurosurgery*, 2013;73(Suppl 2):261-270.

[28] Cinar, C, Bozkaya, H, Parildar, M, Oran, I. Endovascular management *Interv Neuroradiol*, 2013;19:102-109.

[29] Dolenc, VV, Lipovsek, M, Slokan, S. Traumatic aneurysm and carotid-cavernous fistula following transsphenoidal approach to a pituitary adenoma: treatment by transcranial operation. *Br J Neurosurg*, 1999;13:185-188.

[30] Ghatge, SB, Modi, DB. Treatment of ruptured ICA during transsphenoidal surgery. Two different endovascular strategies in two cases. *Interv Neuroradiol*, 2010;16:31-37.

[31] Kim, BM, Jeon, P, Kim, DJ, Kim, DI, Suh, SH, Park, KY. Jostent covered stent *J Neurosurg*, 2015;122:1223-1228.

[32] Harris, FS, Rhoton, AL. Anatomy of the cavernous sinus. A microsurgical study. *J Neurosurg*, 1976;45:169-180.

[33] Nagatani, T, Wakabayashi, T. Endoscopic endonasal transsphenoidal approach for the removal of pituitary adenomas based on basis of microsurgical anatomy. *Jpn J Neurosurg (Tokyo)*, 2013;22:362-369.

[34] Rejas Ugena, E, Trinidad Ruiz, G, Alvarez Domínguez, J, Carrasco Claver, F, Pino Rivero, V, Blasco Huelva, A. Utility of the surgical treatment for severe epistaxis by endoscopic approach of sphenopalatine and ethmoidal arteries. *Acta Otorrinolaringol Esp*, 2006;57:228-234.

[35] Yano, S, Hide, S, Shinoshima, N, Kuratsu, J. Usefulness of indocyanin green fluorescence endoscopy in endoscopic skull base surgery. *Jpn J Neurosurg (Tokyo)*, 2015;24:85-91.

[36] Kassam, AB, Prevedello, DM, Carrau, RL, Snyderman, CH, Thomas, A, Gardner, P, et al. Endoscopic endonasal skull base *J Neurosurg*, 2011;114:1544-1568.
[37] Dusick, JR, Esposito, F, Kelly, DF, Cohan, P, de Salles, A, Becker, DP, et al. The extended direct endonasal transsphenoidal approach for nonadenomatous suprasellar tumors. *J Neurosurg*, 2005;102:832-841.
[38] Zada, G, Kim, AH, Governale, LS, Laws, ER. Midline filum of the sellar dura, a useful landmark during endoscopic transsphenoidal pituitary surgery. *Neurosurgery*, 2010; 67(Suppl 2):391-394.
[39] Rhoton, AL. Diagnosis and management of pituitary tumors: Anatomy of the pituitary gland and sellar region. In Thapar K, Kovacs K, Scheithauer B, Lloyd RV (editors): Diagnosis and Management of Pituitary Tumors. Springer Science+Business Media New York 2001, pp 13-40.
[40] Perondi, GE, Isolan, GR, de Aguiar, PH, Stefani, MA, Falcetta, EF. Endoscopic anatomy of sellar region. *Pituitary*, 2013;16:251-259.
[41] Fujii, K, Chanmbers, SM, Rhoton, AL Jr. Neurovascular relationships of the sphenoid sinus. A microsurgical study. *J Neurosurg*, 1979;50:31-39.
[42] Vescan, AD, Snyderman, CH, Carrau, RL, Mintz, A, Gardner, P, Branstetter, B 4th, et al. Vidian canal: analysis and relationship to the internal carotid artery. *Laryngoscope*, 2007;117:1338-1342.
[43] Kassam, AB, Vescan, AD, Carrau, RL, Prevedello, DM, Gardner, P, Mintz, AH, et al. Expanded endonasal approach: vidian canal as a landmark to the petrous internal carotid artery. *J Neurosurg*, 2008;108:177-183.
[44] Banerji, D, Behari, S, Tyagi, I, Pandey, T, Jain, VK, Chhabra, DK. Extended frontobasal approach to the skull base. *Neurol India*, 2001;49:253-261.
[45] Inamasu, J, Guiot, BH. Iatrogenic carotid artery injury in neurosurgery. *Neurosurg Rev*, 2005;28:239-247.
[46] Cavallo, LM, Messina, A, Esposito, F, de Divitiis, O, Dal Fabbro, M, de Divitiis, E, et al. Skull base reconstruction in the extended endoscopic transsphenoidal approach for suprasellar lesions. *J Neurosurg*, 2007;107:713-720.
[47] Dehdashti, AR, Ganna, A, Witterick, I, Gentili, F. Expanded endoscopic endonasal approach for anterior cranial base and suprasellar lesions: indications and limitations. *Neurosurgery*, 2009;64:677-689.
[48] Vanninen, RL, Manninen, HI, Rinne, J. Intrasellar iatrogenic carotid pseudoaneurysm, endovascular treatment with a polytetrafluoroethylene-covered stent. *Cardiovasc Intervent Radiol*, 2003;26:298-301.
[49] Kai, Y, Hamada, J, Nishi, T, Ushio, Y. Successful treatment *No Shinkei Geka*, 2001;29: 241-245.
[50] Puri, AS, Zada, G, Zarzour, H, Laws, E, Frerichs, K. Cerebral vasospasm after transsphenoidal resection of pituitary macroadenomas: report of 3 cases and review of the literature. *Neurosurgery*, 2012;71(Suppl 1):173-181.
[51] Kasliwal, MK, Srivastava, R, Sinha, S, Kale, SS, Sharma, BS. Vasospasm after transsphenoidal pituitary surgery: a case report and review of the literature. *Neurol India*, 2008;56:81-83.
[52] Nishioka, H, Ito, H, Haraoka, J. Cerebral vasospasm following transsphenoidal removal of a pituitary adenoma. *Br J Neurosurg*, 2001;15:41-47.

[53] Cappabianca, P, Cavallo, LM, Esposito, F, De Divitiis, O, Messina, A, De Divitiis, E. Extended endoscopic endonasal approach to the midline skull base *Adv Tech Stand Neurosurg*, 2008;33:151-199.

[54] Kitano, M, Taneda, M, Shimono, T, Nakao, Y. Extended transsphenoidal approach for surgical management *J Neurosurg*, 2008;108:26-36.

[55] Kitano, M, Taneda, M. Extended transsphenoidal approach with submucosal posterior ethmoidectomy for parasellar tumors *J Neurosurg*, 2001;94:999-1004.

[56] Yamasaki, T, Moritake, K, Nagai, H, Kimura Y. Integration of ultrasonography and endoscopy into transsphenoidal surgery with a "picture-in-picture" viewing system--Technical note. *Neurol Med Chir (Tokyo)*, 2002;42:275-278.

[57] Litvack, ZN, Zada, G, Laws, ER. Indocyanine green fluorescence endoscopy for visual differentiation of pituitary tumor surrounding structures. *J Neurosurg*, 2012;116:935-941.

[58] Rhoton, AL. Jr. The sellar region. *Neurosurgery*, 2002;51(Suppl 4) :S335-374.

[59] Couldwell, WT, Weiss, MH, Rabb, C, Liu, JK, Apfelbaum, RI, Fukushima, T. Variations on the standard transsphenoidal approach to the sellar region, with emphasis on the extended approaches and parasellar approaches: surgical experience in 105 cases. *Neurosurgery*, 2004;55:539-550.

[60] Dolenc, VV, Lipovsek, M, Slokan, S. Traumatic aneurysm and carotid-cavernous fistula following transsphenoidal approach to a pituitary adenoma: treatment by transcranial operation. *Br J Neurosurg*, 1999;13:185-188.

[61] Fukushima, T, Maroon, JC. Repair of carotid artery perforations during transsphenoidal surgery. *Surg Neurol*, 1998;50:174-177.

[62] Matsuno, A, Yoshida, S, Basugi, N, Itoh, S, Tanaka, J. Severe subarachnoid hemorrhage during transsphenoidal surgery for pituitary adenoma. *Surg Neurol*, 1993; 39:276-278.

In: Pituitary Adenoma
Editor: Dimitrios N. Kanakis

ISBN: 978-1-63484-985-2

Chapter 13

TRANSSPHENOIDAL SURGERY FOR PITUITARY ADENOMAS GUIDED BY INTRAOPERATIVE MAGNETIC RESONANCE IMAGING (IMRI)

Sven Berkmann*[*], *MD, and Javier Fandino, MD
Department of Neurosurgery, Kantonsspital Aarau, Tellstrasse, Aarau, Switzerland

ABSTRACT

Transsphenoidal surgery is the first-line treatment in the majority of symptomatic sellar tumors. The goals are cure of endocrinological syndromes (e.g., acromegaly), neurological deficits (e.g., optic chiasm compression syndrome), restoration of pituitary function and long-term tumor control. With the evolution of the transsphenoidal approach, several tools like the X-ray intensifier, cisternography, sonography, computed tomography, the endoscope, and the intraoperative MRI (iMRI) have been used to increase visualization of the tumor and thereby to make surgery safer and to increase the extent of resection.

The iMRI has been used since 20 years in combination with a microscopic or endoscopic approach and numerous studies have shown the efficacy of iMRI-controlled transsphenoidal surgery, as well as identified the indications and drawbacks of the various setups and subtypes. Based on our own peer-reviewed clinical studies and by reviewing the literature we will present critical insights in the use of this fascinating technology for transsphenoidal pituitary adenoma surgery.

Keywords: pituitary adenoma, transsphenoidal surgery, intraoperative MRI

1. INTRODUCTION

Transsphenoidal surgery is the first-line treatment in the majority of symptomatic sellar tumors. The goals are cure of endocrinological syndromes (e.g., acromegaly), relief of

[*] Corresponding author: Sven Berkmann, MD, Department of Neurosurgery, Kantonsspital Aarau, Tellstrasse, 5001 Aarau, Switzerland, +41 62 838 41 41, E-mail: sven.berkmann@ksa.ch.

neurological deficits (e.g., optic chiasm compression syndrome), restoration of pituitary function and long-term remission. Nevertheless, due to the narrow access to the *sella turcica* and its adjacent compartments, the rate of unsuspected – and further resectable - tumor remnants after surgery may be high. While gross total resection (GTR) of hormonally active pituitary adenomas is mandatory for cure of endocrinological syndromes, most remnants of hormonally inactive tumors may regrow within 5 years after resection and eventually cause local compression symptoms again [1]. Nevertheless, aggressive probing for tumor remnants may lead to severe complications due to the proximity of the optic nerves, the internal carotid arteries and the cavernous sinus. Visualization of the tumor and safe exploration of the surgical site is therefore the key to successful transsphenoidal surgery.

Lars Leksell advocated the philosophy that no technique in neurosurgery could be too refined, particularly in reference to the ability to localize lesions [2]. This is especially true for pituitary surgery. The first transsphenoidal tumor resection was performed by Hermann Schloffer (1886-1937) on March 16th 1907 in Innsbruck, Austria [3]. After a number of modifications culminating in the description of the oronasal rhinoseptal approach with a sublabial gingival incision by Albert Edward Halstead (1869-1926), Harvey Cushing (1869-1939) adopted this technique and performed 231 such procedures from 1910 to 1925. Ultimately Cushing abandoned the transsphenoidal approach. He reverted to the transcranial technique because he believed that the optical structures may thereby be more readily decompressed. Ultimately, this was a direct consequence of the non-existing possibility to sufficiently visualize the surgical site by the transsphenoidal approach. Due to Cushing's influence at the time, many surgeons followed his example. The transsphenoidal approach to the pituitary was mostly neglected for 40 years and it was only in the middle of the 60s with the birth of micro-neurosurgery and the introduction of the operating microscope when the renaissance of the transsphenoidal approach began.

Various tools for a better visualization of the tumor and its adjacent structures and for tailoring the transsphenoidal approach have been introduced during the subsequent 50 years. Principally, the further evolution of pituitary surgery was paralleled by the improvement of intraoperative imaging [4, 5]. In 1965 Hardy introduced the use of radiofluoroscopy in combination with the operating microscope [6]. Nevertheless, as the X-ray intensifier only allowed depiction of the skull base and the metal instruments introduced, there were further attempts in conjunction with cisternography to assess the suprasellar extension of the tumor [7]. In 1993 intraoperative computerized tomography was proposed as a more progressive tool to appraise the extent of tumor resection. At this time it was suggested that intraoperative CT scanning would probably remain the preeminent modality for conventional intraoperative image-guided surgery because of the enhanced access to the operating field and its instrument compatibility as compared to the iMRI, which almost evolved at the same time [8]. Nevertheless, use of radiation, fixed slice orientation, and especially the poor soft-tissue contrast limited the benefit [9]. Other attempts [10-12] to further localize the surrounding anatomical structures included ultrasonography and the color Doppler system, however, none of these tools reached a high level of acceptance as an independent method to assess the extent of resection [13-15].

During the past 15 years the evolution of image-guided neuronavigation based on preoperative datasets referenced to the patient's head began to replace intraoperative fluoroscopy for orientation in the surgical site more and more [16-21]. Because one of the main reasons for incomplete tumor resection is poor exposure of the sellar space, neuronavigation facilitated the optimal tailoring of the approach. In conjunction with intraoperative imaging, real-time assessment of the grade of resection became possible because the neuronavigation datasets could be immediately updated with the new footage.

The intraoperative MRI (iMRI) has been used since 1994 [22]. In the subsequent years a growing number of departments all over the world adapted MRI systems to their operating theaters. In transsphenoidal surgery it allows a quick evaluation of the extent of tumor resection, an update of images for intraoperative navigation, and the exclusion of imminent complications (e.g., hemorrhage or ischemia), before the site is closed. Numerous studies have shown the efficacy of iMRI-controlled transsphenoidal surgery, as well as identified indications and drawbacks. In the first part of this chapter an overview of the different setups and subtypes of iMRI with respect to their pros and cons will be given. In the second part, today's experience in iMRI-controlled transsphenoidal surgery for pituitary adenomas with respect to the different pathological entities will be reviewed, before a critical review of the arguments in favor of and against the use of iMRI is finally given.

2. Technical Systems and Operating Room Setups

The basic problems to be solved when using an iMRI are the following:

1. Electromagnetic interaction and compatibility of electrical devices used by the surgeon and the anesthesiologist
2. Ferromagnetic interaction between the surgical instruments and the scanner, which may not only influence image quality, but also the microsurgical handling of the devices and the safety of the patient and the operation personnel
3. Electromagnetic shielding to avoid loss of image quality caused by exogenous fields
4. Access to the operating field and possibilities for patient positioning. All these problems are directly correlated with the field-strength of the MR-scanner.

Therefore, two basic concepts for the use of iMRI have evolved: operating within the magnet and its associated field or moving the patient to the magnet only for scanning (i.e., "two room concept"). Commonly, the setups which make it possible to operate within the field are using field strengths up to 0.5 Tesla (T). These so-called 'low-field setups' are markedly different from 'high-field setups,' which use magnetic fields from 1.5 to 3 T.

The first truly incorporated MR scanner within an operating room was the Magnetic Resonance Therapy Unit at Brigham and Women's Hospital in Boston, Massachusetts, introduced in 1994 [22]. It was a collaborative project between Peter Black as Head of the Neurosurgical Department, Marvin Fried, Director of the Department of Otorhinolaryngology, and Ferenc Jolesz of the Department of Radiology, and engineers at General Electric Medical Systems (Milwaukee, Wisconsin). In the late 1980s, the closed-configuration of conventional MRI systems prohibited access to the patient, therefore, fundamental changes in magnet and coil design and display methods were necessary. This resulted in a "double donut"-shaped scanner, with a magnetic field of 0.5 T in the space between the two "donut" rings (GE 0.5-T Signa SP). The surgeon was standing in the limited space between the two superconductive magnet coils. Along with the design of the iMRI, many commonly used tools had to be adapted: ferromagnetic surgical instruments were replaced by titanium, the Mayfield head holder device was remodeled from high performance plastic, the power-drill used for e.g., modeling the craniotomy flap was redesigned by the Midas Rex Corporation (Medtronic, Minneapolis, Minnesota) as a non-ferromagnetic tool, the ferromagnetic joints of the operating microscope were replaced by plastic, and finally a bipolar coagulator not interfering with the magnetic field was introduced. Anesthesia and patient monitoring devices that did not emit electronic noise were at that time already in use for performing pediatric MR imaging under anesthesia and could be installed in the iMRI suite.

After the potential of the iMRI and its benefits became obvious, the next step was to optimize its availability and to develop cost-effective units. In Erlangen, Germany, Rudolf Fahlbusch, Michael Buchfelder, and Christopher Nimsky from the neurosurgical Department first developed together with their colleagues from Heidelberg and Siemens Medical (Siemens AG, Erlangen, Germany) a 0.2 T scanner (0.2-T Magnetom Open™, Siemens Medical solutions) in 1996, before moving on to a 1.5 T scanner (Magnetom Sonata Maestro Class™, Siemens Medical Solutions) in 2002. Integral to the new high-field concept was the possibility of simultaneous intraoperative imaging and neuronavigation. The setup was based on a rotatable surgical table (Trumpf, Saalfeld, Germany), which could be locked into various positions and adapted to the scanner to allow for a special surgical MR tabletop. MR-compatible monitoring was installed for control of anesthesia and for wireless 2.4 GHz data transfer from the radiofrequency-shielded cabin. For intraoperative navigation, the patient's head was fixed in a 5-pin head holder (Noras MRI products, Hoechberg, Germany) with an integrated 8-channel coil. This allowed to directly update the intraoperatively acquired datasets for neuronavigation without additional referencing. One shortcoming of this system is that patients can only be positioned in the prone or supine position. The neuronavigation datasets were used in conjunction with a navigation microscope placed inside the 0.5 mT zone. As opposed to the image quality generated by low-field-iMR systems, the quality obtained by high-field-strength scanners compared well to regular diagnostic MR-images. In addition, functional MRI, MR spectroscopy and fiber tracking became possible during surgery. For a regular T1- or T2-scan including the draping the scanning time amounts to about 10 to 15 minutes.

While various other low-field settings have been described [23, 24], one of the most widely used units are the PoleStar™ systems (Medtronic Navigation, Louisville, Colorado). This low-field setup was driven by the Israeli surgeon Moshe Hadani and his group and introduced in 2001 [25]. The initial model PoleStar™ N-10 iMRI consisted of a 0.12 T magnet that required only modest remodeling of the operating room. The actual model, PoleStar™ N20, comes with a 0.15 T-magnet (Figure 1).

The portable device is stored within a small garage next to the operating room and at need installed beneath the operating table. Thus, in contrary to a permanently installed scanner, the use of the operating theater is not dominated by the iMRI. A neuronavigation system (StealthStation TREON™, Medtronic) is integrated in the system, which detects not only the position of the patient but also of the iMR-scanner. During the scans radiofrequency shielding is maintained by a foldable tent (StarShield™, Medtronic), which encloses the magnet and the whole operating table. Although the surgical field is directly above the scanner, the use of ferromagnetic tools is still possible due to the comparably low field strength. Nevertheless, the power drill and the patient monitoring devices still have to be MR-compatible. The titanium head clamp and the space within the magnet allow prone, supine and lateral positioning. As in the high field-setup, the scanning time including the draping amounts to about 15 minutes. One of the major drawbacks compared to the high field-iMRI is the low contrast and resolution of the images when used for pituitary surgery. The optic chiasm, the pituitary stalk and the internal carotid arteries may be readily identified, while invasive tumor in the cavernous sinus may be difficult to differentiate from the venous caverns [26, 27].

3. Outcome of iMRI-Controlled Transsphenoidal Surgery

Since 1994 a growing number of studies addressing the outcome of iMRI-controlled transsphenoidal surgery have been published [1, 26-56]. An overview of the literature is given in *Tables 1* and *2*. While earlier studies mostly aimed at feasibility and technical issues and presented patient groups with mixed pathologies [28, 46], the end points of recent studies have become more specific in reporting the outcome of the individual pituitary tumor pathologies, and in assessing the course of symptoms and the long-term outcome [1, 26, 47].

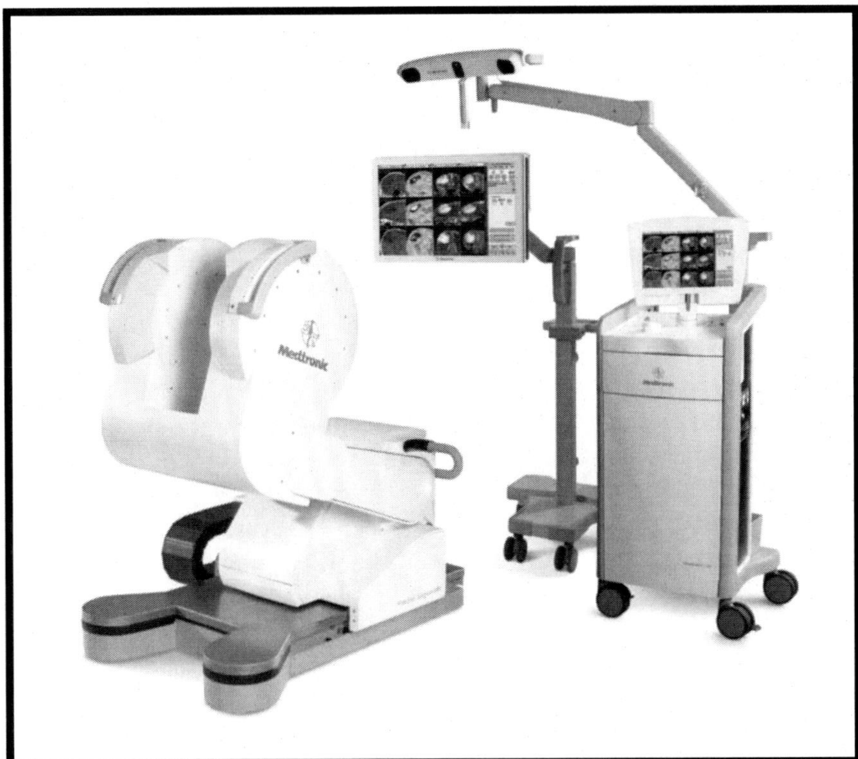

Figure 1. The PoleStar™ N20 unit with integrated neuronavigation system S7. (picture provided by courtesy of Medtronic Switzerland).

3.1. Nonfunctioning Pituitary Adenoma

Transsphenoidal surgery is the first-line treatment in symptomatic hormonally inactive pituitary tumors and histological specimens will show nonfunctioning or so-called silent secreting pituitary adenomas (NFA) in most cases. Serial imaging by MRI is mandatory as a postoperative follow-up routine, as there are no other markers (such as serum hormone levels) to hint for regrowth of tumor remnants or recurrence after GTR before local compression symptoms occur. Roelfsema et al. [57] found a recurrence rate for NFA after transsphenoidal surgery of 0.022 patients/year by analyzing 31 studies. Kaplan-Meier analyses show relapse rates of 23, 47 and 68% at 5, 10 and 15 years, respectively [58].

Therefore, GTR is the highest goal of surgery for NFA. Nevertheless, due to invasive or expansive tumor growth or lack of intraoperative visualization of unsuspected remnants, the final GTR rate may not be as high as could be preoperatively expected. The main reason for a reoperation in these patients is regrowth of tumor remnants [56. 58]. While residual tumors may shrink spontaneously during the first months after surgery, virtually all of the visible remnants do grow during long-term follow-up [1, 59]. The majority of regrowths is detected within 5 years after surgery, however, compared to hormonally active adenomas, up to 50% of these tumors may recur later [1, 57]. Because of invasive growth into the cavernous sinus or the clivus and because of abundant supra- and retrosellar tumor masses surgical resection is sometimes intended to remain incomplete, however if a complete resection seems possible, it is very unfortunate for the patient if tumor is left behind due to limited visualization during surgery. Consequently, this may provoke the discussion whether to re-operate in a patient who has possibly become asymptomatic, or whether to embark for lifelong high-frequent screening for regrowth.

This is the place for using the iMRI in NFA because, as will be shown, it significantly reduces the rate of unexpected remnants. While there was a tendency in the earlier phase to treat as many patients as possible with iMRI-control to gather further experience, latter studies are based on the thereby evolved indications for its use. These criteria include e.g., invasive tumor growth, history of previous transsphenoidal surgery and awkwardly irregular (e.g., dumbbell) shaped tumors. A selection for the use of iMRI in pituitary surgery is often necessary, because of the eventually high caseload of pituitary patients in large centers compared to the operating time capacity in the iMRI, which may also be used, for example, for glioma and epilepsy surgery.

Generally, acquisition of iMRI controls is decided in case GTR is supposed or if incomplete resection is suspected but no further removal seems safely possible. As with several study-designs on the use of intraoperative diagnostics, one may argue that the possibility of visualizing the tumor with iMRI may have weakened the effort to probe for occult remnants. Nevertheless, as control scans are generally time consuming and a final scan before the site is closed is mandatory, most surgeons may avoid supplementary scans. In most cases 2 to 3 scans are needed: the first scan before resection is started as a baseline benchmark for comparison, the second to look for remnants and an eventual third to ensure removal of these remnants.

Table 1. Results of iMRI-controlled pituitary surgery with low-field setups

Author	Ref.	Year	Diagnosis	n	iMRI setup	Field strength (T)	Remnant on 1st iMRI (n)	Additional resection (n)	GTR (n)	Increase of GTR rate by iMRI
Steinmeier et al.	109	1998	misc	16	Siemens Magnetom	0.2	6 (38%)	5 (83%)	13 (81%)	19%, p = NS
Martin et al.	75	1999	misc adenoma	5	General Electric Signa SP	0.5	2 (40%)	2 (100%)	4 (80%)	20%, p = NS
Bohinski et al.	26	2001	misc adenoma	29	Hitachi AIRIS II vertical-field	0.3	19 (66%)	19 (100%)	25 (86%)	52%, p < 0.0001
Fahlbusch et al.	41	2001	misc adenoma	44	Siemens Magnetom	0.2	25 (57%)	15 (60%)	31 (70%)	27%, p = 0.0087
Schwartz et al.	100	2006	misc adenoma	15	Polestar N-10	0.12	3 (20%)	3 (100%)	15 (100%)	20%, p = NS
Ahn et al.	3	2008	misc adenoma	51	Polestar N-20	0.15	13 (25%)	13 (100%)	48 (94%)	20%, p = 0.0062
Gerlach et al.	46	2008	misc adenoma	40	Polestar N-20	0.15	26 (65%)	7 (27%)	15 (38%)	3%, p = NS
Wu et al.	121	2009	misc adenoma	55	Polestar N-20	0.15	23 (42%)	23 (100%)	46 (84%)	26%, p = 0.0029
Baumann et al.	11	2010	giant adenoma	6	Polestar N-20	0.15	5 (83%)	5 (100%)	3 (50%)	33%, p = NS
Bellut et al.	14	2010	acromegaly	37	Polestar N-20	0.15	8 (21%)	8 (100%)	38 (97%)	18%, p = 0.0141
Theodosopoulos et al.	115	2010	misc adenoma	27	Hitachi AIRIS II vertical-field	0.3	9 (33%)	4 (44%)	19 (70%)	7%, p = NS
Vitaz et al.	118	2011	misc	100	General Electric Signa SP	0.5	41 (41%)	41 (41%)	76 (76%)	35%, 0.0077
Ramm-Pettersen	91	2011	misc adenoma	20	General Electric Signa SP	0.5	12 (60%)	11 (92%)	12 (60%)	20%, p = NS
Berkmann et al.	19	2011	misc adenoma	32	Polestar N-20	0.15	15 (47%)	9 (60%)	25 (78%)	25%, p = 0.0321
Berkmann et al.	18	2012	NFA	60	Polestar N-20	0.15	23 (38%)	20 (87%)	51 (85%)	23%, p = 0.0034
Berkmann et al.	17	2012	misc	115	Polestar N-20	0.15	45 (39%)	36 (80%)	94 (82%)	21%, p = 0.0004
Bellut et al.	13	2012	misc adenoma	148	Polestar N-20	0.15	56 (38%)	44 (79%)	106 (72%)	10%, p = NS
Tabakow et al.	113	2012	misc adenoma	18	Polestar N-20	0.15	9 (50%)	6 (67%)	15 (83%)	33%, p = 0.0375
Kim et al.	57	2013	misc adenoma	198	Polestar N-20	0.15	44 (22%)	37 (84%)	184 (93%)	15%, p < 0.0001
Hlavica et al.	51	2013	NFA	104	Polestar N-20	0.15	48 (46%)	44 (92%)	70 (67%)	21%, p = 0.0324

Abbreviations: misc sellar, miscellaneous sellar tumors, misc adenoma, miscellaneous pituitary adenomas, NFA, nonfunctioning pituitary adenoma, GTR, gross total resection, NS, not significant

Table 2. Results of iMRI-controlled pituitary surgery with high-field setups

Author	Ref.	Year	Diagnosis	n	iMRI setup	Field strength (T)	Remnant on 1st iMRI (n)	Additional resection (n)	GTR (n)	Increase of GTR rate by iMRI
Dort et al.	39	2001	misc adenoma	15	Magnex Scientific IMRIS	1.5	9 (60%)	9 (100%)	14 (93%)	33%, p = 0.0026
Fahlbusch et al.	42	2005	acromegaly	23	Siemens Magnetom Sonata Maestro	1.5	13 (57%)	5 (38%)	14 (61%)	18%, p = NS
Nimsky et al.	82	2006	NFA	129	Siemens Magnetom Sonata Maestro	1.5	61 (47%)	47 (77%)	83 (64%)	17%, p = 0.0383
Pamir et al.	87	2011	NFA	42	Siemens Magnetom Trio	3	22 (52%)	10 (45%)	24 (57%)	9%, p = NS
Meng et al.	77	2011	misc adenoma	30	Calgary Crane System, IMRIS	1.5	12 (40%)	10 (83%)	26 (87%)	27%, p = 0.0195
Lang et al.	62	2011	misc	9	Siemens Magnetom Verio IMRIS	3	1 (11%)	1 (100%)	9 (100%)	11%, p=NS
Netuka et al.	81	2011	misc	86	Signa HDx General Electric	3	51 (59%)	31 (61%)	45 (52%)	11%, p = NS
Szerlip et al.	112	2011	misc adenoma	53	Siemens Magnetom Espree	1.5	34 (64%)	28 (82%)	33 (62%)	26%, p = 0.0056
Tanei et al.	114	2013	misc adenoma	14	Siemens Magnetom Symphony	1.5	7 (50%)	5 (71%)	11 (79%)	29%, p = NS
Fomekong et al.	45	2014	misc adenoma	73	Philips Achieve	3	30 (41%)	8 (27%)	53 (73%)	14%, p = 0.05
Berkmann et al.	21	2014	NFA	85	Siemens Magnetom Sonata Maestro	1.5	48 (56%)	40 (83%)	56 (66%)	22%, p = 0.0027
Berkmann et al.	22	2014	NFA recurr	111	Siemens Magnetom Sonata Maestro	1.5	92 (83%)	62 (67%)	54 (49%)	32%, p < 0.0001
Sylvester et al.	111	2014	misc adenoma	156	Siemens Magnetom Espree	1.5	112 (72%)	56 (50%)	59 (38%)	10%, p = 0.0458
Paterno et al.	89	2014	misc adenoma	72	Siemens Magnetom Espree	1.5	42 (58%)	26 (56%)	53 (74%)	32%, p < 0.0001
Coburger et al.	31	2014	misc adenoma	76	Siemens Magnetom Espree	1.5	NA	NA	40 (53%)	NA

Abbreviations: misc sellar, miscellaneous sellar tumors, misc adenoma, miscellaneous pituitary adenomas, NFA, nonfunctioning pituitary adenoma, reop, reoperated, GTR, gross total resection, NS, not significant

The use of iMRI facilitates GTR. This is the common conclusion in studies on iMRI-controlled transsphenoidal surgery. For the pathologies operated with low-field iMRI (Table 1) the mean increase of GTR rates was 22% (range 3-52%). Additional resections based on iMR images were performed in 27-100% (mean 81%) of the patients. For high-field iMRI studies (Table 2) the mean increase of GTR was 21% (range 9-33%) and additional resections were possible in 27-100% (mean 67%) of the patients. The broad range of these results is characterized by the variability of types, sizes and grades of infiltration of pathologies included in these various studies. As mentioned above, some NFA are deemed for intended incomplete resection. The mean GTR rate in the low-field studies (*Table 1*) was 57% (range 17-80%) in the first intraoperative scan and 77% (38-100%) in the postoperative scan. In high-field studies, the initial mean GTR rate was 47% (range 17-89%) and 67% (38-100%) after additional resection. It is noteworthy that a meta-analysis of 5.022 patients with NFA operated without the use of iMRI reported a mean GTR rate of 44% [57]. This reflects nicely the GTR rate detected by the iMRI scans before further resections based on these images were made.

To assure a good outcome, long-term follow-up is the key in NFA, however, there are only few studies with mean follow-ups over 1 year. In a recent series on transsphenoidal surgery for NFA assisted by ultra-low-field MRI, an initial GTR rate of 85% was reported for 60 NFA with a mean volume of 6.8 cm^3. No recurrences were seen during a mean follow-up of 3.2 years (0.5-4.3 years) [27]. Another study with a follow-up of 2.8 years in 104 patients with NFA, who were operated in a PoleStar™-unit, detected recurrences in 3% of the patients [44]. For high-field iMRI, the study [1]. with the currently longest mean follow-up (5.6 years) reported recurrences in 7% of the patients resulting in a comparably low recurrence rate of 0.013 patients/year (as compared to the quoted meta-analysis which reported a rate of 0.022 patients/year) [57]. In the same study, regrowth of known remnants after incomplete resection was noted by follow-up imaging in 64% of the patients. The regrowth rate was 0.114 patients/year. Seventy-nine percent of these patients showed further growth within 5 years after surgery.

In the case of recurrence of NFA after GTR or regrowth of tumor remnants, treatment options include observation, radiotherapy, stereotactic radiosurgery, and transsphenoidal reoperation or craniotomy. Transsphenoidal reoperations for tumor resection may be challenging, due to the varying operative anatomy, frequently invasive growth of these recurring tumors, loss of anatomical landmarks, the effects of radiotherapy and the presence of scarring. While various studies on the use of iMRI also included patients with reoperations in their mixed study groups, a recent study explicitly reports on this subject [56]. The initial GTR rate in these patients was 17%, which correlates well with the rates reported in the literature on transsphenoidal reoperations without iMRI [60]. Further resection based on the updated iMRI sequences was possible in 67% of these patients, resulting in a final GTR rate of 49%. In patients with noninvasive tumors the GTR rate could even be increased from 31% to 75%. Nevertheless, the GTR rate of 49% is still low compared with data from iMRI studies on first-time procedures (*Tables 1 and 2*). The complication rate for reoperations was reported to be significantly higher than for primary surgery [61]. Diabetes insipidus, meningitis and cerebrospinal fluid (CSF) fistulas, as a sequelae that need to be repaired, may be present in up to 25%, 5% and 9% of these patients, respectively. The reported rates for iMRI-controlled resections did not exceed the incidence reported in the literature for primary procedures [62,

63]. Persistent diabetes insipidus was found in 3%, reoperations for CSF leaks were indicated in 4% of these cases and 2% of the patients suffered from postoperative meningitis [56].

Even if not completely resectable and as stated, this may be e.g., more often the case in reoperations of recurrent tumors or in invasive tumors the iMRI may facilitate remnant volume reduction [1, 56]. This is essential if further therapy options like conventional or stereotactic irradiation have to be indicated. Tumor control rates of 90% were reported for fractionated radiotherapy [64, 65], as well as for stereotactic irradiation such as Gamma Knife radiosurgery [66-69]. The peak of tumor size reduction is seen about 3 years after radiotherapy, and volume reductions of 50% have been described within 5 years [70, 71]. Additionally, radiosurgery may be an option for local control in patients with pituitary adenomas who have already undergone radiotherapy [72]. Tumor volume is one of the most important issues for indicating radiosurgery. The main factor influencing the incidence of tumor regrowth or the induction of neurological deficits by radiosurgery is a tumor volume greater than 5 cm^3 [68, 73]. Therefore, even if complete resection may not be possible, additional iMRI guided reduction may achieve smaller remnant volumes and thereby enhance the efficiency and at the same time reduce the morbidity of radiotherapy.

3.2. Outcome of Compression Syndromes

If not detected incidentally by MRI or CT imaging, indicated for non-pituitary related disorders, pituitary adenomas and typically NFA may grow extensively. With time they lead to damage of the anterior visual pathway, such as visual field (VF) defects or decline of visual acuity (VA) as described by Harvey Cushing in 1935 [74, 75]. Oculomotor and facial sensibility disturbances may be seen in the case of parasellar extension to the cavernous sinus, and even obstructive hydrocephalus may occur when the third ventricle is compressed. For ophthalmological symptoms, early decompression of the chiasm and the optic nerves significantly improves visual outcomes [76, 77]. In the case of rapid VA decline caused by pituitary tumor apoplexy transsphenoidal decompression may even be indicated as an emergency procedure [78]. Nevertheless, in case of abundant suprasellar extension of macro- or giant-adenomas, the risk for leaving behind remnants is high. These residual masses may prolong symptoms and thereby reduce the possibility of the optic fibers to recover. Remnants may typically be hidden in descending folds of the sellar diaphragm and visualization by the microscope or the endoscope may be difficult [11]. Furthermore, possibly unnecessary manipulations of the diaphragm, which is often thinned due to the distension caused by the tumor, may lead to CSF leaks. Ultimately, blind probing into the suprasellar space may directly harm the optic nerves.

Through the use of iMRI these limitations in visualizing remnants which compress the optic nerves may be overcome. Generally, the suprasellar structures are more distinctively depicted, while primarily in low-field imaging intra- and parasellar remnants may be more difficult to detect. The specificity for low-field iMRI to detect remnants was reported to be about 90% and the sensitivity 100% [26, 27]. For high-field iMRI, a specificity and a sensitivity as high as 100% was reported [1]. In a study explicitly addressing the issue of early visual recovery after iMRI-controlled tumor resection in a low-field setting, 60% of the patients with residual tumors had persistent optic nerve compression on the first iMRI control scans [26]. An additional resection was possible in 56% of these patients. Ultimately the optic apparatus was decompressed in 84% of the patients. The positive predictive values for VF and for VA recoveries if a decompressed optic chiasm was depicted by iMRI were both as high as 96%. For high-field settings, long-term data show improvement of VF and VA in up to 100% of the patients [1]. In iMRI-controlled reoperations VF and VA recovery were 86% and 74%, respectively [56]. One of the reasons for the lower rate in reoperated patients may be the longer duration of symptoms caused by persistent compression of the optic nerve structures, however, until now there is no controlled data supporting this thesis. Basically, a randomized trial may be able to compare the differences in the ophthalmological outcome caused by the use of iMR imaging, however, it may be questionable to which extent this could withhold the overt benefit of iMR imaging to these patients.

Deterioration of vision is one of the severe complications of transsphenoidal surgery. It was described by different authors, also after procedures guided by iMR imaging [30, 35, 48, 56]. Based on the reported rates in the studies summarized in Tables 1 and 2, the apparent incidence of postoperative decline of visual function may be below 1%, however, the comparison with study groups not using iMRI imaging remains difficult. It may be biased due to the different techniques applied and the variability of factors such as size, consistency and invasiveness of the tumors and duration of symptoms of the patients included. Nevertheless, while an incidence for ophthalmic function decline of 3% has been reported in a study using iMRI [79], the incidence in other studies without iMRI seems to be similar to those using iMRI [16, 20, 80-82].

3.3. Outcome of Hormonal Function

The dominant mechanisms of hypopituitarism are interruption of the hypophyseal portal vessels, compression of the pituitary stalk, and increased intrasellar pressure caused by tumor growth [83-87]. Therefore, surgical decompression of the pituitary gland and its stalk may lead to recovery of hypopituitarism. Predictive factors for better recovery rates include younger age, absence of arterial hypertension, lack of intraoperative CSF leak, pre-operative hyperprolactinemia and smaller tumor size [83, 88, 89]. The detection of gross total resection on postoperative imaging is a significant factor for postoperative hormonal recovery [90]. On the other hand, loss of pituitary function may be a complication of pituitary surgery. The rate of postoperative hypopituitarism in series on transsphenoidal tumor resections is commonly below 20% [63, 88, 89, 91-94]. Nevertheless, higher rates have been described [95-97], especially in the case of larger or hormonally inactive tumors [88-90, 98] or pituitary apoplexy [99, 100].

Series of transsphenoidal surgery for pituitary adenomas with iMRI controls report an incidence of new hypopituitarism of 0-29% [27, 34, 36, 47, 48]. When comparing patients with NFA, who were operated in the iMRI to matched controls, the benefit in increasing GTR again becomes obvious. In a study focusing on endocrinological outcome, the first low-field iMRI scan showed GTR in 62% of the patients, which corresponds well to the results of postoperative MRI in the control group showing a GTR rate of 69% [27]. Additional tumor resection significantly increased the GTR rate in the iMRI-group to 85%. The question whether a possibly aggressive additional resection based on iMRI controls puts pituitary function at harm could be denied in this and in subsequent studies [1, 27, 56]. While the differences of new hormonal deficits (iMRI-group 29%, control group 45%), which was generally high in this study, including mainly large and invasive NFA, did not reach statistical significance, there was however a tendency towards a smaller hormonal complication rate of iMRI-controlled surgery. Considering the recovery rates of tumor-induced hypopituitarism, a similar tendency towards a beneficial effect of iMRI was reported. As 59% of the patients in the iMRI-group showed some restoration of pituitary axis function, this was only detected in 45% of the controls. Predictive factors for a lower risk of pituitary function loss when the iMRI was used were age below 65 years, absence of cardiovascular risk factors (e.g., arterial hypertension and tobacco smoking) and pre-existing partial hypopituitarism [27]. Additionally, long-term data of patients operated in a high-field setting show quite dynamic results of the endocrinological outcome in those with NFA [1]. The development of hypopituitarism was detected in 11% of the patients 1 week after surgery, however, further loss was diagnosed in another 15% during a mean follow-up time of 5.6 ± 1.9 years. On the other hand, hormonal recovery was seen in 29% of the patients 1 week postoperatively and in another 48% of the patients at the end of follow-up. Radiotherapy-induced pituitary damage [101] may have influenced these results to some extent as 27% of the patients with late onset hypopituitarism were irradiated. This points out to the conclusion that repetitive testing of hormonal function is mandatory not only in iMRI-controlled, but in all NFA patients possibly suffering from hypopituitarism, as recovery or loss of function may happen not only in the initial but also in the later course after surgery [1, 102].

While reoperations may be a risk factor for loss of pituitary axes function, the reported rates for iMRI-controlled surgery do not exceed this range [56, 61]. In reoperated NFA with use of iMRI, endocrinological follow-up testing showed postoperative loss and recovery of hormonal axes in 12% and 15% of patients, respectively [56]. This recovery rate seems comparably low to series on primary surgeries, however, this may correlate with the lower GTR rate in reoperations as previously discussed [90].

In patients with intraoperative CSF leaks, craniopharyngiomas or Rathke's cleft cysts as well as transient or permanent diabetes insipidus may be detected more often [103]. The use of iMRI did not significantly influence the incidence of postoperative diabetes insipidus or syndrome of inadequate antidiuretic hormone secretion in a comparative cohort study including patients with NFA [27]. Nevertheless, the reported rates of diabetes insipidus (8%) and SIADH (5%) were comparably small when compared to the incidence in the general literature (18-30%) [62, 103-107].

3.4. Functioning Pituitary Adenoma

Acromegaly is caused by a growth hormone (GH)-producing pituitary adenoma. If excessive output of GH is not normalized, cardiovascular and metabolic disturbances as well as cosmetic and orthopedic deformities will result. Depending on the criteria for remission, transsphenoidal surgery in acromegaly leads to cure of the condition in 50-60% of the patients [41, 108-115]. Indeed, the size matters, as 75-95% of the patients with microadenomas, but only 40-70% of the patients with macroadenomas will show normalization of growth hormone excess. High preoperative growth hormone levels and invasive tumor growth configuration are two other significant predictors of an incomplete resection [108]. Persistent postoperative acromegaly may be accompanied by larger visible, either resectable or unresectable tumor remnants. Re-operations are reasonable only when tumor remnants that seem to be resectable are detected. Nevertheless, due to postoperative changes in early MR-imaging, the sensitivity for detecting remnants is low during the first 3 months after surgery. While early imaging within 3 days postoperatively may still prove helpful [116], later images may become difficult to "read" due to scarring, fluid retention and changes of grafts applied for closure [117]. While growth hormone levels decrease rather rapidly within days, if surgery was successful, IGF-1 may decrease only after 1-2 weeks. That is why normally at the time when persisting acromegaly becomes probable, an immediate MRI to indicate an early reoperation before scarring takes place may not be helpful. Therefore, the results of iMRI scans, performed before the site is closed, may be valuable.

Intraoperative image quality is crucial for the evaluation of the intrasellar structures, and it was therefore postulated that the high-field setup would have definitive advantages over the low-field setups [47]. The only study, exclusively focusing on the outcome of growth hormone excess after transsphenoidal resection in a high-field setting, included 23 patients [47]. In 78% of the patients, complete tumor removal was intended, however, iMRI scans revealed tumor remnants in 44% of the operated cases, leading to an extended resection in 28% of them. This increased the rate of complete tumor removal and endocrine normalization from 33% to 44% using the consensus criteria [118], and improved endocrine outcome in another 17%. The comparability between postoperative MRI after three months and iMRI was excellent as none of the patients with remnants depicted on iMRI met the criteria for remission. In all cases with suspected cavernous sinus infiltration on iMRI, postoperative imaging after 3 months confirmed the parasellar remnants. If iMRI showed complete removal and no full endocrine remission was achieved, postoperative MRI after 3 months neither showed a remnant.

Surgery for GH-producing pituitary adenoma, applying an ultra-low-field iMR imaging modality, showed an overall remission rate of 67% [37]. In patients with primary surgery the remission rate was 74%, however, in previously operated patients the rate dropped to 20%. The remission rate was increased by 5% by additional resections based on iMRI scans. The patients' characteristics of the already performed studies using high-field [47] or low-field iMRI [37] do not seem to be well comparable, thus, deductions which modality may be superior cannot be drawn from these results.

While there are studies including miscellaneous subtypes of functioning pituitary adenomas [41, 54], there is no study up to now reporting results on iMRI-controlled transsphenoidal surgery exclusively for Cushing's disease or prolactinoma in a reasonable large patient group.

3.5. iMRI in Combination with Endoscopy

As stated above, visualization of the tumor and the related anatomy of the operating field is the key to successful transsphenoidal surgery. While the results of iMRI-controlled operations have been presented in this chapter, other techniques which may be used as a sole modality or in conjunction with iMRI have to be mentioned. As an additional tool for transsphenoidal surgery, the endoscope has been used more and more during the past decade. Numerous studies reported technical details, surgical results and its value in tumor visualization. In this context, several reports of endoscopicaly-assisted procedures, as an adjunct to low-field and to high-field iMRI-guidance for resection control, have been published [1, 32, 38, 52, 56]. Considering tumor visualization, sensitivity and specificity for detection of remnants by high-field iMRI were reported to be 100% compared to postoperative MRI [1]. The endoscopical assessment of the resection rate before an iMRI-control scan was acquired in the same patients yielded a sensitivity of only 21% and a specificity of 78%. The remnants depicted by iMRI were found in the following localizations: lateral of the sella/cavernous sinus, 48%, suprasellar space, 28%, retrosellar space/clivus, 12%, in the sella, 12%. An additional resection based on the iMR images was made in 73% of these patients. Thereby the difference between the GTR rate (66%) on the postoperative MRI and the GTR rate (35%) detected by iMRI after endoscopicaly-assisted resection became very significant ($p < 0.0001$, OR 5.4, 95% CI 2.3-13.0).

In transsphenoidal reoperations the endoscopic assessment of GTR may even be more difficult, e.g., due to scarring and lack of anatomical landmarks. A study on transsphenoidal reoperations, which included a small subgroup of patients operated with endoscopical assistance used in a high-field iMRI-setting, reported that GTR was assumed in 40% of the patients based on the endoscopic assessment [56]. In another 40% of the patients partial resection was detected by the endoscope but further tumor removal did not seem possible. In the remaining 20% no definite statement about the extent of resection could be given. All of these patients showed tumor remnants on the subsequent iMRI control scans even those who were thought to be without remnants based on the endoscopic visualization. The localization of the remnants on the iMRI scans was as follows: lateral/in the cavernous sinus, 60%, suprasellar, 50%, intrasellar, 10%. Notably, an additional iMRI-guided resection was possible in 80% of these cases.

Previous studies raised similar points concerning false negative endoscopical findings, and uniformly reported an increase of GTR rates after further tumor visualization by iMRI [32, 38]. In contrast to the direct inspection by the endoscope, iMRI allows the evaluation of hidden structures which are not accessible by direct visualization (e.g., by being hidden in invaginations of the descending diaphragm or in the suprasellar space). The identification of tumor remnants may be even more facilitated by the possibility of comparing pre- and intraoperative images that are acquired in the same position of the device. Compared to the iMRI, the endoscope may be less cost intensive. Nevertheless, the benefit of a complete resection in these mostly benign tumors weakens arguments about costs. While most studies on iMRI were not weighed towards the analysis of cost efficiency, the significantly higher GTR rate made possible by iMRI controlled surgery resulting in a lower rate of reoperations or additional therapies (e.g., radiotherapy) is indeed noteworthy.

4. Pros and Cons

4.1. Specificity and Sensitivity of Tumor Detection

Visualization is the key, however, the surgeon has to remind himself that not everything that he detects with whatever tool used to visualize tumor remnants is really what it seems to be. False-positive iMRI findings may provoke unnecessary probing for remnants and increase the risk of hypopituitarism and CSF leakage. Both the specificity and sensitivity of iMRI for detection of residual sellar lesions were subject of debate in several studies [1, 26, 27, 30, 31, 35, 56, 119]. The following reasons for misinterpretations have been reported:

1. The iMRI fails to give sufficient imaging results due to "noise"
2. Gadolinium enhancement is poor
3. Image layering misses the tumor
4. Poor resolution due to low field strength
5. There is difficulty in differentiating remnants of sellar tumor from intrasellar blood products and blood within the venous sinus. Specificity and sensitivity reported for both low- and high-field iMRI are commonly in the range of 90-100% and 75-100%, respectively.

It seems that most often coagula may be misinterpreted as residual tumor. In low-field settings pituitary adenoma and blood products often have an isointense aspect in non-enhanced T1- and T2-weighed images. If gadolinium is administered a difference may be observed during the first control scan. Nevertheless, in the case of repeat imaging the accumulated blood may be mixed with contrast agent and reliable differentiation may not be possible anymore. There are several technical tricks to facilitate image interpretation. Pooling of blood may be prevented by applying bone wax as a temporary reconstruction of the sellar floor [31]. In small adenomas the resection cavity may be filled with a small wax ball and the localization and extent of the ball may be compared to the tumor localization on the scans acquired before resection. Another technique to enhance the contrast is packing of the tumor resection cavity with contrast-soaked cotton pledgets and filling the remainder of the space with gauze [45].

4.2. Time and Cost Efficiency

One of the common arguments used by sceptics against iMRI-controls in transsphenoidal surgery is the additional time needed for the scans. Nevertheless, the duration of the control scans is often overestimated. Most devices provide short scanning sequences to verify the scanner's correct position before a longer sequence is started. For the Medtronic PoleStar™-unit there is e.g., the eSteady sequence, which is acquired in 24 seconds. The Siemens Magnetom Sonata™ provides a shortcut via the HASTE sequence, which takes 20 seconds. In case of a remnant already depicted by these sequences, surgery may be continued without further detailed time-consuming imaging. More detailed scan sequences (e.g., the T1-weighed contrast enhanced 3mm scan of the Medtronic PoleStar™unit or the T2-scan of the Siemens Magnetom Sonata™) will take about 10 minutes and may be immediately transferred to the neuronavigation sequences without further referencing. Thus, the mean duration for draping, scanning and return to the surgical field is about 15 minutes. Depending on the number of intraoperative scans needed, the use of an iMRI will prolong the procedure by 15-30 minutes in most cases [36, 56]. Nevertheless, the operating time will also be prolonged by the consecutive additional resections, which obviously would not have been made without the use of iMRI. Thus, the operating times of procedures with and without iMRI may not be well comparable. Until now, no tendency of an increased complication rate caused by the prolonged operation time was detected [12]. Ultimately the surgeon has to ask the question whether the goal is to increase the chances for a GTR during the first procedure which will take some extra time or whether the operating time is better used for the reoperation if a resectable remnant keeps on growing.

Due to the additional time needed, in case this technology is used, it may be reasonable to use selection criteria for indicating the use of iMRI in transsphenoidal pituitary surgery. This may even be mandatory in high-impact centers, as operative capacity in the iMRI may be lower than the number of patients asking for treatment. A proposal which patients benefit from iMRI-controlled procedures has been made and includes the following points [1]:

1. History of previous transsphenoidal surgery (e.g., with presence of massive scarring and loss of anatomical landmarks)
2. Invasive tumor growth pattern (e.g., into the clivus or the cavernous sinus, Knosp grades 3 or 4)
3. Abundant suprasellar or retrosellar tumor growth (modified Hardy's grades 3 or 4) [6, 120] with consecutive high probability of incomplete resection and/or persisting symptomatic remnants (e.g., dumbbell-shaped tumors)
4. Tumors that need extended transsphenoidal approaches (e.g., subfrontal, transclival).

An additional drawback for the use of iMRI is the considerable equipment cost. This may be an issue more dominated by medico-economic arguments, than influenced by the results of the individual operative procedures which, as has been shown in the previous pages, are significantly enhanced by the use of iMRI. Of course the iMRI suites are not exclusively used for transsphenoidal surgery. Concurrent with the quoted results of its use for pituitary tumors, numerous studies have reported the benefit in several other cranial procedures. Promising results have e.g., been reported for iMRI-controlled resection of low and high grade glioma [121-123] and in epilepsy surgery [124, 125]. Depending on the case load and case mix of a department, the concept of an iMRI may be very reasonable. Given by the fact that informed patients often seek treatment in specialized departments with availability of intraoperative imaging techniques, the thereby provoked increase in cases may once more improve the affordability of such a device.

The true value of iMRI in transsphenoidal pituitary surgery may ultimately only be determined by randomized studies. Ironically, due to the excellent results provided by the studies presented above, this will be difficult to accomplish. Surgeons as well as patients with tumors suitable for iMRI-controlled procedures will want to use this technology and artificially withholding an obvious benefit is simply not justifiable.

References

[1] Berkmann S, Schlaffer S, Nimsky C, Fahlbusch R, Buchfelder M. Follow-up and long-term outcome of nonfunctioning pituitary adenoma operated by transsphenoidal surgery with intraoperative high-field magnetic resonance imaging. *Acta Neurochir* (Wien) 2014;156:2233-2243.

[2] Lunsford LD, Kondziolka D, Bissonette DJ. Intraoperative imaging of the brain. *Stereotact Funct Neurosurg* 1996;66:58-64.

[3] Schloffer H. Erfolgreiche Operation eines Hypophysentumors auf nasalem Wege (In German). *Wien Klin Wochenschr* 1907;20:621-624.

[4] Buchfelder M. Treatment of pituitary tumors: surgery. *Endocrine* 2005;28:67-75.

[5] Maartens NF. The history of the treatment of pituitary adenomas. *Endocrine* 2005;28:9-26.

[6] Hardy J, Wigser SM. Trans-sphenoidal surgery of pituitary fossa tumors with televised radiofluoroscopic control. *J Neurosurg* 1965;23:612-619.

[7] Nesbakken R, Reinlie S, Eldevik OP. Intraoperative gas cisternography and gas dissection in the operative treatment of pituitary tumors. A methodological description. *Eur Surg Res* 1984;16 Suppl 2:73-79.

[8] Lunsford LD, Kondziolka D, Maitz A, Flickinger JC. Black holes, white dwarfs and supernovas: imaging after radiosurgery. *Stereotact Funct Neurosurg* 1998;70 Suppl 1:2-10.

[9] Okudera H, Takemae T, Kobayashi S. Intraoperative computed tomographic scanning during transsphenoidal surgery: technical note. *Neurosurgery* 1993;32:1041-1043.

[10] Sylvester PT, Evans JA, Zipfel GJ, Chole RA, Uppaluri R, Haughey BH, et al. Combined high-field intraoperative magnetic resonance imaging and endoscopy increase extent of resection and progression-free survival for pituitary adenomas. *Pituitary* 2015;18:72-85.

[11] Paterno V, Fahlbusch R. High-Field iMRI in transsphenoidal pituitary adenoma surgery with special respect to typical localization of residual tumor. *Acta Neurochir* (Wien) 2014;156:463-74.

[12] Coburger J, Konig R, Seitz K, Bazner U, Wirtz CR, Hlavac M. Determining the utility of intraoperative magnetic resonance imaging for transsphenoidal surgery: a retrospective study. *J Neurosurg* 2014;120:346-356.

[13] Arita K, Kurisu K, Tominaga A, Kawamoto H, Iida K, Mizoue T, et al. Trans-sellar color Doppler ultrasonography during transsphenoidal surgery. *Neurosurgery* 1998;42:81-86.

[14] Atkinson JL, Kasperbauer JL, James EM, Lane JI, Nippoldt TB. Transcranial-transdural real-time ultrasonography during transsphenoidal resection of a large pituitary tumor. Case report. *J Neurosurg* 2000;93:129-131.

[15] Doppman JL, Ram Z, Shawker TH, Oldfield EH. Intraoperative US of the pituitary gland. Work in progress. *Radiology* 1994;192:111-115.

[16] Elias WJ, Chadduck JB, Alden TD, Laws ER, Jr. Frameless stereotaxy for transsphenoidal surgery. *Neurosurgery* 1999;45:271-277.

[17] Jane JA Jr., Thapar K, Alden TD, Laws ER Jr. Fluoroscopic frameless stereotaxy for transsphenoidal surgery. *Neurosurgery* 2001;48:1302-1308.

[18] Kacker A, Komisar A, Huo J, Mangiardi J. Transsphenoidal surgery utilizing computer-assisted stereotactic guidance. *Rhinology* 2001;39:207-210.

[19] Lasio G, Ferroli P, Felisati G, Broggi G. Image-guided endoscopic transnasal removal of recurrent pituitary adenomas. *Neurosurgery* 2002;51:132-137.

[20] Thomale UW, Stover JF, Unterberg AW. The use of neuronavigation in transnasal transsphenoidal pituitary surgery. *Zentralbl Neurochir* 2005;66:126-132.

[21] Walker DG, Ohaegbulam C, Black PM. Frameless stereotaxy as an alternative to fluoroscopy for transsphenoidal surgery: use of the InstaTrak-3000 and a novel headset. *J Clin Neurosci* 2002;9:294-297.

[22] Black PM, Moriarty T, Alexander E 3rd, Stieg P, Woodard EJ, Gleason PL, et al. Development and implementation of intraoperative magnetic resonance imaging and its neurosurgical applications. *Neurosurgery* 1997;41:831-845.

[23] Lewin JS, Nour SG, Meyers ML, Metzger AK, Maciunas RJ, Wendt M, et al. Intraoperative MRI with a rotating, tiltable surgical table: a time use study and clinical results in 122 patients. *AJR Am J Roentgenol* 2007;189:1096-1103.

[24] Darakchiev BJ, Tew JM, Jr., Bohinski RJ, Warnick RE. Adaptation of a standard low-field (0.3-T) system to the operating room: focus on pituitary adenomas. *Neurosurg Clin N Am* 2005;16:155-164.

[25] Hadani M, Spiegelman R, Feldman Z, Berkenstadt H, Ram Z. Novel, compact, intraoperative magnetic resonance imaging-guided system for conventional neurosurgical operating rooms. *Neurosurgery* 2001;48:799-809.

[26] Berkmann S, Fandino J, Zosso S, Killer HE, Remonda L, Landolt H. Intraoperative magnetic resonance imaging and early prognosis for vision after transsphenoidal surgery for sellar lesions. *J Neurosurg* 2011;115:518-527.

[27] Berkmann S, Fandino J, Muller B, Remonda L, Landolt H. Intraoperative MRI and endocrinological outcome of transsphenoidal surgery for non-functioning pituitary adenoma. *Acta Neurochir* (Wien) 2012;154:639-647.

[28] Steinmeier R, Fahlbusch R, Ganslandt O, Nimsky C, Buchfelder M, Klaus M, et al. Intraoperative magnetic resonance imaging with the magnetom open scanner: concepts, neurosurgical indications, and procedures: a preliminary report. *Neurosurgery* 1998;43:739-748.

[29] Martin CH, Schwartz R, Jolesz F, Black PM. Transsphenoidal resection of pituitary adenomas in an intraoperative MRI unit. *Pituitary* 1999;2:155-162.

[30] Bohinski RJ, Warnick RE, Gaskill-Shipley MF, Zuccarello M, van Loveren HR, Kormos DW, et al. Intraoperative magnetic resonance imaging to determine the extent of resection of pituitary macroadenomas during transsphenoidal microsurgery. *Neurosurgery* 2001;49:1133-1144.

[31] Fahlbusch R, Ganslandt O, Buchfelder M, Schott W, Nimsky C. Intraoperative magnetic resonance imaging during transsphenoidal surgery. *J Neurosurg* 2001;95:381-390.

[32] Schwartz TH, Stieg PE, Anand VK. Endoscopic transsphenoidal pituitary surgery with intraoperative magnetic resonance imaging. *Neurosurgery* 2006;58(Suppl 1) :ONS44-51.

[33] Ahn JY, Jung JY, Kim J, Lee KS, Kim SH. How to overcome the limitations to determine the resection margin of pituitary tumours with low-field intra-operative MRI during trans-sphenoidal surgery: usefulness of Gadolinium-soaked cotton pledgets. *Acta Neurochir* (Wien) 2008;150:763-771.

[34] Gerlach R, du Mesnil de Rochemont R, Gasser T, Marquardt G, Reusch J, Imoehl L, et al. Feasibility of Polestar N20, an ultra-low-field intraoperative magnetic resonance imaging system in resection control of pituitary macroadenomas: lessons learned from the first 40 cases. *Neurosurgery* 2008;63:272-285.

[35] Wu JS, Shou XF, Yao CJ, Wang YF, Zhuang DX, Mao Y, et al. Transsphenoidal pituitary macroadenomas resection guided by PoleStar N20 low-field intraoperative magnetic resonance imaging: comparison with early postoperative high-field magnetic resonance imaging. *Neurosurgery* 2009;65:63-71.

[36] Baumann F, Schmid C, Bernays RL. Intraoperative magnetic resonance imaging-guided transsphenoidal surgery for giant pituitary adenomas. *Neurosurg Rev* 2010;33:83-90.
[37] Bellut D, Hlavica M, Schmid C, Bernays RL. Intraoperative magnetic resonance imaging-assisted transsphenoidal pituitary surgery in patients with acromegaly. *Neurosurg Focus* 2010;29:E9.
[38] Theodosopoulos PV, Leach J, Kerr RG, Zimmer LA, Denny AM, Guthikonda B, et al. Maximizing the extent of tumor resection during transsphenoidal surgery for pituitary macroadenomas: can endoscopy replace intraoperative magnetic resonance imaging? *J Neurosurg* 2010;112:736-743.
[39] Vitaz TW, Inkabi KE, Carrubba CJ. Intraoperative MRI for transphenoidal procedures: short-term outcome for 100 consecutive cases. *Clin Neurol Neurosurg* 2011;113:731-735.
[40] Ramm-Pettersen J, Berg-Johnsen J, Hol PK, Roy S, Bollerslev J, Schreiner T, et al. Intra-operative MRI facilitates tumour resection during trans-sphenoidal surgery for pituitary adenomas. *Acta Neurochir* (Wien) 2011;153:1367-1373.
[41] Berkmann S, Fandino J, Muller B, Kothbauer K, Henzen C, Landolt H. Pituitary surgery: experience from a large network in Central Switzerland. *Swiss Med Wkly* 2012;142:w13680.
[42] Bellut D, Hlavica M, Muroi C, Woernle CM, Schmid C, Bernays RL. Impact of intraoperative MRI-guided transsphenoidal surgery on endocrine function and hormone substitution therapy in patients with pituitary adenoma. *Swiss Med Wkly* 2012;142:w13699.
[43] Tabakow P, Czyz M, Jarmundowicz W, Lechowicz-Glogowska E. Surgical treatment of pituitary adenomas using low-field intraoperative magnetic resonance imaging. *Adv Clin Exp Med* 2012;21:495-503.
[44] Hlavica M, Bellut D, Lemm D, Schmid C, Bernays RL. Impact of ultra-low-field intraoperative magnetic resonance imaging on extent of resection and frequency of tumor recurrence in 104 surgically treated nonfunctioning pituitary adenomas. *World Neurosurg* 2013;79:99-109.
[45] Kim EH, Oh MC, Kim SH. Application of low-field intraoperative magnetic resonance imaging in transsphenoidal surgery for pituitary adenomas: technical points to improve the visibility of the tumor resection margin. *Acta Neurochir* (Wien) 2013;155:485-493.
[46] Dort JC, Sutherland GR. Intraoperative magnetic resonance imaging for skull base surgery. *Laryngoscope* 2001;111:1570-1575.
[47] Fahlbusch R, Keller B, Ganslandt O, Kreutzer J, Nimsky C. Transsphenoidal surgery in acromegaly investigated by intraoperative high-field magnetic resonance imaging. *Eur J Endocrinol* 2005;153:239-248.
[48] Nimsky C, von Keller B, Ganslandt O, Fahlbusch R. Intraoperative high-field magnetic resonance imaging in transsphenoidal surgery of hormonally inactive pituitary macroadenomas. *Neurosurgery* 2006;59:105-114.
[49] Pamir MN. 3 T ioMRI: the Istanbul experience. *Acta Neurochir Suppl* 2011;109:131-137.
[50] Meng XH, Xu BN, Wei SB, Zhou T, Chen XL, Yu XG, et al.[High-field intraoperative magnetic resonance imaging suite with neuronavigation system: implementation and preliminary experience in the pituitary adenoma operation with transsphenoidal approach] *Zhonghua Wai Ke Za Zhi* 2011;49:703-706.

[51] Lang MJ, Kelly JJ, Sutherland GR. A moveable 3-Tesla intraoperative magnetic resonance imaging system. *Neurosurgery* 2011;68:168-179.

[52] Netuka D, Masopust V, Belsan T, Kramar F, Benes V. One year experience with 3.0 T intraoperative MRI in pituitary surgery. *Acta Neurochir Suppl* 2011;109:157-159.

[53] Szerlip NJ, Zhang YC, Placantonakis DG, Goldman M, Colevas KB, Rubin DG, et al. Transsphenoidal resection of sellar tumors using high-field intraoperative magnetic resonance imaging. *Skull Base* 2011;21:223-232.

[54] Tanei T, Nagatani T, Nakahara N, Watanabe T, Nishihata T, Nielsen ML, et al. Use of high-field intraoperative magnetic resonance imaging during endoscopic transsphenoidal surgery for functioning pituitary microadenomas and small adenomas located in the intrasellar region. *Neurol Med Chir* (Tokyo) 2013;53:501-510.

[55] Fomekong E, Duprez T, Docquier MA, Ntsambi G, Maiter D, Raftopoulos C. Intraoperative 3T MRI for pituitary macroadenoma resection: Initial experience in 73 consecutive patients. *Clin Neurol Neurosurg* 2014;126:143-149.

[56] Berkmann S, Schlaffer S, Nimsky C, Fahlbusch R, Buchfelder M. Intraoperative high-field MRI for transsphenoidal reoperations of nonfunctioning pituitary adenoma. *J Neurosurg* 2014;121:1166-1175.

[57] Roelfsema F, Biermasz NR, Pereira AM. Clinical factors involved in the recurrence of pituitary adenomas after surgical remission: a structured review and meta-analysis. *Pituitary* 2012;15:71-83.

[58] Reddy R, Cudlip S, Byrne JV, Karavitaki N, Wass JA. Can we ever stop imaging in surgically treated and radiotherapy-naive patients with non-functioning pituitary adenoma? *Eur J Endocrinol* 2011;165:739-744.

[59] Berkmann S, Schlaffer S, Buchfelder M. Tumor shrinkage after transsphenoidal surgery for nonfunctioning pituitary adenoma. *J Neurosurg* 2013;119:1447-1452.

[60] Benveniste RJ, King WA, Walsh J, Lee JS, Delman BN, Post KD. Repeated transsphenoidal surgery to treat recurrent or residual pituitary adenoma. *J Neurosurg* 2005;102:1004-1012.

[61] Jahangiri A, Wagner J, Han SW, Zygourakis CC, Han SJ, Tran MT, et al. Morbidity of repeat transsphenoidal surgery assessed in more than 1000 operations. *J Neurosurg* 2014;121:67-74.

[62] Black PM, Zervas NT, Candia GL. Incidence and management of complications of transsphenoidal operation for pituitary adenomas. *Neurosurgery* 1987;20:920-924.

[63] Ciric I, Ragin A, Baumgartner C, Pierce D. Complications of transsphenoidal surgery: results of a national survey, review of the literature, and personal experience. *Neurosurgery* 1997;40:225-237.

[64] Boelaert K, Gittoes NJ. Radiotherapy for non-functioning pituitary adenomas. *Eur J Endocrinol* 2001;144:569-575.

[65] Zierhut D, Flentje M, Adolph J, Erdmann J, Raue F, Wannenmacher M. External radiotherapy of pituitary adenomas. *Int J Radiat Oncol Biol Phys* 1995;33:307-314.

[66] Losa M, Valle M, Mortini P, Franzin A, da Passano CF, Cenzato M, et al. Gamma knife surgery for treatment of residual nonfunctioning pituitary adenomas after surgical debulking. *J Neurosurg* 2004;100:438-444.

[67] Sheehan JP, Kondziolka D, Flickinger J, Lunsford LD. Radiosurgery for residual or recurrent nonfunctioning pituitary adenoma. *J Neurosurg* 2002;97:408-414.

[68] Sheehan JP, Starke RM, Mathieu D, Young B, Sneed PK, Chiang VL, et al. Gamma Knife radiosurgery for the management of nonfunctioning pituitary adenomas: a multicenter study. *J Neurosurg* 2013;119:446-456.

[69] Pollock BE, Carpenter PC. Stereotactic radiosurgery as an alternative to fractionated radiotherapy for patients with recurrent or residual nonfunctioning pituitary adenomas. *Neurosurgery* 2003;53:1086-1094.

[70] Kopp C, Theodorou M, Poullos N, Jacob V, Astner ST, Geinitz H, et al. Tumor shrinkage assessed by volumetric MRI in long-term follow-up after fractionated stereotactic radiotherapy of nonfunctioning pituitary adenoma. *Int J Radiat Oncol Biol Phys* 2012;82:1262-1267.

[71] Sasaki R, Murakami M, Okamoto Y, Kono K, Yoden E, Nakajima T, et al. The efficacy of conventional radiation therapy in the management of pituitary adenoma. *Int J Radiat Oncol Biol Phys* 2000;47:1337-1345.

[72] Verma J, McCutcheon IE, Waguespack SG, Mahajan A. Feasibility and outcome of re-irradiation in the treatment of multiply recurrent pituitary adenomas. *Pituitary* 2014;17:539-545.

[73] Starke RM, Williams BJ, Jane JA, Sheehan JP. Gamma Knife surgery for patients with nonfunctioning pituitary macroadenomas: predictors of tumor control, neurological deficits, and hypopituitarism. *J Neurosurg* 2012;117:129-135.

[74] Losa M, Donofrio CA, Barzaghi R, Mortini P. Presentation and surgical results of incidentally discovered nonfunctioning pituitary adenomas: evidence for a better outcome independently of other patients' characteristics. *Eur J Endocrinol* 2013;169:735-742.

[75] Cushing H. The chiasmal syndrome of primary optic atrophy and bitemporal field defects in adults with a normal sella turcica. *Arch Ophthalmol* 1935;3:505-551.

[76] Cohen AR, Cooper PR, Kupersmith MJ, Flamm ES, Ransohoff J. Visual recovery after transsphenoidal removal of pituitary adenomas. *Neurosurgery* 1985;17:446-452.

[77] Suri A, Narang KS, Sharma BS, Mahapatra AK. Visual outcome after surgery in patients with suprasellar tumors and preoperative blindness. *J Neurosurg* 2008;108:19-25.

[78] Muthukumar N, Rossette D, Soundaram M, Senthilbabu S, Badrinarayanan T. Blindness following pituitary apoplexy: timing of surgery and neuro-ophthalmic outcome. *J Clin Neurosci* 2008;15:873-879.

[79] Sandeman D, Moufid A. Interactive image-guided pituitary surgery. An experience of 101 procedures. *Neurochirurgie* 1998;44:331-338.

[80] Burkey BB, Speyer MT, Maciunas RJ, Fitzpatrick JM, Galloway RL, Jr., Allen GS. Sublabial, transseptal, transsphenoidal approach to the pituitary region guided by the ACUSTAR I system. *Otolaryngol Head Neck Surg* 1998;118:191-194.

[81] Jagannathan J, Prevedello DM, Ayer VS, Dumont AS, Jane JA, Jr., Laws ER. Computer-assisted frameless stereotaxy in transsphenoidal surgery at a single institution: review of 176 cases. *Neurosurg Focus* 2006;20:E9.

[82] Zhao Y, Yu S, Wang R, Zhao J. Clinical application of a neuronavigation system in transsphenoidal surgery of pituitary macroadenoma. *Neurosurg Rev* 2006;29:306-312.

[83] Arafah BM. Reversible hypopituitarism in patients with large nonfunctioning pituitary adenomas. *J Clin Endocrinol Metab* 1986;62:1173-1179.

[84] Arafah BM, Kailani SH, Nekl KE, Gold RS, Selman WR. Immediate recovery of pituitary function after transsphenoidal resection of pituitary macroadenomas. *J Clin Endocrinol Metab* 1994;79:348-354.
[85] Arafah BM, Prunty D, Ybarra J, Hlavin ML, Selman WR. The dominant role of increased intrasellar pressure in the pathogenesis of hypopituitarism, hyperprolactinemia, and headaches in patients with pituitary adenomas. *J Clin Endocrinol Metab* 2000;85:1789-1793.
[86] Randall RV, Scheithauer BW, Laws ER, Jr., Abbound CF, Ebersold MJ, Kao PC. Pituitary adenomas associated with hyperprolactinemia: a clinical and immunohistochemical study of 97 patients operated on transsphenoidally. *Mayo Clin Proc* 1985;60:753-762.
[87] Zayour DH, Selman WR, Arafah BM. Extreme elevation of intrasellar pressure in patients with pituitary tumor apoplexy: relation to pituitary function. *J Clin Endocrinol Metab* 2004;89:5649-5654.
[88] Fatemi N, Dusick JR, Mattozo C, McArthur DL, Cohan P, Boscardin J, et al. Pituitary hormonal loss and recovery after transsphenoidal adenoma removal. *Neurosurgery* 2008;63:709-719.
[89] Nomikos P, Ladar C, Fahlbusch R, Buchfelder M. Impact of primary surgery on pituitary function in patients with non-functioning pituitary adenomas - a study on 721 patients. *Acta Neurochir* (Wien) 2004;146:27-35.
[90] Webb SM, Rigla M, Wagner A, Oliver B, Bartumeus F. Recovery of hypopituitarism after neurosurgical treatment of pituitary adenomas. *J Clin Endocrinol Metab* 1999;84:3696-3700.
[91] Abosch A, Tyrrell JB, Lamborn KR, Hannegan LT, Applebury CB, Wilson CB. Transsphenoidal microsurgery for growth hormone-secreting pituitary adenomas: initial outcome and long-term results. *J Clin Endocrinol Metab* 1998;83:3411-3418.
[92] Barker FG 2nd, Klibanski A, Swearingen B. Transsphenoidal surgery for pituitary tumors in the United States, 1996-2000: mortality, morbidity, and the effects of hospital and surgeon volume. *J Clin Endocrinol Metab* 2003;88:4709-4719.
[93] Cappabianca P, Cavallo LM, Colao A, de Divitiis E. Surgical complications associated with the endoscopic endonasal transsphenoidal approach for pituitary adenomas. *J Neurosurg* 2002;97:293-298.
[94] Comtois R, Beauregard H, Somma M, Serri O, Aris-Jilwan N, Hardy J. The clinical and endocrine outcome to trans-sphenoidal microsurgery of nonsecreting pituitary adenomas. Cancer 1991;68:860-866.
[95] Baskin DS, Boggan JE, Wilson CB. Transsphenoidal microsurgical removal of growth hormone-secreting pituitary adenomas. A review of 137 cases. *J Neurosurg* 1982;56:634-641.
[96] Faria MA, Jr., Tindall GT. Transsphenoidal microsurgery for prolactin-secreting pituitary adenomas. *J Neurosurg* 1982;56:33-43.
[97] McPherson CM, Bohinski RJ, Dagnew E, Warnick RE, Tew JM. Tumor resection in a shared-resource magnetic resonance operating room: experience at the University of Cincinnati. *Acta Neurochir Suppl* 2003;85:39-44.
[98] Colao A, Cerbone G, Cappabianca P, Ferone D, Alfieri A, Di Salle F, et al. Effect of surgery and radiotherapy on visual and endocrine function in nonfunctioning pituitary adenomas. *J Endocrinol Invest* 1998;21:284-290.

[99] Randeva HS, Schoebel J, Byrne J, Esiri M, Adams CB, Wass JA. Classical pituitary apoplexy: clinical features, management and outcome. *Clin Endocrinol* (Oxf) 1999;51:181-188.

[100] Semple PL, Webb MK, de Villiers JC, Laws ER Jr. Pituitary apoplexy. *Neurosurgery* 2005;56:65-73.

[101] Littley MD, Shalet SM, Beardwell CG, Ahmed SR, Applegate G, Sutton ML. Hypopituitarism following external radiotherapy for pituitary tumours in adults. *Q J Med* 1989;70:145-160.

[102] Berg C, Meinel T, Lahner H, Mann K, Petersenn S. Recovery of pituitary function in the late-postoperative phase after pituitary surgery: results of dynamic testing in patients with pituitary disease by insulin tolerance test 3 and 12 months after surgery. *Eur J Endocrinol* 2010;162:853-859.

[103] Nemergut EC, Zuo Z, Jane JA Jr, Laws ER Jr. Predictors of diabetes insipidus after transsphenoidal surgery: a review of 881 patients. *J Neurosurg* 2005;103:448-454.

[104] Adams JR, Blevins LS Jr., Allen GS, Verity DK, Devin JK. Disorders of water metabolism following transsphenoidal pituitary surgery: a single institution's experience. *Pituitary* 2006;9:93-99.

[105] Olson BR, Gumowski J, Rubino D, Oldfield EH. Pathophysiology of hyponatremia after transsphenoidal pituitary surgery. *J Neurosurg* 1997;87:499-507.

[106] Robinson AG, Verbalis JG. Diabetes insipidus. *Curr Ther Endocrinol Meta*b 1994;5:1-6.

[107] Singer PA, Sevilla LJ. Postoperative endocrine management of pituitary tumors. *Neurosurg Clin N Am* 2003;14:123-138.

[108] Nomikos P, Buchfelder M, Fahlbusch R. The outcome of surgery in 668 patients with acromegaly using current criteria of biochemical 'cure'. *Eur J Endocrinol* 2005;152:379-387.

[109] Shimon I, Cohen ZR, Ram Z, Hadani M. Transsphenoidal surgery for acromegaly: endocrinological follow-up of 98 patients. *Neurosurgery* 2001;48:1239-1245.

[110] Beauregard C, Truong U, Hardy J, Serri O. Long-term outcome and mortality after transsphenoidal adenomectomy for acromegaly. *Clin Endocrinol* (Oxf) 2003;58:86-91.

[111] Laws ER, Vance ML, Thapar K. Pituitary surgery for the management of acromegaly. Horm Res 2000;53(Suppl 3):71-75.

[112] Kreutzer J, Vance ML, Lopes MB, Laws ER Jr. Surgical management of GH-secreting pituitary adenomas: an outcome study using modern remission criteria. *J Clin Endocrinol Metab* 2001;86:4072-4077.

[113] Kaltsas GA, Isidori AM, Florakis D, Trainer PJ, Camacho-Hubner C, Afshar F, et al. Predictors of the outcome of surgical treatment in acromegaly and the value of the mean growth hormone day curve in assessing postoperative disease activity. *J Clin Endocrinol Metab* 2001;86:1645-1652.

[114] De P, Rees DA, Davies N, John R, Neal J, Mills RG, et al. Transsphenoidal surgery for acromegaly in wales: results based on stringent criteria of remission. *J Clin Endocrinol Metab* 2003;88:3567-3572.

[115] Ludecke DK, Abe T. Transsphenoidal microsurgery for newly diagnosed acromegaly: a personal view after more than 1,000 operations. *Neuroendocrinology* 2006;83:230-239.

[116] Yoon PH, Kim DI, Jeon P, Lee SI, Lee SK, Kim SH. Pituitary adenomas: early postoperative MR imaging after transsphenoidal resection. *AJNR Am J Neuroradiol* 2001;22:1097-1104.

[117] Kremer P, Forsting M, Ranaei G, Wüster C, Hamer J, Sartor K, et al. Magnetic resonance imaging after transsphenoidal surgery of clinically non-functional pituitary macroadenomas and its impact on detecting residual adenoma. *Acta Neurochir* (Wien) 2002;144:433-443.

[118] Giustina A, Barkan A, Casanueva FF, Cavagnini F, Frohman L, Ho K, et al. Criteria for cure of acromegaly: a consensus statement. *J Clin Endocrinol Metab* 2000;85:526-529.

[119] Hirschl RA, Wilson J, Miller B, Bergese S, Chiocca E. The predictive value of low-field strength magnetic resonance imaging for intraoperative residual tumor detection. Clinical article. *J Neurosurg* 2009;111:252-257.

[120] Shou XF, Li SQ, Wang YF, Zhao Y, Jia PF, Zhou LF. Treatment of pituitary adenomas with a transsphenoidal approach. *Neurosurgery* 2005;56:249-256.

[121] Kubben PL, ter Meulen KJ, Schijns OE, ter Laak-Poort MP, van Overbeeke JJ, van Santbrink H. Intraoperative MRI-guided resection of glioblastoma multiforme: a systematic review. *Lancet Oncol* 2011;12:1062-1070.

[122] Livne O, Harel R, Hadani M, Spiegelmann R, Feldman Z, Cohen ZR. Intraoperative magnetic resonance imaging for resection of intra-axial brain lesions: a decade of experience using low-field magnetic resonance imaging, Polestar N-10, 20, 30 systems. *World Neurosurg* 2014;82:770-776.

[123] Pamir MN, Özduman K, Yıldız E, Sav A, Dinçer A. Intraoperative magnetic resonance spectroscopy for identification of residual tumor during low-grade glioma surgery: clinical article. *J Neurosurg* 2013;118:1191-1198.

[124] Levivier M, Wikler D, Massager N, Legros B, Van Bogaert P, Brotchi J. [Intraoperative MRI and epilepsy surgery] *Neurochirurgie* 2008;54:448-452.

[125] Sommer B, Grummich P, Coras R, Kasper BS, Blumcke I, Hamer HM, et al. Integration of functional neuronavigation and intraoperative MRI in surgery for drug-resistant extratemporal epilepsy close to eloquent brain areas. *Neurosurg Focus* 2013;34:E4.

ABOUT THE EDITOR

Dimitrios N. Kanakis, MD, PhD
Senior Lecturer
Department of Pathology, Medical Faculty,
Democritus University of Thrace, Greece

Dimitrios Kanakis was born on 18th of April 1973, in Thessaloniki/Greece. He began his studies in Medicine at Ernst-Moritz-Arndt University of Greifswald/Germany and completed them in July 2001, at the University of Novi Sad/Federal Republic of Yugoslavia. In October 2004, Dr. Kanakis was awarded with the PhD Title from Otto-von-Guericke University of Magdeburg/Germany, after successful accomplishment of his PhD Thesis, with the Theme "Mutation Analysis in the Promoter of Human Pituitary Tumor Transforming Gene 1 (hPTTG-1) in Pituitary Adenomas". He received the Specialty of Neuropathology from the Medical Corp of Nordrhein in Düsseldorf/Germany (September 2011) and the Specialty of General Pathology from the General Directorate of Public Health and Social Welfare of the Region of Thessaly in Larissa/Greece (January 2013). Currently, he holds the academic position of Senior Lecturer at the Department of Pathology, Medical Faculty of Democritus University of Thrace in Alexandroupolis/Greece.

INDEX

A

C

D

E

Q

R

S

T

V

W